The Failed Back Syndrome

Etiology and Therapy

Second Edition

Harold A. Wilkinson

The Failed Back Syndrome

Etiology and Therapy

Second Edition

With 108 Figures in 209 Parts

Springer-Verlag
New York Berlin Heidelberg London Paris
Tokyo Hong Kong Barcelona Budapest

Harold A. Wilkinson, M.D., Ph.D.
Professor and Chairman
Division of Neurosurgery
University of Massachusetts Medical School
Worcester, Massachusetts 01655
USA

Library of Congress Cataloging in Publication Data
Wilkinson, Harold A.
The failed back syndrome : etiology and therapy / Harold A. Wilkinson. — 2nd ed.
p. cm.
Includes bibliographical references and index.
ISBN 0–387–97617–5 (alk. paper). — ISBN 3–540–97617–5 (alk. paper)
1. Back—Diseases—Etiology. 2. Back—Diseases—Treatment. 3. Back—Surgery. I. Title.
[DNLM 1. Back—surgery. 2. Backache—diagnosis. 3. Backache—surgery. 4. Lumbosacral Region. 5. Postoperative Complications—etiology. WE 755 W686f]
RD768.W435 1992
617.5′6—dc20
DNLM/DLC
for Library of Congress 91-4926
CIP

Printed on acid-free paper.

Production managed by Terry Kornak and coordinated by Faye Zucker Editorial Service.
Manufacturing supervised by Rhea Talbert.
Typesetting by The Composing Room of Michigan, Grand Rapids, MI.
Printed and bound by Edwards Brothers, Ann Arbor, MI.
Printed in the United States of America.

9 8 7 6 5 4 3 2 1

ISBN 0-387-97617-5 Springer-Verlag New York Berlin Heidelberg
ISBN 3-540-97617-5 Springer-Verlag Berlin Heidelberg New York

Preface to the Second Edition

In the eight years since the first edition of this book several marvelous technical advances have become available clinically for the care of patients with "failed back syndromes." High resolution MRI scans, three dimensional CT scans, and percutaneous discectomy are notable technological advances. Overall, however, the problem of "the failed back" remains as complex and poorly understood as ever. A discouraging amount of what we claim to be our knowledge of the pathophysiology and appropriate therapy for the complex of disorders that constitute the failed back syndrome remains unvalidated by careful scientific study.[1] The discussions of pathophysiology, diagnosis, and therapy put forth in the first edition for the most part remain equally as valid or as controversial as they were eight years ago. The first edition was well received by numerous physicians and other health care givers from a variety of disciplines and through them the book seems to have contributed usefully to many of those who suffer the unpleasant maladies of "the failed back." I hope this second edition will likewise prove to be a positive contribution.

The timing of the publication of this second edition is significant in several ways in the context of the current medicolegal climate in the United States. Unquestionably the failed back syndrome, and its consequences in terms of human suffering and loss of productivity, are extremely important medicolegally both in matters concerning qualification for disability compensation and in matters concerning claims of medical malpractice. If the concepts put forth in this book are well accepted, they may help to set new standards of medical practice which require tailored, diverse, and flexible care and ongoing responsibility especially on the part of the operating surgeon. Even more importantly, however, it is my hope that this book will provide greater options and optimism for those who suffer from the failed back syndrome by helping to stem the tide of doctor flight from involvement in the care of failed back patients. Especially in the Northeast, where I practice, but increasingly throughout the United States, neurosurgeons and orthopedists are turning away from accepting professional responsibility for patients who have previously undergone lower back surgery. The increasingly adversarial, regulatory, and even punitive climate in which doctors must practice has driven these specialists to attempt to reduce their own personal liability, distress and "hassle" (to borrow a term from the U.S. federal government) by turning away from the treatment of these patients, many of whom will never again be fully "well" or productive, many of whom are therefore chronically unhappy with their condition and medical care, and many of whom are litigious by choice or necessity. Unfortunately this doctor flight has further aggravated the problem of obtaining ongoing care for their lower back condition, which many patients encounter after lower back surgery has failed to cure them. Once the patient has been operated upon, many nonsurgeons decline to treat what becomes designated as "a surgical disease," and many surgeons, who recognize that further surgery is not likely to be productive, do not offer nonsurgical treatment. This book hopes to help bridge that gap by encouraging neurosurgeons and orthopedists to offer more varied and effective nonsurgical care and by encouraging nonsurgeons to offer the nonsurgical care that most of these patients need, even though they bear surgical scars on their backs and on their work records.

WORCESTER, MASSACHUSETTS HAROLD A. WILKINSON

Preface to the First Edition

Initially, my patients with the "failed back syndrome" were those I had personally operated upon, but in recent years an increasing percentage of these patients have been referred to me by other surgeons who know of my interest in this field. I have never attempted to make the management of the failed back syndrome my major therapeutic effort, but I have consistently recognized it as a major intellectual and technical challenge and a major responsibility for me as a physician. I am aware that more than one surgical resident has been angered by my refusal to permit him to operate on a patient with a virgin lumbar disc rupture until after he had assisted me with several such operations—even though I might have allowed him to operate on a malignant brain tumor or perform other "more glamorous" operations with me as his assistant. My reasoning for this is simple. The patient with the lumbar disc rupture is likely to live for many years following his operation. If he fails to achieve an optimum result from his first operation, his chances of achieving success decline sharply with each subsequent operative intervention that is required.

I also make no claim to omniscience or perfection in this field but continue to approach the menagerie of the diseases of the lower back with inquisitive respect. I offer none of my patients the guarantee of success, only a guarantee that I will work with them stubbornly in an effort to help them overcome their painful disability. I have not withdrawn from the challenge of the failed back syndrome into a state of pessimism, for I have seen much good come from my efforts in this field. I am humbled by my failure to bring relief and wounded by the occasional damaging complications that I produce, but I am also sensitive to the misery and pain of my patients. Deciding whom to treat or not to treat, when to treat, which treatment to employ, and whether the potential benefit of the treatment indeed acceptably outweighs the risk of failure and complication sorely taxes the skill, intelligence and art of the physician—but should not discourage him from rational efforts to help his patients.

I hope that *The Failed Back Syndrome* will serve several purposes. First, I hope it will stimulate others in the health care field to a greater interest in and understanding of the broad range of disorders that affect the lumbar spine. Because the management of these problems requires surgical intervention only for a relatively small number of these patients, it is imperative that nonsurgical health care professionals become actively involved in the effort to help these patients. With this goal in mind I have adopted a style of writing that attempts to minimize technical jargon and to maximize explanations of basic concepts without jeopardizing the factual content of this text. This monograph is not intended to be a scholarly and exhaustive, but formidable compendium; rather it is intended to be a recounting of my experiences in this field and my approaches to the problems of the failed back syndrome. Only a few references have been included, and these are offered more as guides to additional reading than as scholarly documentation.

Second, by attempting to outline and categorize a list of diagnostic and therapeutic possibilities, I hope to encourage surgeons and other health care professionals to approach these problems in a thoughtful, logical, flexible and versatile way. With a health care problem of such magnitude, more physicians, including neurosurgeons, orthopedists, internists and family practitioners should develop a broad expertise in this field. Seeing a patient with low back pain and sciatica should not elicit a "knee jerk reaction" of early operative intervention, but neither should the patient be denied timely surgical intervention if careful and thoughtful evaluation suggests that this would be the optimum course of action. Patients who suffer from the failed back syndrome require continuing and often long-term care. Ideally, this care should be rendered by the same physicians and surgeons who were actively involved in the patient's initial low back illness and initial surgery. Neurosurgeons or orthopedic surgeons who "do backs" (i.e., who operate on problems of the lower back) should also continue to treat those patients who develop a failed back syndrome despite their surgical efforts. Shipping these patients off to a "back specialist" in a distant city is unfair to both patient and specialist, because a meaningful, integrated and extended therapeutic relationship cannot be adequately established in a distant city.

Neurosurgeons are trained to deal with the physical and mental complexities of chronic pain and of nervous system diseases, and orthopedic surgeons are trained to deal with the dynamic interactions of bones, joints and ligaments. More neurosurgeons and orthopedists should develop an expertise in and willingness to undertake the therapy of those chronic sufferers who have failed to obtain relief from back surgery. After all, surgery on the lumbar disc was jointly pioneered by neurosurgeons and orthopedic surgeons, even though the field was long dominated by neurosurgeons.

Finally, I hope that this text will help to improve the lot of some patients who are painfully disabled by the failed back syndrome, either by helping to bring them relief or at least by reassuring them through those who are attempting to care for them that there is much that can be done for the failed back syndrome.

HAROLD A. WILKINSON, 1983

Acknowledgments

No text would be complete without giving recognition to those persons whose assistance and support have made *The Failed Back Syndrome* a reality. For the first edition I am particularly indebted to my professors and colleagues who taught me much of what I now attempt to pass on to others. Among these is Dr. Joseph Abate, a talented and thoughtful practicing orthopedic surgeon with whom I was privileged to work for over a decade, while we jointly learned about the care of low back diseases. Valuable assistance was provided in reviewing and preparing textual material by Dr. Tracy Miller, Professor of Pharmacology, University of Massachusetts Medical School; Dr. Joseph Zito, former Chief of the Division of Neuroradiology, University of Massachusetts Medical School; and Mr. Rob Measley, a medical student, who spent long hours helping to review my clinical material.

Preparation of the manuscript would not have been possible without the dedicated assistance of my secretary, Mrs. Mollie Dufresne; the creative and constructive editorial assistance of our Departmental Medical Writing Specialist, Ms. Sheryl Blaire; the artistic efforts of our Departmental Medical Artist, Ms. Kathy Powell; and the patience and accuracy of the workers in the Word Processing Unit who tolerated countless manuscript revisions. None of this, of course, would have been possible without the support and tolerance of my wife, Alice, and my sons, Arthur and Edward, who suffered months of deprivation while I devoted long hours to this project.

For the second edition of this book I am especially dedicated to my hard working, long-suffering, highly efficient, and dedicated Secretary and Divisional Manager, Mrs. Nancy Gove. Her perseverance with this project over many long hours, during which she also ran a busy clinical office and academic division, proved that the nearly impossible can be achieved.

HAROLD A. WILKINSON

Contents

1

Introduction: Etiology, Diagnosis, and Therapy

Management of a patient with a *failed back* following unsuccessful back surgery poses a serious problem to all health practitioners who attempt to aid these unfortunate sufferers. Neurosurgeons, orthopedists, psychiatrists, family practitioners, physical therapists, nurses, and even marriage counselors all too often find themselves frustrated in their therapeutic efforts. Many of these patients fail to respond to prolonged therapy, but the situation is certainly not hopeless. The list of therapeutic possibilities is, in fact, quite long and varied. Unfortunately, in many instances the failure to achieve success must be attributed to a lack of flexibility and versatility in the therapeutic efforts expended on these patients. One's approach to these problems must be based on a systematic awareness of the potential therapies available and careful tailoring of therapeutic efforts to the patient's specific symptoms, physical findings, and psychologic makeup.

Etiology

It has been suggested that the *failed back syndrome* should actually be called the *failed back surgery* syndrome. By definition, all failed back syndrome patients have undergone back surgery without improvement, but this should not be misconstrued to imply that the operation that was performed was done incorrectly or inadequately. In many instances, the syndrome results following a well-performed operation on a patient who may have fared better with a different operation or with no operation at all. One naturally tends to assume that the surgeon was at fault for having undertaken an unsuccessful operation. This may indeed be the case if a surgeon fails to evaluate a patient properly preoperatively or is not sufficiently versed in the diagnosis and management of the myriad disorders and variations that afflict the lumbar spine. It would also be accurate to assume that the surgeon was at fault if he or she proceeded to the operating room before pursuing an adequate and reasonable trial of nonoperative therapy, especially if the surgeon was insufficiently familiar with the range of nonoperative therapies that are available for the treatment of low back disorders. Yet the surgeon should not be blamed for all therapeutic failures that result in the failed back syndrome. Unfortunately, our knowledge of the diseases of the lower back and of their proper therapy is woefully incomplete.[1] Even the most knowledgeable and experienced surgeon will encounter patients who remain painfully disabled despite the application of what should have been an adequate series of nonoperative therapies and who then seem to be reasonable candidates for surgical intervention—yet fail to achieve the hoped-for relief following surgery. Even more troublesome is the frequently encountered situation in which the diagnosis remains imprecise, despite the best diagnostic and therapeutic efforts, and in which surgical intervention is offered to an informed patient, as a calculated risk, on the reasonable expectation that it may be the optimum mode of therapy for that patient. No therapeutic maneuver known to modern medicine is uniformly and invariably successful and, on occasion, denying a patient surgical intervention on the basis of a less than ideal probability of success may do more harm than proceeding with a carefully executed surgical effort on the basis of a reasonable probability of success.

Diagnostic and Therapeutic Approach

During the nearly two decades that I have attempted to deal diagnostically and therapeutically with patients with low back disorders, I have evolved an increasingly complex reaction toward these problems, and I find myself relying more and more cautiously on surgical intervention. I was trained neurosurgically during the heyday of Mixter and Barr's "triumph," when surgical excision of ruptured lumbar discs seemed to be a heaven-sent answer to a nation of back pain sufferers. Since those early experiences, I have encountered a rising number of disappointed patients and surgeons and have increasingly been called upon to deal with the failed back syndrome. From this experience, I have evolved what I hope is a reasonable and systematic approach to these challenging problems.[2,3,4]

I have found it useful to approach failed back patients initially by attempting to place them in *diagnostic general categories,* based largely on their *symptoms.* This has been useful, since many effective forms of therapy can be initiated on the basis of this general categorization alone, without the need for more *precise diagnosis.* If these more nonspecific and generally lower-risk therapies fail, precise diagnosis of the pathophysiologic basis of the patient's disabling disorder becomes more important. At times, a careful physical examination will confirm the specific diagnosis. If not, a sequence of diagnostic aids is available, although I continue to be disappointed upon encountering patients whose neurosurgeon or orthopedist has relegated them to a "hopeless" category without employing those diagnostic aids that may have led to a precise, and perhaps treatable, diagnosis.

Therapy also *must be tailored* to the disorder that afflicts the individual patient. Prescribing muscle relaxers to a patient whose back pain stems from arthritis is illogical—unless an acute episode of painful muscle spasm has been superimposed. Many therapies may have a beneficial effect on more than one disorder. These therapies can be applied in a somewhat nonspecific manner, but their logical application requires at least a general diagnostic categorization. Other therapies, especially the invasive therapies, are tailored to specific disorders, and precise diagnosis is required. Not all of the therapies that I apply are universally accepted, and scientifically valid proof of efficacy and even of safety is unavailable for most of the therapies employed in managing lower back problems, even therapies that are widely employed and generally accepted.[1] Nevertheless, I apply these therapies, and wish to recommend them to others, because in my practice they have been of benefit to at least some patients. Some of the therapies that I prescribe are generally accepted, yet are frequently improperly applied or too seldom employed. One of the most outstanding examples of underuse of therapy is the prescription of anti-inflammatory drugs for patients with chronic back pain, although their effectiveness is often striking when they are properly applied.[5]

I am at all times acutely aware of both the *risks and the limitations* of the therapies that I recommend. But an awareness of these risks and limitations on the part of the therapist is not enough. For patients to benefit fully, they must be made a part of the decision-making and therapeutic processes. Patients must be allowed to assist in deciding when the severity of their symptoms is sufficient to justify the risks of a specific therapy. They must also reasonably comprehend the aims, limitations, and alternatives to a specific therapy to ensure their full and effective participation in the therapeutic process. After all, medicines left in a bottle do little good, improperly performed exercises may do harm, and no surgery will be deemed successful if the patient's expectations are unrealistic. Surgery is also unlikely to be successful if patients are principally disabled by psychologic problems.

The *psychological aspects* of the failed back syndrome are indeed formidable, both diagnostically and therapeutically. Conventional psychotherapy is too rarely successful, and too few psychotherapists are comfortable dealing with patients with both physical disabilities and psychopathology. Nonetheless, a constant awareness of and sensitivity to the patient's psychologic makeup is a basic ingredient in the successful therapy of the failed back syndrome.

This text has *three chief messages.* The first is that not all failed backs fail because of "recurrent discs"; a *variety of conditions* are responsible for the many failures that are encountered. Second, just as there are a variety of causes of the failed back syndrome, there are also a *variety of available therapies*. Surgical therapy should account for only a minority of the treatment rendered these patients, but patients should not be denied proper and logically dictated surgical therapy. Diagnostic and therapeutic needle procedures are often of great benefit to failed back syndrome sufferers, yet are woefully underused by most physicians who attempt to deal with these patients. Last, this book is intended to emphasize that the great bulk of therapy for failed back syndrome sufferers *can and should be carried out* by neurosurgeons, orthopedists, and other health care practitioners *near to the patient's home*. Only rarely should it be necessary to refer patients to specialists in distant cities, and such referrals should be made only on the basis of a specific diagnosis that requires specific, specialized therapy.

2

The Role of Improper Surgery in the Etiology of the Failed Back Syndrome

In the United States, approximately two thirds of all patients enrolled in chronic pain centers suffer from the failed back syndrome. Neurosurgeons perform 100,000 operations for lumbar disc disease every year, and orthopedic surgeons perhaps perform a similar number.[6] It is estimated that between 20% and 40% of these operations are unsuccessful and result in the failed back syndrome. Dr. William Sweet, former Professor and Chairman of Neurosurgery at the Massachusetts General Hospital, has estimated that, in contrast, only approximately 10% of patients enrolled in European pain clinics suffer from the failed back syndrome.[7] The reasons for this discrepancy are likely to be multiple, including, perhaps, Europeans' greater stoicism and a less supportive acceptance of disability and nonproductivity. But it is indisputable that a far greater number of lumbar disc operations per 100,000 population are performed in the United States than in European countries, even though there is little or no evidence to suggest a major dissimilarity in the frequency, severity, or type of low back disease encountered on the two continents. Thus, the conclusion that many American failed back syndromes result from excessive surgical intervention seems difficult to avoid.

Incorrect Diagnosis

Even carefully executed surgery is doomed to failure if it is performed for an *incorrect diagnosis*. Without detracting from the luster justly due to Mixter and Barr for their major contribution to the understanding of a painful condition that has been one of the true scourges of humanity, one must keep in mind that all that glitters is not gold and all that hurts the back is not disc disease.[8] I will make no attempt to put forth an exhaustive review of the differential diagnoses of conditions causing back pain and sciatica that may mimic virginal lumbar disc disease, but some samples of the spectrum of these diseases deserve special mention.

Perhaps the most worrisome of the alternative diagnoses is the possibility of a *misdiagnosed neoplasm,* either malignant or benign. Of the patients with metastatic cancer to the spine who are seen by neurosurgeons, approximately 20% will present with spinal metastasis as the first indication of metastatic disease. Spinal metastases are more common in the thoracic region, although metastases to the lumbar spine are far from rare. Local tenderness to percussion more than palpation may help to distinguish this condition from disc disease. Intraspinal benign tumors, primarily ependymomas at the lumbar or lumbothoracic level, may also mimic lumbar disc disease. They may cause a combination of back and radiating leg pain that is aggravated by activity. Characteristically, however, these tumors cause considerably more neurologic deficit than lumbar disc ruptures, although they cause an equivalent amount of pain. A distinguishing feature between the symptoms caused by intraspinal tumors and those caused by lumbar disc ruptures is the phenomenon of "chair sleep." Lumbar disc patients almost universally obtain some relief by recumbency in bed. On the other hand, this position may cause painful upward displacement of a spinal tumor, so that symptoms may be aggravated during recumbency. As a result, tumor patients may describe themselves as being more comfortable while sleeping sitting up in a chair (Fig. 2.1).

The combination of overweight and underexercise, so common in affluent countries today, is undoubtedly the most common cause of back pain in modern society—even more common than lumbar disc disease. Nonetheless, this so-called *flabby back syndrome* is usually not considered a disease per se.

The disease state, or group of diseases, most likely to be misdiagnosed as lumbar disc disease is *arthritis*—a condition that is extremely unlikely to be benefited by disc excision. Arthritis that mimics lumbar disc disease usually causes pain in the lower back or hip, but pain may be referred to the posterior thigh and may be confused with sciatica. Arthritis in younger patients may be more easily overlooked or misdiagnosed than the degenerative arthritis seen most commonly in patients of middle age or older. Degenerative arthritis is usually associated with striking radiographic changes: bone spurs, interspace narrowing and lipping, and sclerosis of facet joints. This form of arthritis may cause significant back pain that is unrelieved or even aggravated by removal of an intervertebral disc. However, the mere presence of radiographic changes of arthritis does not confirm that this is the cause of a patient's persistent back pain. Some degree of degenerative change is a part of the normal aging process, and many patients whose radiographs demonstrate degenerative changes have no symptoms of back disease (Fig. 2.2).

Ankylosing spondylitis is a disease of young men, especially those with serotype HLA-B27.[9,10] It

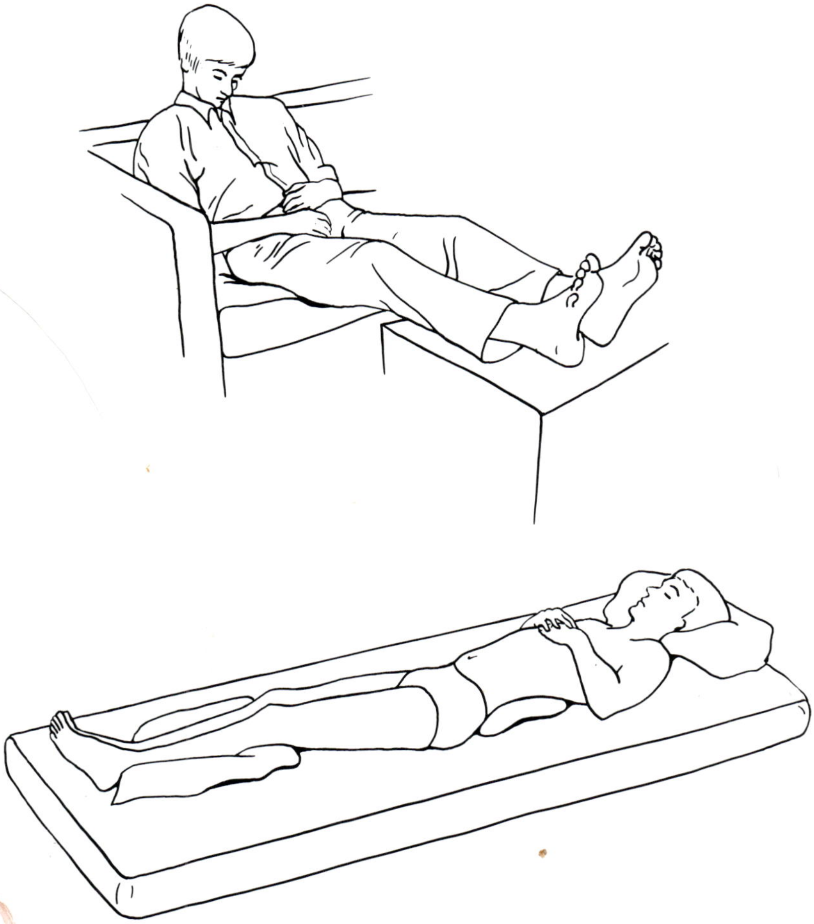

FIGURE 2.1. Patients with benign intraspinal tumors often sleep more comfortably sitting up. Patients with lumbar disc disease almost universally are more comfortable while recumbent. Supports under the calves and lumbar spine may add to the patient's comfort while recumbent.

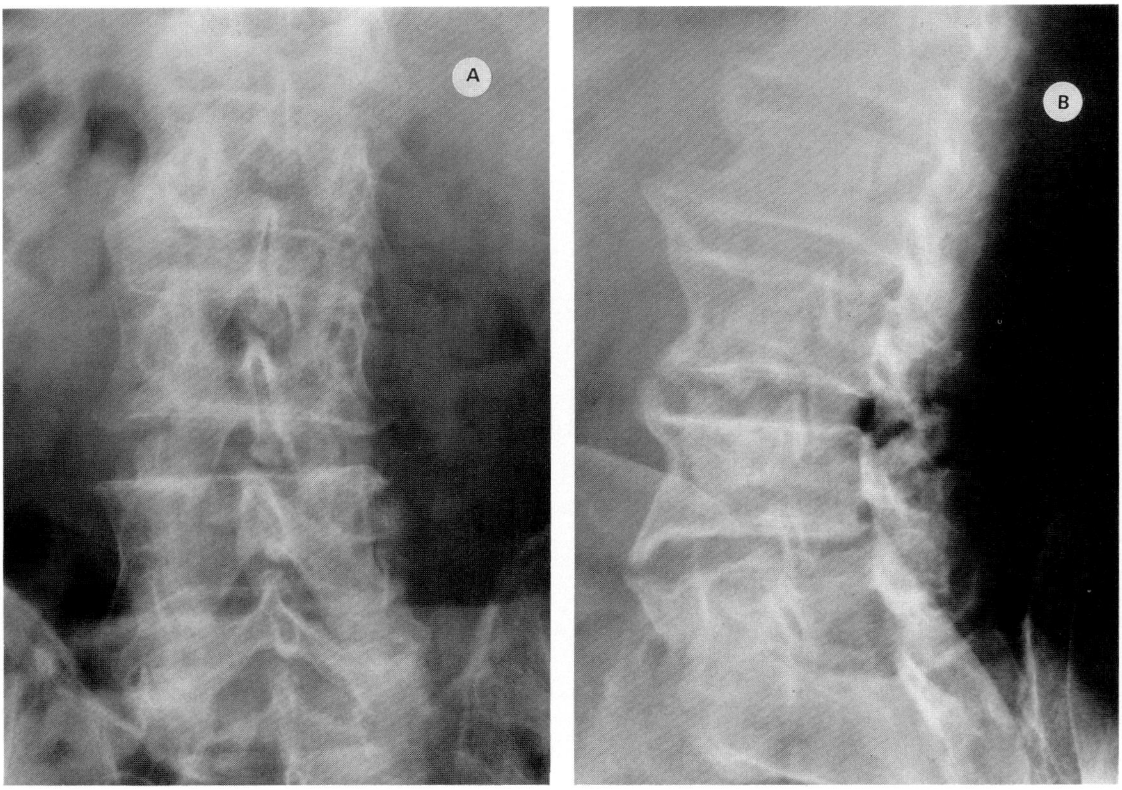

FIGURE 2.2. Degenerative arthritis in the lumbar spine is part of the normal aging process, as seen on the PA (**A**) and lateral (**B**) lumbar spine radiographs. Many patients are found to have long-standing degenerative arthritic changes in their lumbar spine, yet have not been bothered by back pain. This man's leg pain and claudication-like symptoms were proven to be due to vascular insufficiency rather than spinal stenosis.

causes an insidious form of nagging lower backache that often becomes severe before radiographic changes become obvious. The characteristic *arthritis "double peak" of pain* may not always be present. This double-peaked pattern is characterized by painful stiffness of the back and extremities on first arising in the morning, some improvement following initial activity, but recurrence of discomfort following continued activity during the course of the day. Ankylosing spondylitis is not limited to the lumbar spine, and, in fact, one helpful diagnostic maneuver is measurement of chest expansion. This is often sharply limited in patients with this disease, even early in its course.

In young women, *osteitis condensans* may cause a similar aching lower back pain, most commonly seen during pregnancy. Here too, the radiographic changes may not be striking, but careful study of radiographs may yield diagnostic information.

Unnecessary Surgery

Even if the diagnosis of lumbar disc disease is correctly made, surgery may be improper if it is unnecessary. A significant percentage of patients with lumbar disc disease, even those with sciatica and nerve root compression, will respond quite adequately to *nonoperative therapy.* The introduction of chymopapain discolysis led to some of the most careful studies of the therapy of lumbar disc ruptures ever performed, yet the most important finding of these studies is rarely quoted.[11,12] Five double-blind studies on three continents were done on patients with clinical pictures typical of lumbar disc rupture causing sciatica, with objective clinical findings and confirmatory imaging studies and with a failure of conventional nonoperative therapy. These patients were considered to be surgical candidates and were randomized to receive either chymopapain discolysis or placebo (different placebos were used in different studies). The most important finding of these studies is not that chymopapain discolysis benefited many patients, but that in each of the five studies *approximately 50% of the placebo group also recovered,* even though conventional nonoperative therapy had failed. This indictment of our concept of adequate nonoperative therapy has been more recently reaffirmed in a multicenter trial of a carefully formulated physical and pharmacologic therapy for patients with confirmed lumbar disc ruptures. More than 90% of these patients were relieved of their symptoms and were returned to work without surgery.[13]

The presence of *sensory loss or moderate weakness* does not mandate early surgical intervention. If active nonoperative therapy rapidly relieves the patient of pain, neurologic recovery is quite likely to follow at the same slow pace that neurologic recovery takes following successful surgery. Bruised or compressed nerves still require time to recover, so that even following surgical decompression, return of motor and sensory functions is often delayed by several weeks or even months. Pain relief generally occurs much sooner following nerve decompression than does return of motor and sensory function—a distinction that is true for both surgical and nonoperative decompression. Therapy that results in prompt improvement of pain is probably effective, at least as long as progressive sensory loss is not the basis for the observed pain relief. Many back conditions, of course, will respond to *nonoperative therapy* but will fail to respond to operative therapy. Patients with acute muscle spasms or with chronic back weakness and lack of exercise will be much better served by vigorous nonoperative therapy than by surgical intervention. This does not imply, however, that patients with severe or progressive neurologic deficits, or patients whose less severe deficits do not rapidly improve, should be denied appropriate surgical decompression, since failure to operate may leave the patient with permanent and potentially avoidable neurologic deficits.

But even though it may be unnecessary, is carefully performed lumbar disc surgery likely to be *harmful?* Many optimistic series of lumbar disc operations suggest that the chance of a patient's condition actually being made worse following surgery is in the range of 1% or 2%. However, Fager and Freidberg reviewed a series of patients with the failed back syndrome (admittedly a strongly biased group) who were referred to the Lahey Clinic and concluded that over 10% of these patients had been rendered significantly worse by their back surgery and that many of these operations were, in their opinion, unnecessary.[14] It seems obvious that removing the nucleus pulposus from a normal disc is likely to do little good and is likely to create some instability of the back and malalignment of the facet joints. As a result, an increased incidence of *chronic back pain* following this surgical procedure would be expected. The addition of a foramenotomy, with interruption of facet joints unilaterally, would reasonably be expected to compound the induced *instability.* But what if surgical exploration is confined to the epidural space and a lumbar disc that is discovered intraoperatively to be normal is not resected? Carelessly or roughly performed surgery can directly *injure nerve roots,* even to the point of nerve root avulsion. The *dura may be lacerated* by careless or rough handling or may tear quite easily in the presence of preexisting epidural adhesions. If the defect is not repaired, nerve roots may herniate through to become strangulated at a later date. If the arachnoid is also torn, cerebrospinal fluid (CSF) leakage may result, causing a CSF fistula with the risk of meningitis or perhaps delayed formation of a painful pseudomeningocele. Even carefully performed surgery may be followed by delayed *wound infection* or *hemorrhage.* The latter may not only cause severe pain and neurologic deficits in the early postoperative phase, but may well be a prelude to delayed formation of severe adhesions. Are *epidural adhesions* and *intradural arachnoiditis* likely to occur even following carefully executed and uncomplicated disc surgery, with or without disc excision? There are authors who ascribe the etiology of these two conditions almost exclusively to surgical intervention, but certainly both conditions are encountered repeatedly in patients who have never previously undergone surgery or even myelography. The studies done by Mayfield and his coworkers on the laminectomy membrane support the contention that symptomatic adhesions may follow even carefully executed surgery.[15]

I find it inescapable to conclude that lumbar disc surgery, no matter how radically or meticulously performed, carries with it some inherent risk of leaving patients worse than they were before surgery. If the surgery was unnecessary, the patients have been placed in jeopardy with no significantly improved chance of obtaining relief of their back conditions.

Improper or Inadequate Surgery

Even if patients escape from their back surgery without harm and even if the surgery was clearly indicated, improper surgery may still lead to the failed back syndrome. One fairly common form of improper surgery is disc excision performed at the *wrong level*. Considerable differences of opinion exist among neurosurgeons and orthopedists about what constitutes an adequate determination of the level of disc rupture. Some are willing to operate without myelography on the basis of clinical findings alone, but most now obtain at least a computerized tomography (CT) scan or magnetic resonance imaging (MRI) scan. Clinical features do localize the level of disc rupture with fair accuracy: L5-S1 disc ruptures cause loss of ankle reflex, plantar flexor ankle weakness, and lateral calf and foot sensory loss; L4-L5 disc ruptures cause loss of the rarely detectable tibialis anterior reflex, dorsiflexor ankle weakness, and anterior shin and dorsal foot sensory loss; L3-L4 disc ruptures cause loss of knee reflex, weakness of knee extension, and medial knee and calf sensory loss (Fig. 2.3). Two types of *unreliability of clinical features* may be encountered. Occasionally, patients will have anomalous nerve root exit levels, especially patients with lum-

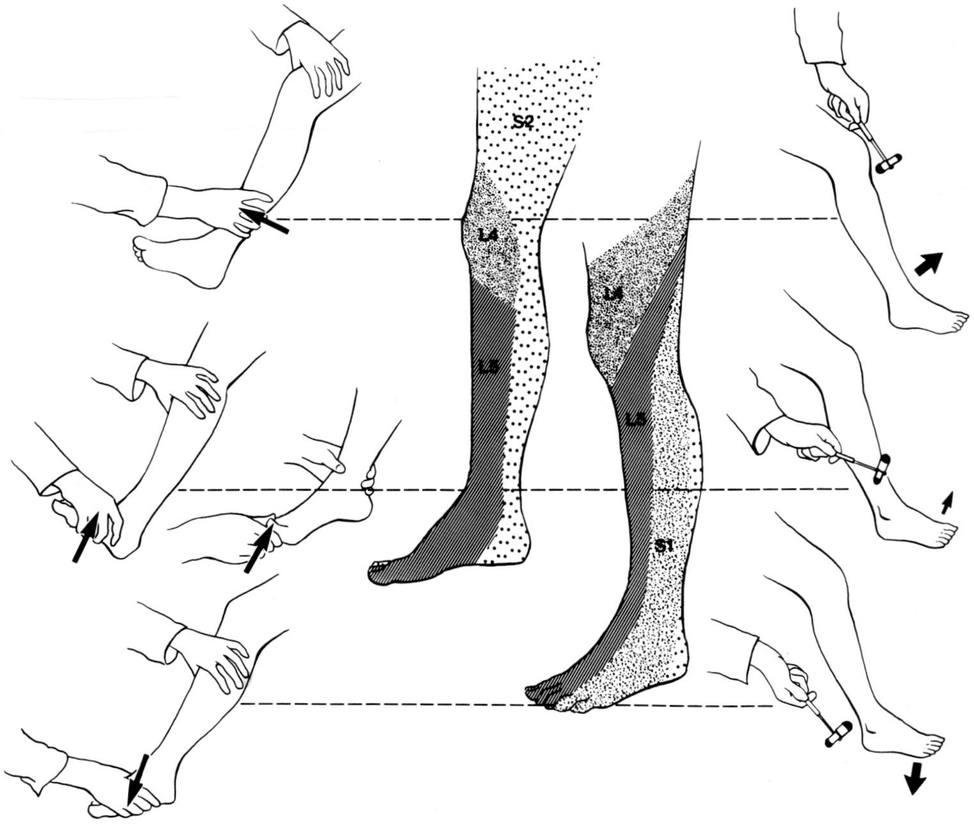

FIGURE 2.3. The neurologic examination should reveal characteristic changes with dysfunction of individual lumbosacral nerve roots. The type of motor weakness **(left),** the cutaneous pattern of sensory loss **(center),** and the loss of deep tendon reflex **(right)** most commonly seen with dysfunction of these nerve roots are shown here. L4 root findings are shown interconnected by the horizontal line at the top, L5 root findings are shown by the middle horizontal line, and S1 root findings are shown by the lower horizontal line. Arrows on the left denote the direction of voluntary motion by the patient against the physician's hand or thumb. Arrows on the right denote reflex movement of the limb in response to deep tendon stretching.

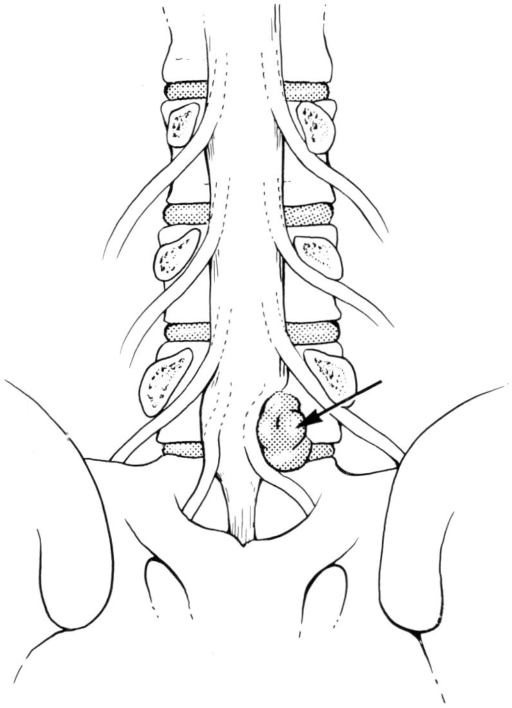

FIGURE 2.4. Disc ruptures commonly compress the nerve root exiting at the interspace level below the level of disc rupture. The L5 root, which exits at the lumbosacral junction or L5-S1, usually does not cross the L5-S1 interspace and therefore escapes compression by an L5-S1 disc rupture (arrow). Instead, the S1 nerve root, which exits at the S1-S2 level, is compressed by an L5-S1 disc rupture.

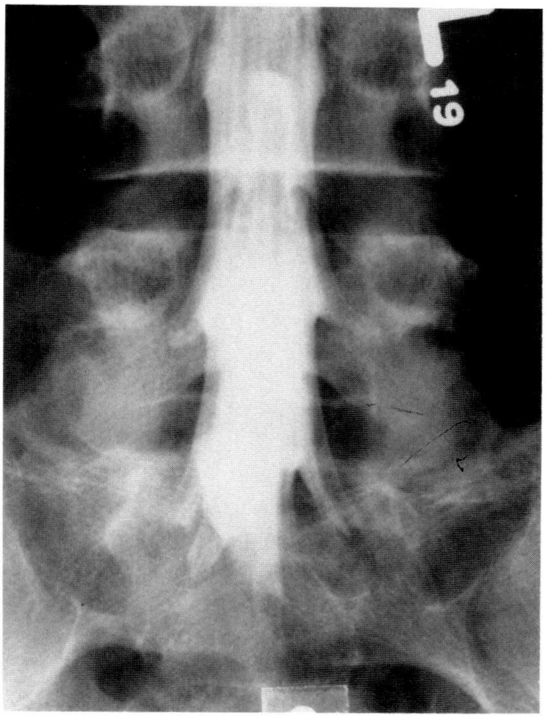

FIGURE 2.5. Anomalous nerve roots, such as the ones seen in this myelogram film, may confuse clinical localization when disc ruptures occur at the level of anomaly. They can also be confusing to the operating surgeon, especially if myelography has not been performed.

barized or sacralized vertebrae. In these patients, the nerve root exiting between the lowest lumbar vertebra and the upper sacrum (and therefore most likely to be entrapped by a disc rupture at the next highest level) may be either the S1 or the L4 nerve root, rather than the normal L5 root. The other source of unreliability is the exact location of the disc rupture relative to the spinal canal. Most disc ruptures occur through the posterolateral annulus at the point where the pedicles prevent a longitudinal continuation of the posterior or lateral longitudinal spinal ligaments. At this point, the nerve root exiting at that spinal level has already passed laterally around the superior pedicle, which attaches to the vertebral body rostral to its center and so does not pass over the disc at that level (Fig. 2.4). The most vulnerable nerve root at this level is the nerve root that exits through the neuroforamen at the next lower interspace level, but that penetrates the dura and is therefore relatively fixed in position at that level. The widespread introduction of lumbar CT scanning documented that "far-lateral" (i.e., lateral to the pedicle) disc ruptures occur more commonly than was previously imagined. These far-lateral disc ruptures compress the nerve root exiting at the same interspace and thus give a clinical picture like that which would be expected with a more customary, more medial disc rupture at the level of the next highest spinal motion segment. Patients are occasionally encountered in whom the point of dural penetration of the nerve root is anomalously high or in whom nerve roots are unusually long or redundant, and in these patients a disc rupture may compress the nerve root that exits from the neuroforamen two levels below or may compress the nerve root that exits from the same interspace level as the disc rupture (Fig. 2.5). A more medially placed disc rupture may compress the nerve roots that exit more than one interspace level below the disc rupture, even though the root remains intradural at the level

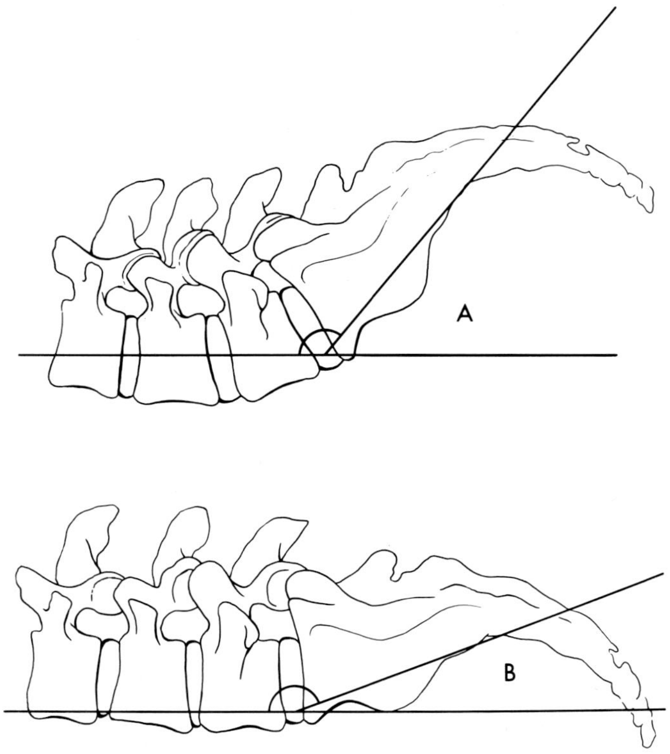

FIGURE 2.6. **A:** The more commonly encountered sacral angle. **B:** A "flat" sacral angle may confuse operative localization of the lumbosacral interspace. Because identification of the lumbosacral interspace is commonly relied on for localization of other lumbar interspaces intraoperatively, failure to identify the lumbosacral junction correctly may lead to surgery at an incorrect interspace level.

of disc rupture. On the other hand, a disc rupture that results in a free fragment may cause nerve root compression at some distance from the point of rupture of the fragment through the posterior longitudinal ligament. If such a fragment moves upward or laterally, the nerve root that exits through the neuroforamen at the level of disc rupture may not be spared, but may be compressed by the migrating fragment within the spinal canal, over the superior vertebral body, or within the neuroforamen.

Inadequate imaging can lead to unnecessary and improper surgery if the surgeon fails to detect a *spinal tumor* that clinically mimics a disc rupture. Especially problematic is the situation in which the operating surgeon finds a modest bulge, perhaps combined with some arthritic spurring, at the level of surgical intervention. This may be presumed to be a symptomatic disc rupture when, in fact, removal of this disc (in actuality not a symptomatic rupture) may divert attention away from an intradural tumor at the thoracolumbar junction, compressing a lower lumbar or sacral nerve root. Routine CT scans and many lumbar MRI scans do not image the thoracolumbar area, and CT scans without contrast usually cannot discriminate tumor from normal intraspinal tissues. Myelography or MRI scans should include the low thoracic area, especially in patients with obvious neurologic deficits. Even though myelography or scans disclose abnormalities of one or more lower lumbar discs, these may be asymptomatic, and benign spinal tumors may be overlooked unless the possibility of their presence is included in the initial differential diagnosis. This possibility, of course, becomes even greater in the patient with neurologic deficits who failed to improve following resection of what a radiologist enigmatically reported as a "bulging disc."

Anatomical variation may frustrate a surgical attempt to achieve improvement in the patient's condition in still another way. The possibility of *lumbarization or sacralization of spinal segments* has been referred to earlier. In these conditions, especially if they are unrecognized preoperatively, accurate spinal level localization at the time of surgical exposure may prove to be difficult. The sloping angle of the sacrum is a useful guide to the lumbosacral interspace, but in a number of patients the sacral/lumbar angle may be relatively flat (Fig. 2.6). Disc ruptures high in the lumbar area, L3-L4 or even L4-L5, require particular attention to localization. Now that a "microsurgical approach" to disc ruptures (done with or without a microscope) is in vogue, the possibility of operating at the wrong spinal level is even greater than before. When operating on a disc rupture at these levels, the surgeon should always confirm his surgical exposure level by tunnelling downward to the sacrum, which he can identify by its shape, its angle, its deeper tone on percussion, or a combination of these factors. If he elects not to expose the sacrum, the surgeon would do well to depend on intraoperative radiography for interspace localization. Surgeons who plan to practice microsurgery and who do not wish to use intraoperative radiography would do their patients and themselves a service by leaving behind a radiographically opaque metallic marker, either in the interspace or dorsal to the site of laminectomy, for later radiographic confirmation of the accuracy of the localization of the surgical intervention. Metal marking clips should not be placed on the cut posterior longitudinal ligament adjacent to the nerve root because they can induce severe local scarring and nerve root adhesions.

Even if the level of disc rupture is accurately identified and correctly operated upon, a failed back syndrome may result, especially in the presence of *free rupture of disc material* through the posterior longitudinal ligament. As mentioned earlier, fragments of disc material may migrate laterally into the neuroforamen, up or down the epidural space in the lateral gutter, or ventral to the dura. During the course of exposure of the major fragment, including retraction of the nerve root and placement of cottonoids rostrally and caudally to tamponade extradural bleeding, these secondary fragments may be further displaced. If they are not carefully sought, located, and removed, they may be the source of persistent or later-developing symptoms. If the retained fragment continues to cause nerve root compression, neurologic symptoms will persist. If the fragment has now been displaced to compress a nerve root other than the one primarily affected, the postoperative clinical picture may be different from that which existed preoperatively. Even if the fragment does not cause persistent nerve root compression, it may form a focus for later development of severe extradural scarring or intradural arachnoiditis and, therefore, may lead to delayed onset of severe symptoms and the failed back syndrome.

Careful excision of a frankly ruptured disc with due care to prevent damage to nerve roots and dura and to prevent overlooking free fragments may still yield a failed back syndrome if the surgery performed is *inadequate to correct associated bony abnormalities* in the area of the disc rupture. Sciatica may persist if a lateral recess stenosis is not adequately unroofed to decompress the nerve root from overhanging bone as it passes around the pedicle on its way to leave the spinal canal. A diffuse form of back and leg pain, perhaps with claudication-like pain on activity, may persist if disc excision does not include an adequately wide laminectomy to decompress a coexistent spinal stenosis. Chronic back pain may persist if simple discectomy is performed in the face of spondylolisthesis or, in some cases, if disc excision is not followed by spinal fusion.

The question of when simple disc excision should be coupled with spinal fusion continues to defy accurate preoperative prediction and is an area in which the considerable flame of controversy is frequently based on the individual surgeon's personal opinions, often bearing no more weight than the smoke that accompanies most flaming arguments (see Chapter 7). Even among those who advocate spinal fusion for some, or all, lumbar disc and other back problems there is no uniformity of opinion about the proper application of the various types of lumbar fusion: posterior fusion, lateral fusion, interbody fusion, and interbody-facet fusion. Nor is there uniformity of opinion about the selection of patients who should have lumbar spinal fusion in addition to a discectomy. For some surgeons, spinal fusion seems desirable in the patient obliged to return to heavy physical work. Spinal arthritis, including facet arthritis, is at times given as an indication for spinal fusion (especially if facet nerve blocks have documented pain relief), but at other times the presence of lumbar degenerative arthritis is viewed as a contraindication to spinal fusion because it is feared that painful arthritic degeneration will then be more likely to develop at the adjacent interspace. Even for patients with documented spondylolisthesis, agreement on the precise indications for spinal fusion is more the exception than the rule. Most surgeons agree that extreme subluxations, especially with associated neurologic deficits as well as pain, should be treated with spinal fusion. However, some surgeons feel that patients with minimal slippage and only back pain can be adequately treated nonoperatively or by decompression without spinal fusion. Other surgeons advocate that initial lumbar disc excision should rarely be coupled with spinal fusion, but that spinal fusion should be considered as a second operative procedure if back pain persists despite simple discectomy. For still other surgeons, this approach seems inadvisable. Instead, they advocate including spinal fusion at the time of initial discectomy for patients who suffer exclusively, or even predominantly, from back pain rather than leg pain. With the avowed indications for spinal fusion varying so widely, it is little wonder that valid and interpretable conclusions can rarely be drawn from the many conflicting reports in the medical literature about the clinical outcome following lumbar spinal fusion.

3

Symptomatic Diagnosis

A systematic, symptomatic approach to a patient with the failed back syndrome is equally important in determining a diagnosis and in recommending therapy. Not all therapy requires a specific diagnosis, especially the more nonspecific, noninvasive therapy; but it is important to analyze the *general diagnostic category* for each patient before recommending any form of treatment. Some forms of treatment can be predicted to have a very small chance of success for certain diagnostic categories. An initial assessment of the general category of disorder from which a patient suffers can be obtained by combining a careful evaluation of the patient's symptoms, as delineated by accurate history taking, with a thoughtfully performed physical examination. These basic diagnostic techniques are also important in arriving at a precise diagnosis and will be examined in more detail in Chapter 4. I feel it is useful first to consider the major categories of symptoms that one is likely to encounter, since accurate history taking is considerably enhanced by having a categorization of symptoms in mind before beginning the history-taking process.

My experience in dealing with patients with back problems has led to the evolution of a *symptomatic categorization* of disorders that I have found to be clinically useful in my practice. Nearly all patients with the failed back syndrome can be placed, largely on the basis of their symptoms, into one or more of the following three categories: low back pain, fusion problems, and leg pain. Many patients, in addition, have a significant component of psychogenic factors, and in some patients this is the paramount diagnostic category. I have also recognized a specific disease state as a general diagnostic category, partly because of my specific interest in this disease and partly because the symptoms that it produces differ significantly from any of the above categories. This diagnostic category is lumbar adhesive arachnoiditis.

Low Back Pain

When one encounters a patient with the failed back syndrome who suffers predominantly from back pain, a specific group of diagnostic possibilities comes to mind (Table 3.1). These possibilities include preexisting but misdiagnosed or improperly treated conditions, properly treated but uncorrected and persistent problems, and newly acquired problems. Most of these conditions are different from those that cause primarily sciatica or leg pain. Postdiscectomy patients whose back pain stems from a spinal neoplasm or misdiagnosed disc disease at a level other than the operative level will often give a history of *transient improvement* following the initial disc excision. In retrospect, this usually results from the period of enforced bed rest, in addition to liberal application of analgesic medications during the early postoperative period. However, once these patients attempt to resume normal activity, their back pain recurs and it is apparent that they have achieved no lasting benefit.

Spinal Neoplasms

Benign intraspinal neoplasms are more likely to cause severe sciatica, with back pain as a less severe complaint. Patients with neoplasms who persist

TABLE 3.1. Diagnosis and therapy of failed back syndrome patients with low back pain as their principal complaint—Based on a symptomatic approach.

Initial presumptive diagnosis (on basis of history)	Initial diagnostic tests	Initial therapy	Confirmatory diagnostic tests	Extended therapy
Flabby back syndrome	History and examination only	Enforced activity, anti-inflammatory, muscle relaxers	X-ray, myelogram (?), CT, or MRI scan to exclude other causes	Physical therapy, psychosomatic psychotherapy, pain clinic
Epidural scar, irritation	History and examination only	Anti-inflammatory	Myelogram, CT, or MRI scan, epidural anesthetic block	Epidural/intrathecal steroids, surgical lysis
Pseudomeningocele, arachnoidal cyst	Examination, CT, MRI scan, or myelogram	Surgery	—	—
Discitis or aseptic interspace inflammation	Sedimentation rate, WBC, x-ray, CT, or MRI scan	Anti-inflammatory, enforced inactivity, bracing	Contrast/anesthesia discogram and culture, isotope scan	Intradiscal steroid, surgical fusion
Disc infection or osteomyelitis	Sedimentation rate, WBC, x-ray, CT, or MRI scan	Antibiotics, enforced inactivity, bracing	Disc aspriation and culture, isotope scan	Surgical debridement
Painful disc degeneration without rupture	X-ray, CT, or MRI scan	Anti-inflammatory, bracing, enforced inactivity (if acute)	Contrast/anesthesia discogram, myelogram (?)	Intradiscal steroid, surgical fusion, disc resection without fusion (?)
Facet syndrome	X-ray, CT scan	Anti-inflammatory, bracing	Facet nerve anesthetization, steroid, surgical fusion	Facet neurectomy, intrafacet steroid
Acute or fixed muscle spasm	History and examination only	Muscle relaxers, topical therapy, enforced inactivity, limbering exercises	Local anesthesia	Hospital bed rest, anti-inflammatory, traction
Trigger point, ischiogluteal bursitis, fasciitis	History and examination only	Local steroid injection or prolotherapy	Local anesthesia	Local resection of trigger points
Fibromyalgia	History and examination only	Anti-inflammatory, amitriptyline, topical, exercises	—	—
Transaponeurotic fat herniation	History and examination only	Local steroid or sclerosing solution injection	Local anesthesia	Local resection and repair (?)
Spondylolysis, spondylolisthesis	X-ray, CT scan	Bracing, anti-inflammatory, enforced inactivity (if acute)	Bracing	Spinal fusion
Trauma: contusions, sprain, muscle spasms, compression fracture, microfracture	History and examination, x-ray, CT scan	Enforced inactivity, bracing, anti-inflammatory	Isotope scan	Spinal fusion
Benign neoplasm	Neurologic loss on examination, myelogram, MRI scan	Excision	—	—

TABLE 3.1. (*Continued*)

Metastatic neoplasm	Percussion tenderness, x-ray, myelogram, CT, or MRI scan	Surgery, x-ray therapy, chemotherapy	—	—
Arthritis	Blood tests, x-ray, CT scan (?)	Anti-inflammatory, enforced activity, enforced inactivity (if acute)	Rheumatology consult, radioisotope scan	—
Cervical disc disease	X-ray, examination	Traction, collar, heat, rest, anti-inflammatory, antineuralgia	Myelogram, CT, or MRI scan	Surgery
Osteoporosis	X-ray	Enforced inactivity, bracing, anti-inflammatory (if acute)	Specialty referral	—

with back pain more than sciatica are likely to harbor a *metastatic lesion* in their vertebrae. These patients, of course, rarely go undiagnosed for very long because of the progressive nature of their disease—which sooner or later makes itself obvious. A helpful diagnostic maneuver on physical examination of patients suspected of having metastatic spinal disease is the detection of pain on spinal percussion. Percussion usually elicits a greater amount of pain than is elicited by local palpation only. The shock wave produced by percussion transmits more stress to deep structures than simple surface pressure. Therefore, percussion is more likely to elicit pain in conditions that affect the vertebrae and discs primarily—diseases such as metastatic cancer, disc space infection or inflammation, and osteomyelitis. Stressing the affected region with bending maneuvers is also characteristically painful, both in patients with metastatic spinal tumors and in patients with persistent disc disease.

Cervical Disc Disease

An uncommon cause of low back pain is *cervical disc disease* or *tumor*.[16,17] This phenomenon has been recognized for many years, and recently an active school of enthusiastic proponents has advocated therapy of the cervical spine for patients with low back disease. The converse situation, neck pain and headache associated with low back disease, is extremely common. The mass of paraspinal muscles that attaches at one end to the sacrum attaches at its rostral end to the neck and base of the skull. When painful problems arise in the lower back, this entire mass of paraspinal muscle tissue commonly develops increased protective muscle tension and may even go into severely painful muscle spasm. Secondary pain centers may become focal at the point of muscle attachments at the other end of the muscle mass (i.e., in the cervical spine and suboccipiut with low back problems, and at the iliac crest and lumbar spine with cervical problems). The number of documented cases of objective cervical disc disease or cervical spinal tumors in which lower back complaints have ceased following correction of the cervical problem is limited. Although I have encountered a number of patients with simultaneous cervical disease and lower back pain, I can recall only the following instance in which the lumbar pain improved following definitive cervical surgery:

Case 1

A 48-year old homemaker had suffered for 3 1/2 years with progressively increasing pain in her neck. This radiated vaguely to the posterior aspect of her shoulders (right greater than left) and was severely aggravated by activity. She had previously undergone two myelograms, each showing no obvious abnormality in the cervical or lumbar area. Cervical spine radiographs showed focal interspace narrowing at C5-C6 and minimal spurring at C6-C7. She had been treated for many months with cervical traction, collar, and anodynes prior to being referred to me.

A series of anti-inflammatory drugs was either not well tolerated or produced only insignificant improvement in pain and range of neck movements. Cervical contrast discography was quite normal at C4-C5. However, injections of 0.3 ml at C5-C6 and 0.5 ml at C6-C7 of 76% diatrizoate meglumide/sodium (Renograftin-76) caused intense neck and interscapular pain. Anesthesia discography consisting of intradiscal injection of equal volumes of lidocaine (Xylocaine) and bupivacaine (Marcaine) gave prompt and almost total relief of neck pain that lasted a number of hours. Intradiscal injections of methylprednisolone acetate (Depo-Medrol), 40 mg (0.5 ml) at each interspace gave good but imperfect relief that lasted nearly two months. When neck pain recurred, methylprednisolone acetate was reinjected at C5-C6 and C6-C7. On this occasion, only partial relief that lasted four weeks was obtained. At the end of this interval, the patient discussed with me the chronic, diffuse, aching low back discomfort that had plagued her for two or more years.

At the time of anterior cervical surgery, an extremely narrowed and arthritic disc space was encountered at C5-C6. Less severe degenerative changes were found at C6-C7. Both levels were fused anteriorly. She responded rapidly, was ambulatory the following day, and was discharged in a cervical collar three days later. At the time of her discharge and on six weeks follow-up, she spontaneously observed that her lower back discomfort seemed to have cleared completely. Unfortunately, four months later some local back aching had again become evident, even though her cervical situation remained quite satisfactory.

The lower back discomfort that is usually described in association with cervical disc disease or tumor is a more diffuse aching or burning discomfort that spreads throughout the lumbar region, both buttocks, and both posterior thighs. Characteristically, these patients do not exhibit signs of nerve root entrapment on physical examination.

Arthritis, Arthralgia, and Osteoporosis

Arthritis (destructive changes in joints) and *arthralgia* (pain arising from joints) are other easily overlooked or misdiagnosed causes of back pain in the failed back syndrome sufferer.[13] *Degenerative osteoarthritis* in older patients usually produces dramatically obvious radiographic changes, but radiographic changes may be much more easily overlooked in other forms of arthritis, such as *rheumatoid arthritis, ankylosing spondylitis,* or *osteitis condensans.*[9,10] These latter forms of arthritis are more common in younger patients, who are also more susceptible to lumbar disc disease. Thus, the risk of mistakenly diagnosing these forms of arthritis as lumbar disc disease is high, unless specific confirmatory laboratory studies have been obtained. Degenerative changes may not be obvious when the sacroiliac joint is involved, especially without specific oblique radiographic views. Of course, degenerative osteoarthritis is not necessarily associated with severe back pain. Many patients who demonstrate marked radiographic changes may have little or no back trouble, while many patients with disabling back pain secondary to arthritis may have limited radiographic changes. Lumbar disc ruptures seem to occur commonly in association with disc degeneration, and preexisting arthritic pain from the disc may be sharply aggravated following disc rupture and disc excision. Severe degenerative changes may later develop at the site of disc rupture (Fig. 3.1). Two acquired forms of localized arthritis, *discitis* and the *facet syndrome,* will be discussed in more detail later.

Historically, patients suffering from arthritis are more likely to describe the *double peak* of arthritis pain. These patients usually awaken with stiffness and aching in their lower backs, buttocks, or occasionally in their posterior thighs. This aching then seems to improve somewhat with morning activity but again increases in severity with the passage of hours to a crescendo of discomfort in late afternoon or evening. Attempted relaxation may be initially quite uncomfortable but then brings considerable relief. Physical examination is characterized by pain on back motion with relatively little tenderness. In the absence of arthritis of the hip, which can also produce symptoms that mimic back pain and sciatica, testing hip motion by straight and bent leg raising should cause pain only when the range of hip motion is carried sufficiently far to cause pelvic flexion or extension and distortion of the intervertebral spaces.

Arthritis is not the only degenerative disease that may be overlooked or misdiagnosed as a cause of chronic back pain in the failed back syndrome patient. Back pain secondary to *osteoporosis* classically develops in postmenopausal women who develop sudden, sharp back pain on minor exertion and whose radiographs show partial collapse of a lumbar or lower thoracic vertebral body. At times, however, the degree of vertebral collapse may be relatively slight, and the initiating event

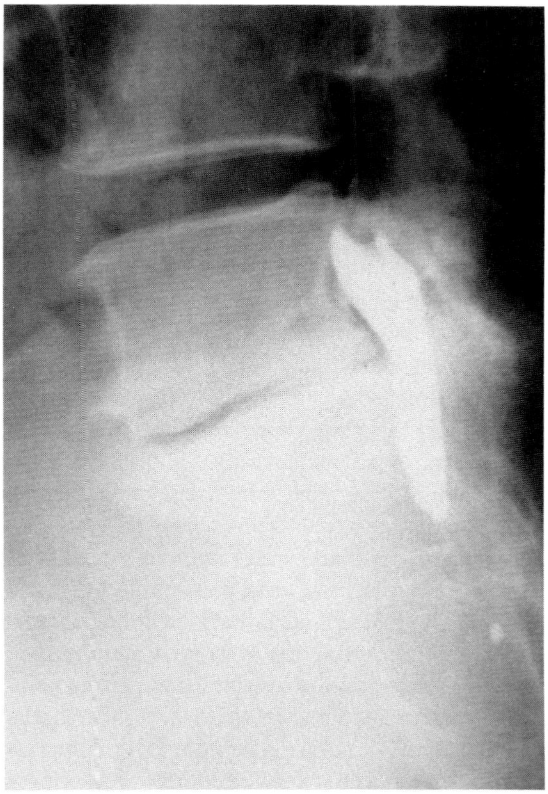

FIGURE 3.1. Degeneration of the intervertebral disc goes hand-in-hand with degenerative arthritis of the spine. Surgical removal of a disc may lead to further collapse, angulation, and instability of that disc level. Years later, severe degenerative arthritis may develop focally at that interspace, as it did in the man whose radiograph is pictured here.

may have been sufficiently inconspicuous to have escaped recognition. In these patients, radiographs should show significant osteoporosis, physical examination should show limitations of back motion and pain on deep percussion, and isotope bone and joint scans may be focally abnormal at sites of even limited stress fractures.

Trauma

Another cause of persistent low back pain is *trauma*. Acute or recent trauma should cause little etiologic, diagnostic difficulty, but failed back patients tend to fall rather frequently, especially when their legs "give way" during abrupt pains. Persistent low back pain following trauma in a failed back syndrome patient may be due to one or more of several different types of injury. Acute *bruising* or *contusion* and *muscle stretching* or *strain* accounts for much of the short term pain that follows back trauma. These aspects of trauma usually respond to local topical therapy combined with systemic analgesics or muscle relaxants and usually subside within a week or so. Pain that persists for many weeks or months makes it necessary to consider other potential types of injury caused by the trauma. *Tearing of muscles or ligaments,* or *avulsions of scar tissue or adhesions* (in actuality only misplaced scar tissue) may result in areas of local tenderness and pain that persists for many weeks. These regions may require prolonged immobilization, systemic anti-inflammatory drugs, or local injection therapy before they finally resolve. Similarly, *tiny fractures* may develop and may be difficult to detect on plain radiographs.[18] These may involve minor compression fractures of the vertebral bodies or tiny linear fractures of posterior spinal elements (Fig. 3.2).

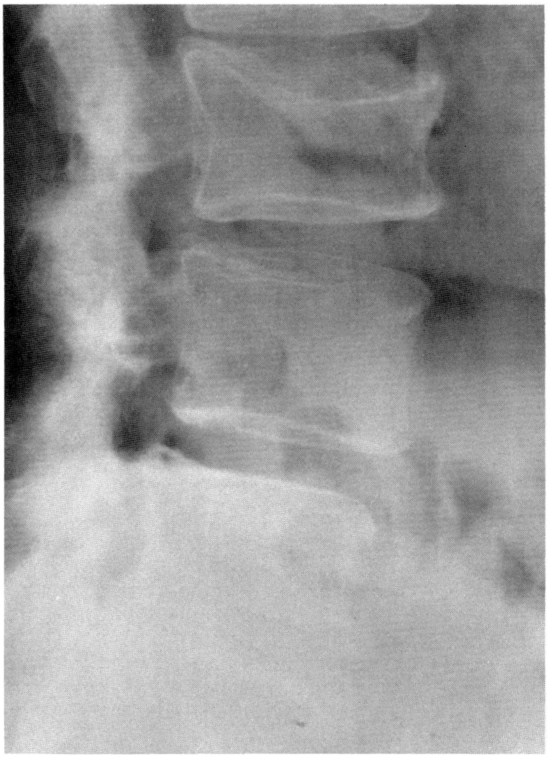

FIGURE 3.2. This man was suspected of having a recurrent disc problem at a previously resected L5-S1 interspace when he returned with severe low back pain after a fall. Instead, he was discovered to have a compression fracture of the L3 vertebral body, as this radiograph documents.

Such small fractures may result either from a single episode of clearly defined injury or from the stress of everyday trauma of lifting, bending, and other activity. When small fractures are not readily visualized on radiographs or when chronic tears or avulsions of soft tissues cause no radiographic changes, isotope bone scans may be diagnostically helpful in delineating the source of the patient's pain.

Flabby Back Syndrome

A more insidious and pervading form of degenerative back disease has been termed the *flabby back syndrome* or *disuse hypoplasia of the back*. This common affliction has apparently increased in frequency as human existence has increased in complexity, luxury, and leisure. Patients who have previously suffered from low back disease, especially if they have undergone back surgery, are at a particularly high risk of developing this syndrome at some point prior to or following back surgery. The avoidance of back muscle exertion and prolonged, enforced bed rest, necessitated by and prescribed in the treatment of low back derangements, rapidly add to a deteriorating tone and strength in the back mechanism. Exactly why this flabby back syndrome causes pain has been the subject of repeated debate, with flabby muscles, weakened ligaments, and slipping joints all being implicated. In talking with patients, I frequently employ a simplistic explanation, as follows: If a normal set of back muscles can lift a 100 pound weight easily, those muscles will experience no discomfort when called to lift a 75-pound weight—whether this weight is external to the body or is merely the upper half of the body during flexion. On the other hand, if these muscles are allowed to weaken to the point that they can exert a maximum force of only 50 pounds, calling upon them to lift 75 pounds will seriously overtax them and will lead to pain. No matter what the precise cause of discomfort in this syndrome, the clinical presentation is one of diffuse back discomfort. This type of back discomfort is usually aggravated by nearly all forms of activity and is commonly associated with diffuse and nonspecific tenderness of the lower back.

Meningeal Irritation

acquired causes of low back pain fol- ccessful back surgery is the develop- *ized meningeal irritation*. This may be associated with *localized epidural* or *intradural scar formation*. When this is coupled with a similar inflammation of nerve roots, sciatica is also a prominent symptom. Histologically and by cerebrospinal fluid (CSF) examination, there is usually little or no evidence of active inflammation, and leukocytes are rarely present. The precise cause of pain in this disorder is unclear, but it is not difficult to imagine a process of repetitive dural stretching or irritation when focal segments of the dura are held in place by scar, while the rest of the dural scar migrates or expands with changes in activity or posture. The patient with this disorder typically complains of increased back pain not only with activity, but with maintenance of an erect posture. In the erect position the lumbar intrathecal spinal fluid pressure is elevated and the spinal sac distends, causing traction on dura and nerves and compression of surrounding scar. Characteristically, coughing and straining sharply aggravate back pain. These maneuvers not only raise the intraspinal pressure but also cause distention of Batson's veins in the epidural space, compounding the local distortion and compression. Occasionally a patient will complain of a variation of this syndrome complex, describing an accentuated, steady pain or a throbbing, pulsating pain in the lower back with recumbency, especially after first lying down. This postural change allows an upward distortion of the dural scar, allows the dural sac to partially collapse, and often exaggerates the normal pulsatile CSF pressure waves transmitted down the spinal canal. Physical examination of patients with localized meningeal irritation usually shows a combination of local tenderness and pain on back movements or movements of the hip sufficient to cause back movement. The tenderness is usually most severe over a site of laminectomy or laminotomy and is usually severe both with direct pressure and with percussion. A sharp aggravation of back pain by coughing is also characteristic, although not diagnostic, of this condition.

Lumbar Pseudomeningocele

Lumbar pseudomeningocele is another complication of back surgery that may lead to the failed back syndrome.[19,20] This uncommon, but surgically correctable, condition develops when a tear in the dura and arachnoid goes undetected or is unsuccessfully treated so that a persistent internal CSF leak develops. Most commonly, patients with pseudomeningoceles will experience some version of the *post–lumbar puncture* headache in the early postoperative period. However, patients who are kept at bed rest for several weeks because of a concomitant spinal fusion may not exhibit the classic exacerbation of headache and backache with erect posture, because they are confined to bed during the period of acute symptoms. If the internal spinal fluid leak persists long enough, a pocket or pseudomeningocele can develop in the area of soft-tissue dissection dorsal to the laminectomy site. With the passage of time a pseudomembrane forms that lines the cyst cavity. These patients may continue to experience headaches reminiscent of the post–lumbar puncture headache, but back pain is the cardinal feature of this disorder. This back pain may be constant, but is usually severely aggravated by the erect posture or by coughing, sneezing, or straining—all activities that cause distention and increased pressure within the pseudomeningocele. Physical examination usually reveals an area of midline tenderness. Only if the cyst is extremely large is it possible to detect tumescence or cystic softening beneath the incision line.

Inflammation of the Lumbar Disc

Postoperative inflammation of the lumbar disc may continue to be a source of lasting pain. When this inflammation is severe, it is frequently associated with a specific elevation of the erythrocyte sedimentation rate (ESR) and is given the name *discitis* or *aseptic interspace inflammation*. The precise frequency of occurrence of this disorder is unknown, but elevation of the ESR lasting more than one or two weeks following discectomy may occur in as many as 5% of patients. Many patients with a less severe or less acute form of this disorder may continue to have pain from an inflamed disc but do not demonstrate an elevation of ESR. Inflammatory discitis may occur spontaneously in children, where it may be misdiagnosed as lumbar disc disease. In adults, the syndrome occurs almost exclusively following disc surgery, with symptoms usually becoming severe within the first few postoperative weeks. The pain caused by this condition usually centers in the lower back, frequently radiating to the posterior aspect of both thighs. On rare occasions, the pain may be chiefly abdominal and may even lead to exploratory laparotomy. Back pain may be associated with local muscle spasms, which in turn may lead to neck and shoulder pain or muscle tension headaches. The back pain is sharply aggravated by activity and slowly relieved by prolonged bed rest, although it may persist despite short periods of bed rest.

Bacterial Disc Infection

Inflammatory discitis must be carefully distinguished from postoperative *bacterial disc infection* or *vertebral osteomyelitis*. Patients with these disorders describe a similar crescendo increase in low back pain over the first few weeks or months following back surgery (see pages 65 and 99). The pain is usually maximal in the lower back, but may radiate into the abdomen, pelvis, or either the anterior or posterior thigh. The findings on physical examination are quite similar to those in patients with inflammatory discitis, with pain on percussion frequently encountered. These patients likewise exhibit an elevated sedimentation rate. But unlike the picture seen with aseptic interspace inflammation, these patients also have a significant elevation in white blood counts (WBCs) and are commonly febrile. Their pain is not improved by protracted bed rest and usually rapidly becomes intolerable.

Instability and the Lumbar Facet Syndrome

Instability of the back is a much abused and much maligned diagnosis, but undoubtedly a disruption in the normal stability and alignment of the back in association with abnormalities of the intervertebral disc (with or without disc excision) may be a cause of back pain. A loss of height of the intervertebral space through degeneration, disc rupture, or disc excision places the facet joints under abnormal strain and alters their normal angle of apposition. This can result in a painful condition known as *lumbar facet syndrome* (Fig. 3.3). Characteristically, this causes maximum pain in the lower back, often predominantly unilateral despite the bilateral facet anatomy. Pain that originates in the facet joint radiates strongly into the posterior aspect of the thigh down to the knee. This radiation of pain should be distinguished from sciatica, which arises from nerves rather than from facet joints. Facet pain radiates to the posterior thigh but rarely, if ever, below the knee. In contrast, sciatic pain is typi
severe distally in the foot, ankle, calf,
even though it commonly projects upwa
posterior thigh, buttock, or back as well

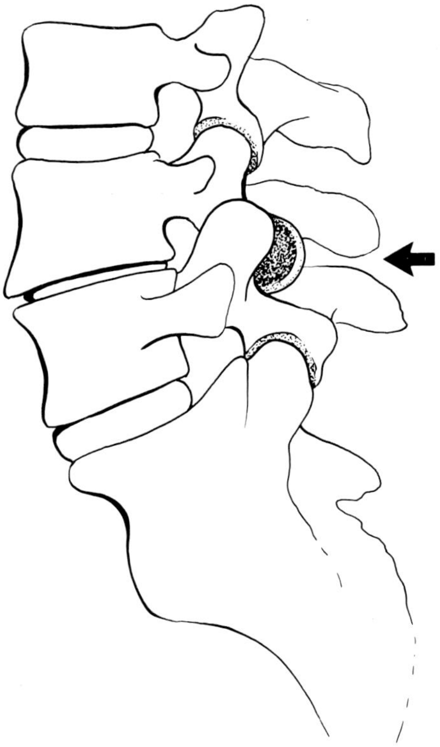

FIGURE 3.3. Degeneration and narrowing of the intervertebral disc causes malalignment of the facet joints **(arrow),** which may lead to the facet syndrome. Narrowing, instability, and facet malalignment may be aggravated following disc excision.

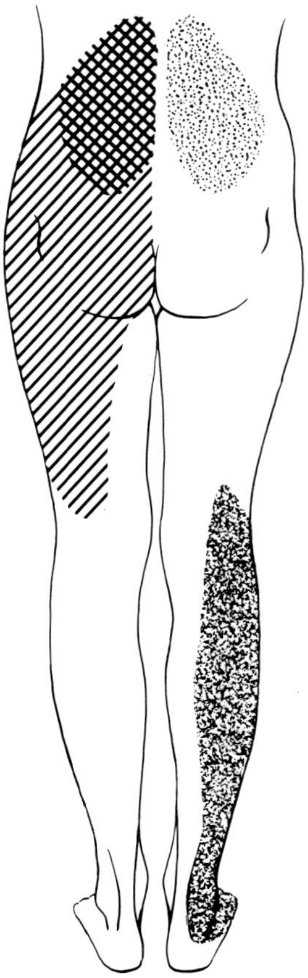

FIGURE 3.4. Pain in the low back and leg may result from nerve root irritation, lumbar disc disease without root involvement, or the lumbar facet syndrome, but the distribution of pain should permit clinical differentiation. Nerve root irritation or sciatica **(right),** causes pain that is more severe **(heavy stippling)** in the lower leg than in the low back. Discogenic and facet pain are more severe in the lower back **(crosshatching, left)** than in the buttock and posterior thigh, but usually the lower leg is spared.

Electrical or mechanical stimulation of the facet joint capsule, which commonly occurs during the performance of facet injections, confirms this pattern of referred pain, eliciting a strong sensation of posterior thigh pain, but rarely eliciting pain below the knee. Discomfort caused by the facet syndrome is clearly aggravated by activity and is partially improved by bed rest or external bracing. On physical examination, lumbago is more consistently elicited by hyperextension of the back than by forward flexion.

Muscle Spasms

Muscle spasms rarely account for chronic and longstanding back pain, but are frequently superimposed upon other conditions that cause back and leg pain. Most patients who have undergone back surgery have also undergone a period of enforced bed rest and physical inactivity that leaves them specifically vulnerable to back muscle spasms. If back muscles become flabby and weakened to the point that they must operate at near maximum effort just to maintain erect posture and ambulation, they will poorly tolerate any additional physical activity, including attempted restorative exercises. A certain amount of backache and discomfort, therefore, should be expected during the period of muscle restoration following disc surgery. Unfortunately, painful muscle spasms may, by themselves, become a disabling disorder. At times, *fixed muscle spasms* develop and cause intense and persistent pain. Once this state has developed, even the addition of muscle relaxing and analgesic medication to break the painful spasm will leave behind a residue of local tenderness and pain that customarily lasts a minimum of five to ten days, and nonsteroidal anti-inflammatory medication should be added to the therapy. Local tenderness of paraspinal muscles, often with visible or palpable tumescence, is a major element in the symptom complex of back muscle spasms, especially fixed or persistent spasms. The patient characteristically complains of a marked intolerance and limitation of back motion.

Trigger Points and Fasciitis

A common phenomenon that is related to that of the fixed back spasm is that of trigger point development. These areas of persistent, focal, exquisite tenderness, with pain both spontaneously and in response to movement, may occur over muscle bodies, but most commonly occur at the periosteal sites of ligamentous attachments to bones (Fig. 3.5). By far, the most common location for *periosteal trigger points* is the site of insertion of lumbodorsal muscles into the posterior medial border of the iliac crest. Similar trigger points can develop in other ligamentous or tendinous areas along the sacrum or iliac crests, over the tips of spinous processes, or in interspinous ligaments. Areas of focal tenderness that develop in the lumbar or gluteal regions are sometimes referred to as *fasciitis*. This term is particularly appropriate when a larger and more diffuse area of tenderness is encountered. As is true of focal meningeal inflammation, fasciitis is not a true inflammatory process, because it is not associated with local leukocytic infiltration or systemic changes in blood or serum characteristic of true inflammation. Because of the lack of pathologic confirmation, the term fasciitis is a controversial one. But challenging the diagnostic terminology will not make this common clinical disorder go away. No matter what the cause of fasciitis and trigger points, many patients suffer from these painful and tender afflictions. Focal tenderness is a cardinal feature of trigger points and fasciitis. Pain is usually maximum at the site of maximum tenderness, but may be referred to the posterior thigh, lateral knee, buttock, or interscapular spine. This pattern of pain referral can often be confirmed by local injection if this initially reproduces the referred pain, then relieves it following anesthetization. This common cause of chronic back pain should always be sought, because despite its disabling severity, it often responds dramatically to nonspecific or local therapy (especially injection therapy), is most often unrelieved by bed rest, and may be made worse by back surgery.

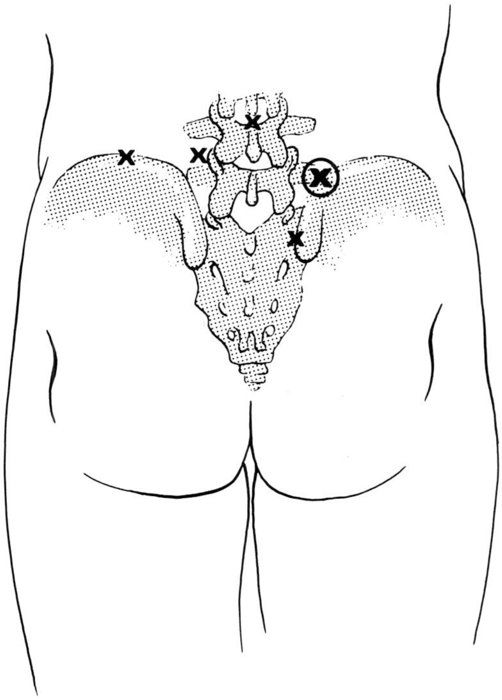

FIGURE 3.5. Lumbosacral periosteal trigger points are found at characteristic locations **(x's)** along or near the bony edges of the sacrum, sacroiliac joint, and spinous processes. The most common site **(circled x)** is at the junction of lumbodorsal and gluteal muscles at the posterior iliac spine.

Fibromyalgia Syndrome

A more diffuse form of periosteal and muscular tenderness and pain has been termed the *fibromyalgia syndrome* or *fibromyositis*.[21] Extensive studies have failed to disclose a precise etiology for this syndrome, but it occurs more often in women than men, and perhaps more often in patients who exhibit overt emotional tension. It is characterized by multiple areas of tenderness and pain over the trunk, limbs, or neck, without evident inflammation. Laboratory findings are nonspecific, and elevations of sedimentation rate or white count and abnormalities of radiographs or isotope scans are not expected. The syndrome does seem to respond to a therapeutic regimen including nonsteroidal anti-inflammatory drugs, persistent limbering and strengthening exercises, and bedtime amitriptyline.

Fat Herniations

Another potential cause of low back pain with local tenderness is fat herniation through the aponeurosis of the transverse abdominal muscle fascia overlying the lower back. The area of this aponeurosis that overlies the lower and most medial "corner" of the lumbosacral paraspinal musculature is normally extremely thin. Because of this distinguishing characteristic it is often given the identifying name of *Petit's triangle*. Nodules of fat, usually ranging from a few millimeters to not more than 2 cm in diameter, may herniate through this thin tissue and become painfully strangulated. They can be palpated as tender lumps of firm, fatty tissue, and their clinical significance can be documented by infiltrating them locally with an anesthetic. Prompt relief of pain and tenderness suggests that the herniated nodule may indeed be a significant cause of the patient's persistent symptoms. I have occasionally encountered this as a convincing entity, although in my experience the vast majority of local tender points in the lumbosacral paraspinal vicinity are the musculoskeletal trigger points that occur along the periosteal margin of the iliac bone.

Ischiogluteal Bursitis

When back pain localizes maximally to the buttock, another quite specific syndrome should be kept in mind—*ischiogluteal bursitis*. This disorder, which has been termed in medical literature "the classical pain in the arse," often goes unrecognized or improperly diagnosed by those lacking expertise in diseases of the back.[22] Local tenderness is a major feature of this disorder, with patients complaining bitterly of pain when they attempt to sit. The pain is frequently unremitting, is sharply aggravated by sitting or walking, and is poorly relieved by bed rest. Physical examination is usually diagnostic, revealing precisely focal tenderness over the ischial tuberosity. This can be palpated best in a patient who is seated or lying on his side with hips flexed, which allows the gluteal muscle to rotate aside and uncover the ischial tuberosity and its bursa (Fig. 3.6). Palpation at the point of contact between the buttocks and the chair elicits extreme tenderness. With the patient prone and hips extended, tenderness is elicited by vertical palpation over the center of the gluteus maximus or by palpation in an upward direction from the buttock crease. Confirmation can

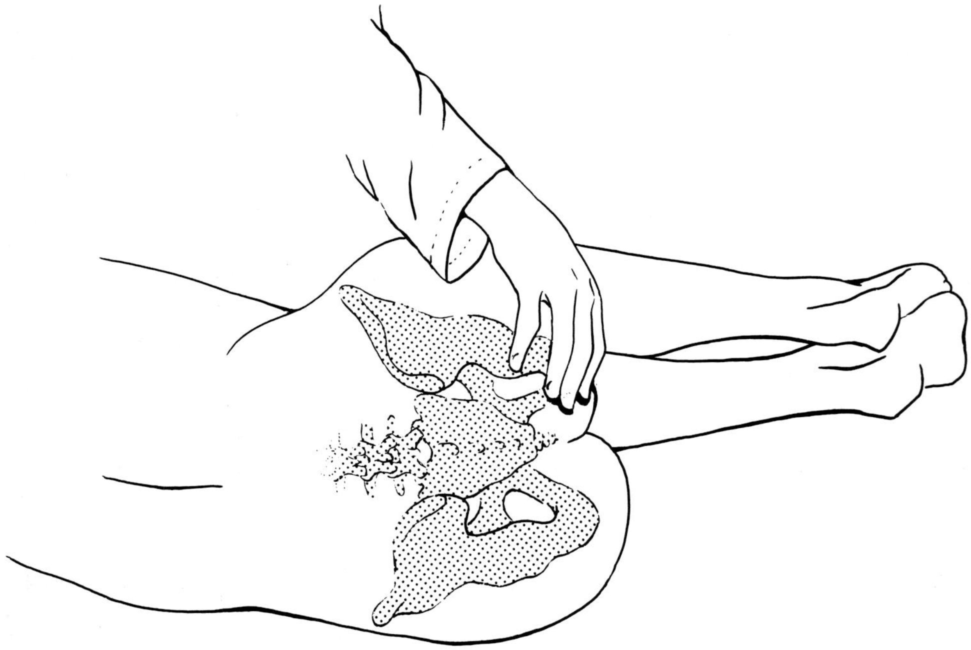

FIGURE 3.6. Ischiogluteal bursitis, the "classical pain in the arse," is diagnosed by palpating the ischial tuberosity with the patient in the decubitus position with hips flexed. This maneuver uncovers the tuberosity from beneath the gluteal muscles. Demonstrating marked local tenderness by palpating at the site of the patient's maximum pain is diagnostic of this not uncommon cause of low back, buttock, and posterior thigh pain.

be obtained from the immediate relief that ensues following anesthetization of the bursa that overlies the ischial tuberosity, the ischiogluteal bursa. As is true of trigger points, the diagnosis of ischiogluteal bursitis as the cause of a patient's chronic back pain should be carefully sought, because it too is a disabling and painful syndrome that frequently responds dramatically to relatively simple therapy and may be exacerbated by further back surgery.

Fusion Problems

The addition of a lumbar spine fusion to simple discectomy may at times be of great benefit to a patient, but this second operation adds the potential for a second series of complications (Table 3.2).

Pseudarthrosis

It has been estimated that *nonunion* or *pseudarthrosis* of a lumbar posterior or posterolateral fusion occurs with a frequency of approximately 20% to 30% for each level fused. That is, a two-level fusion will carry a nonunion rate of 40% to 60%, and a three-level fusion will carry a nonunion rate of 60% to 90%. Failure to achieve a perfect fusion does not guarantee pain. Many painful back conditions that are encountered in patients with pseudarthrosis are not caused by the pseudarthrosis, and the discovery of a pseudarthrosis should not preclude a search for alternative, treatable conditions. Nonetheless, the pseudarthrosis may be painful and may be a cause for continuing disability. A pseudarthrosis typically causes predominantly back pain that is aggravated by activity or bending and is greatly improved by bed rest or external bracing. Occasionally, a pseudarthrosis may also produce severe *persistent sciatica*. Beneath the pseudarthrotic line, hypertrophic scar tissue often develops, causing adhesions to the underlying dura, nerve roots, or both. Following activity, or simply following prolonged standing with distention of the lumbar thecal sac, local nerve root irritation may develop, causing radiating sciatic pain down the posterior or lateral aspect of the

TABLE 3.2. Diagnosis and therapy of failed back syndrome patients with fusion problems as their principal complaint—Based on a symptomatic approach.

Initial presumptive diagnosis (on basis of history)	Initial diagnostic tests	Initial therapy	Confirmatory diagnostic tests	Extended therapy
Pseudarthrosis	X-ray, including flexion/extension and tomography (?), CT scan	Bracing, anti-inflammatory	Facet nerve or fusion anesthesia, isotope scan, bracing, surgical exploration	Repeat fusion or extension of fusion
Kissing pseudarthrosis	X-ray, CT scan	Bracing, anti-inflammatory	Local anesthesia, bracing	Surgical reduction of fusion
Iatrogenic spinal stenosis	X-ray, CT scan	Antineuralgia, intrathecal steroid	Myelogram	Surgical reduction of fusion
Painful bone donor site	History and examination only	Anti-inflammatory, local steroid injection, prolotherapy	Local anesthesia	Local resection
Osteomyelitis of fusion	X-ray, WBC, sedimentation rate, CT scan (?)	Antibiotics, bracing	Aspiration and culture, isotope scan	Surgical debridement
Local trauma (contusion or acute muscle spasm)	History and examination	Heat, liniment, rest, temporary bracing, anti-inflammatory	—	—
Traumatic avulsion of attachments to fusion	History and examination, x-ray	Heat, liniment, temporary bracing, anti-inflammatory	Local anesthetic injection, isotope bone scan	Local steroid injection or prolotherapy
Fracture of fusion	X-ray including flexion/extension, tomography (?), and CT scan	External bracing, anti-inflammatory, heat, liniment, rest (when acute)	Facet nerve or fusion anesthesia, isotope scan, bracing, surgical exploration	Revision of fusion

leg to the ankle or foot. If epidural scarring continues to progress, actual damage to nerve roots can occur, causing unilateral or bilateral weakness, reflex loss, or sensory impairment.

Slipped Fusion Bone

Following interbody fusion, with or without the addition of facet fusion and posterior wiring, the specific problem of intraspinal *posterior slippage of interbody fusion bone* can occur. Such slippage can simply cause failure of fusion, with pseudarthrosis and lumbago. More commonly, though, slippage of more than a few millimeters can cause compression of one or more nerve roots, with intractable sciatica. The sciatica is usually constant, but is commonly aggravated by activity and especially by bending. Examination usually discloses marked signs of nerve root entrapment (see page 45), and there may or may not be evidence of actual nerve root damage with motor, sensory, or reflex loss. This complication is more likely to occur in patients with severely osteoporotic and soft bones, especially postmenopausal women. It also can occur following an episode of severe vomiting or retching in the first days or weeks postoperatively, especially while the patient is resting in bed and not wearing a back support. Computerized tomography (CT) scans are usually diagnostic.

Kissing Pseudarthrosis and Adjacent Degeneration

Even a solid fusion may be a source of pain. If the fusion bone encroaches too closely upon adjacent bones a *kissing pseudarthrosis* may result. In this condition, bony impingement occurs most commonly with hyperextension of the lumbar spine. Local tenderness may develop at this site, usually centered in the area of maximum spontaneous pain.

Even if a kissing pseudarthrosis does not develop, a solid fusion may produce pain in the area above the fusion. With a solid fusion the interspace level above the fusion is called upon to compensate with increased mobility. Over the years, this may result in marked *degenerative changes* at this level, with radiographs demonstrating bone spurring, subluxation, and interspace collapse (Fig. 3.7). Severe pain, predominantly confined to the back, may then develop.

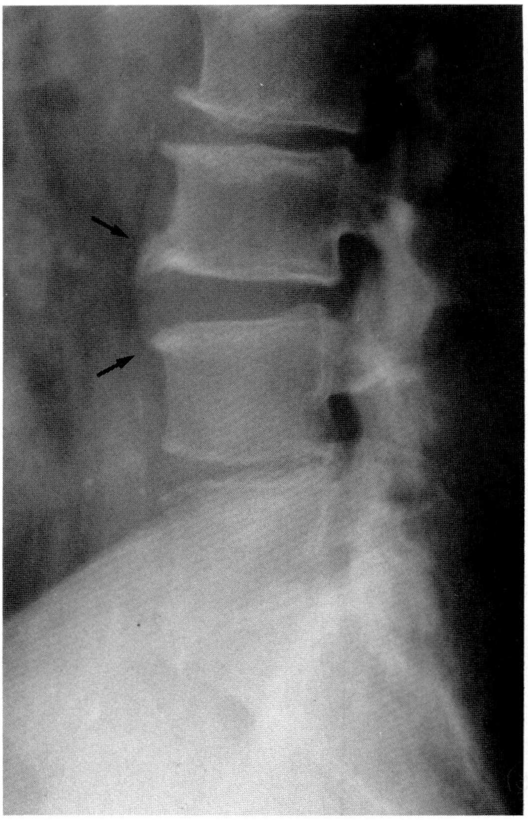

FIGURE 3.7. Fusing the lumbar spine places additional stress and strain on the next highest intervertebral level. Over the years, this can lead to severe degenerative arthritis at this level, as documented in this radiograph of a patient who presented with increasing low back pain after being relieved of similar back pain and sciatica by spinal fusion of L4 to the sacrum. Degenerative spurring above the fusion is marked by arrows.

Osteomyelitis

Low back pain following spinal fusion may also be seen as a result of *osteomyelitis* of the fusion bone. This may or may not be seen in conjunction with acute soft-tissue sepsis, and it sometimes develops in delayed fashion in the absence of acute symptoms of wound infection. The patient usually notes an aching, constant pain at the fusion site that increases progressively in severity. The pain is usually sharply aggravated by motion, especially if the fusion bone has not yet fully healed or if the infection has caused dissolution of a previously relatively stable fusion. Physical examination most often reveals marked local tenderness to palpation or percussion. If the patient has had sufficient time since fusion to permit testing of range of back motion, this will prove to be severely restricted by pain. Pain will be particularly severe if the stability of the fusion has been impaired by the osteomyelitis, but pain on motion may be severe simply due to stressing the fusion bone or stretching ligamentous attachments to the bone. Body temperature is usually elevated significantly only in the face of acute or extensive sepsis. Sedimentation rate and WBCs are usually distinctly abnormal. Plain radiographs are commonly diagnostic, demonstrating dissolution or destruction of the fusion bone. CT scans often demonstrate the area of bone destruction in exquisite detail, and isotope bone and joint scans or white cell scans usually confirm the biological hyperactivity of the area.

Iatrogenic Spinal Stenosis

Spinal fusion can also produce an *iatrogenic spinal stenosis* if the bony fusion mass impinges upon the underlying thecal sac.[23] This is more likely to occur if bilateral laminotomies or extensive laminectomy has been performed, leaving a large exposed area of dorsal dura. This can, however, occur even in an area where the dura remains covered by the ligamentum flavum if bone fragments are too vigorously packed into place during the performance of the fusion. Posterior interbody-facet fusions can produce symptomatic stenosis from bone driven in at the facet fusion site, a failure to recess the interbody fusion bone, or a posterior migration of the interbody fusion bone.

These patients may complain of an aching back that is usually not severe at rest or even with bending. Hyperextension is often more painful than forward flexion, and patients may adopt a stooped posture. Most of these patients complain that attempted activity, especially walking, aggravates their back pain and usually brings on a diffuse aching in both lower extremities that is reminiscent of the pain of claudication. This so-called *neurogenic claudication* is usually rapidly improved by cessation of walking and is differentiated from vascular claudication primarily by the presence of good peripheral pulses on physical examination. Surgical decompression by wide laminectomy at the involved levels usually produces prompt and gratifying relief.

Bone Donor Site

The bone donor site along the posterior iliac crest frequently becomes a cause of pain and local tenderness. Both lumbosacral and gluteal muscles attach along the posterior iliac crest, putting tremendous stress and tension on this region. Even though no major nerves traverse the area, multiple small and *painful neuromata* occasionally develop at this donor site. The pain and tenderness that develop over this site are similar whether the etiology is local neuroma formation, chronic ligamentous sprain or trigger points, or fasciitis.

Trauma

Trauma may initiate back pain in patients with previous fusions through a variety of mechanisms. Direct *contusion* of the lower back and acute muscle strain are usually easily diagnosed by history. These pains are usually of limited duration and respond nicely to local heat, liniments, muscle relaxing medication, brief periods of bed rest, or temporary external bracing. At other times the back pain initiated by trauma may be persistent and may even gradually increase in severity.

Persistent pain with marked, local tenderness over the fusion bone raises the diagnostic possibility of *traumatic avulsion* of adjacent muscles, ligaments, and fascia from the surface of the mass of fusion bone. There are usually no radiographic changes, but isotope bone scans may be positive. The more localized areas of pain and tenderness may be confirmed as avulsion injuries by local anesthetization, and long-term benefit may follow local steroid injection. Anti-inflammatory drugs and prolonged external bracing are useful for many patients.

A *fracture of the fusion* may result from major trauma or even from seemingly relatively minor trauma, depending on the preexisting stability of the fusion itself. Spinal fusions grow into place from collections of small chips of bone that normally fuse into a single mass of bone firmly attached to the underlying vertebral arches or vertebral bodies. Not infrequently, fusion is incomplete, so a fusion may be stable on the basis of limited attachments of adjacent bony fragments to each other or to underlying vertebral structures. As discussed later (page 63), instability or pseudarthrosis of a fusion may be extremely difficult to demonstrate radiographically. This is especially true if the fracture in a previously stable fusion occurs in the form of a separation of overlying fusion bone from underlying vertebral lamina or transverse processes. An isotope bone scan might be helpful if the process is sufficiently large and sufficiently active biologically to produce enough isotope uptake to be readily visible. Anti-inflammatory drug therapy and prolonged bracing, supplemented by local heat and liniments, usually suffice for most of these injuries, but on occasion, open surgical revision of the fractured fusion may become necessary.

Leg Pain

The failed disc patient may suffer from leg pain that fails to subside following laminectomy or that improves transiently but then recurs, either in constant or episodic fashion (Table 3.3). Neurologic loss of a radiculopathic type may accompany radiating sciatic leg pain, but need not be present. Discounting a patient's complaints of pain due to the absence of neurologic loss ignores clinical reality and often does the patient a disservice if it denies the patient adequate therapy for a very real affliction.

Diagnostic Errors and Inadequate Surgery

Leg pain that continues unabated following disc surgery raises the strong possibility of either *diagnostic error* prior to surgery or *improper or inadequate surgery.* Removal of an intervertebral disc will do little to relieve the pain caused by an intraspinal tumor that was missed because only CT and not myelography was employed, and removing a normal L4-L5 disc will fail to benefit the sufferer from an L5-Sl rupture that was occult on myelography. As discussed in more detail later in this chapter, lumbar *adhesive arachnoiditis* can give a myelographic picture and clinical presentation similar to that of lumbar disc rupture, but extradural exploration and disc removal fail to alter either the radiographic picture or the clinical symptoms.

Persistent sciatic pain caused by a *retained disc fragment* following disc surgery is a much talked about, but infrequently encountered, syndrome. Once disc material has ruptured free through the posterior longitudinal ligament, one or more fragments of firm disc material may be encountered in the epidural space. It is possible for one of these fragments to migrate laterally along the epidural "gutter" or into the neural foramen, either spontaneously or as a result of inadvertent displacement during surgery—usually while the surgeon is attempting to gain exposure through retraction. This possibility, of course, is avoidable by careful exploration of the epidural space and the neuroforaminal canal in every case in which perforation of the posterior longitudinal ligament is documented.

A pain-free interval following initial lumbar disc surgery does not completely exonerate the *accuracy of preoperative diagnosis* or *adequacy of surgery.* A partial decompression may be inadequate to give long-term satisfactory relief but may sufficiently reduce the intensity of the initial pain to bring considerable relief by comparison. This is especially true during the early operative recovery period when the patient's activity is limited, when analgesics are freely given, and when the patient is apt to be at bed rest more than usual. Resumption of normal activity and weight bearing may once again escalate persistent leg pain to unbearable severity. At this point, additional fragments of disc material may herniate outward through the now-perforated posterior longitudinal ligament, especially if interspace clean-out has been scanty or hastily performed. The argument over how thoroughly interspace clean-out should be performed continues unresolved, with fierce advocates supporting each position. This is discussed further in Chapter 6.

Far lateral disc ruptures, presenting exclusively in the neuroforaminal canal and not detectable on myelography or surgical exploration of the epidural space, were thought to be quite rare prior to the widespread application of CT and magnetic resonance imaging (MRI) scans (see page 79). These newer imaging modalities have demonstrated that far-lateral disc ruptures are indeed not rare and that they occur most commonly at L3-L4 and L4-L5. Since far-lateral disc ruptures compress nerve roots within the neural foramen, and not at the intraspinal epidural site where posterolateral disc ruptures compress nerve roots, the nerve root affected is one segmental level higher than that normally seen with disc ruptures. Thus a far-lateral rupture at L3-L4 compresses the L3 root, not the L4 root, and an L4-L5 rupture compresses the L4 root, not the L5 root. Surgical resection requires either a *paraspinal exposure* or an *extensive foramenotomy.*

On imaging studies, the major differential diagnostic alternatives to far-lateral disc ruptures are nerve root *neurilemomas* (usually resectable with preservation of the extrinsically compressed nerve root) or *neurofibromas* (entwined within the nerve root, which must be sacrificed at the time of resection). These *nerve root tumors* can cause the acute

TABLE 3.3. Diagnosis and therapy of failed back syndrome patients with leg pain as their principal complaint—Based on a symptomatic approach.

Initial presumptive diagnosis (on basis of history)	Initial diagnostic tests	Initial therapy	Confirmatory diagnostic tests	Extended therapy
Retained disc fragment or far lateral rupture, unresected disc rupture	X-ray, myelogram, CT, or MRI scan	Antineuralgia, anti-inflammatory, enforced inactivity	Epidurography, epidural venogram, nerve root anesthetic block (?), electromyography (?)	Surgical removal of disc rupture
Retained foreign body (postoperative)	X-ray, myelogram, CT, or MRI scan	Surgical removal, anti-inflammatory	—	—
Nerve root fibrosis	History and examination only	Antineuralgia, anti-inflammatory, enforced inactivity (if acute)	Myelogram, CT or MRI scan, nerve root anesthetic block	Epidural or intrathecal steroid, surgical epidural neurolysis, nerve root sensory interruption, or surgical section
Arachnoiditis	X-ray, myelogram, MRI scan (?)	Antineuralgia, anti-inflammatory, enforced inactivity (if acute)	Spinal or nerve root anesthetic block	Intrathecal steroid, surgical lysis or arachnoiditis, nerve root sensory interruption or surgical section, dorsal column stimulator
Arachnoidal cyst (postoperative)	Myelogram or MRI scan	Antineuralgia, anti-inflammatory	—	Surgical repair, intrathecal steroid
Nerve root cyst, synovial cyst	X-ray, CT or MRI scan, myelogram	Antineuralgia, anti-inflammatory	Nerve root anesthetic block	Surgical resection/plication of cyst (?)
Spinal stenosis	X-ray, CT scan	Antineuralgia, bracing	Myelogram	Intrathecal steroid, surgical decompression
Lateral recess stenosis	X-ray, CT scan	Antineuralgia, bracing	Myelogram	Epidural or intrathecal steroid, surgical decompression
Viral neuritis, diabetic mononeuritis, herpetic nerve root involvement	WBC, sedimentation rate, blood sugar, serum viral titers	Antineuralgia, control diabetes	Electromyography and nerve root anesthetic block	Nerve root sensory interruption or surgical section (rarely)
Benign spinal neoplasm	X-ray, myelogram, MRI, or CT scan	Surgical resection	—	—

or rapidly progressive onset of sciatic pain or neuropathy following trauma or heavy exertion through the initiation of localized edema and swelling within the confines of the neural foramen. The imaging uncertainty can be resolved if intravenous contrast enhancement of the lesion is strongly apparent on CT or MRI scans or if contrast discography is performed, especially supplemented by postdiscography CT scanning. Patients frequently respond to nonsurgical therapy, and in these instances surgery may be deferred since (1) most nerve root tumors grow slowly and the symptoms may have resulted from reversible effects of trauma to the tumor, (2) tumor resection may involve sacrificing the motor and sensory function of the involved nerve root if the tumor is a neurofibroma, and (3) at least 50% of frank disc ruptures respond satisfactorily to nonsurgical therapy. If surgery is elected, distinction can be made between neurilemoma and neurofibroma only at the time of dissection. If a neurofibroma is found, the patient and surgeon must have decided in advance of surgery whether to undertake resection of the intertwined tumor and nerve root or to settle instead for surgical decompression only—which may provide many years of relief of symptoms and deficits.

Hypertrophic Scarring

Hypertrophic scarring of three major types may cause sciatic pain to develop after a relatively pain-free interval. Scar tissue that develops primarily in the lateral epidural space is called *nerve root fibrosis.* Although this primarily involves perineural scarring, intraneural scarring may also develop, especially in a nerve root that has been injured by the previous disc rupture or at the time of surgery. Following intraoperative nerve root injury, pain and neurologic loss are likely to appear de novo following surgery and to persist, although a gradual increase may be experienced later. The causes of nerve root fibrosis are unclear but are frequently attributed to the quality of the surgery itself, often being aggravated by limited exposure of the swollen and displaced nerve root due to inadequate bone removal or a macho attempt at minimal-exposure microsurgery. Extensive epidural monopolar coagulation, vigorous nerve root retraction, vigorous packing of cottonoids in the lateral epidural gutter, or inadequate protection of the nerve root during repeated mechanical instrumentation for removal of the nucleus pulposus may all result in direct nerve injury. On the other hand, failure to control extradural bleeding meticulously may lead to postoperative hematoma formation with severe sciatica—which may develop early in the postoperative period, then partially resolve, only to be followed by later development of severe nerve root fibrosis. Several careful studies, notably those by Mayfield and his group, have implicated the "postlaminectomy membrane" in the formation of epidural adhesions and nerve root fibrosis.[15] They found that exposure of the dura to overlying fibrous tissue tended to result in exuberant adhesions, but that this could largely be prevented by interposition of a layer of autogenous fat in the dorsal epidural space at the conclusion of surgery. This technique seems to be superior to simple gelatin foam placement and has been my routine surgical practice for many years. Two decades ago, we were taught to mark the surgical site for future radiographic reference (to ensure surgical excision of the proper disc and so on) by placing a metal clip on the cut edges of the posterior longitudinal ligament. Now I strongly condemn this practice, because these metal clips elicit a fibrous reaction that is quite dramatic when reoperation is performed for lysis of the nerve root fibrosis that commonly forms in these patients. If metal marking clips are to be placed, and their use seems quite valid, they should preferably be attached to the anulus within the interspace or placed dorsal to the epidural fat pad.

The second form of postoperative scarring occurs within the dural sac as *arachnoiditis* and will be discussed in more detail later. It has already been mentioned that this condition may develop subsequent to surgery, perhaps caused by disc rupture itself, and may cause a delayed onset of severe leg pain, back pain, or both.

As alluded to earlier, a third form of epidural scarring may be seen following spinal fusion in situations of *pseudarthrosis.* In these patients the leg pain that develops is almost always accompanied by a significant degree of back pain as well.

Wound Infections

Leg pain that develops following back surgery may have an infectious etiology. Wound infections most often are relatively superficial and are easily detected by examination of the wound as well as by observation of fever and progressive elevation of WBCs. Temperature is often mildly elevated for several days following uncomplicated and uninfected back surgery, and an elevation is predictable if spinal fusion has been included. WBCs usually show less of a rise and should return to normal within a few days. Occasionally, patients will present with *deep wound infections,* characteristically becoming symptomatic two to five days postoperatively. A bacterial infection in the *epidural space* causes intense local pain with strong sciatic radiation, whereas infection chiefly localized to the *intervertebral disc space* initially causes pain that is most severe in the lower back. *Painful viral neuritis* or *diabetic mononeuritis* may rarely occur by chance association in a patient suffering from the failed back syndrome, but one specific form of viral neuritis infrequently occurs as a direct sequela of nerve injury caused by disc rupture or back surgery. Herpetic nerve root involvement may develop after back surgery, just as it may complicate disc rupture without back surgery. The temporal onset is more unpredictable than that for bacterial wound infection, but severe burning leg pain results. In nearly every case a typical herpetic, papular, pruritic rash develops in the cutaneous distribution of the affected nerve root shortly after the onset of the leg pain.

Nerve Root Cysts

Congenital lumbar nerve root cysts are occasionally implicated as a source of sciatic pain.[24] These cysts are also known as *Tarlov cysts* in honor of the neurosurgeon who described their clinical significance.[25] These cysts are outpouchings of arachnoid and dura that occur along the proximal nerve roots within the spinal canal. They are much more common in the lumbar region than at other spinal levels and usually communicate with the subarachnoid space. On myelography they fill either immediately or after a delayed interval and can easily be seen. Multiple nerve root cysts in a single patient are common. They become symptomatic presumably due to local pressure effects, but it is difficult in a given patient to know when a documented cyst is indeed symptomatic. The surgical treatment involves surgical reduction of the cyst or plication of its wall. Because the nerve root usually lies in the wall of the cyst, it is rarely possible to completely excise these structures, and surgical decompression allows further enlargement of the cyst with even greater stretching and irritation of the nerve root. Surgery is at times quite beneficial, but not predictably so, as the following case report documents (Fig. 3.8):

Case 2

This 56-year-old homemaker fell on her coccyx in 1971, initiating a protracted course of pain in her coccyx and buttock. Over a period of several years, pains gradually began to radiate into the right posterior thigh and calf. In 1978, a myelogram at another hospital revealed a large nerve root cyst involving the right S1 nerve root. The upper sacrum was unroofed surgically and a portion of the cyst wall was resected to reduce the size of the cyst. Immediately after surgery she was pain free, but over the next three months sciatic pain gradually recurred. I examined her in 1980 because of persistent severe pain that rendered her bedridden and completely dependent on opiate narcotics. Repeat myelography showed persistence of several lumbar cysts, but no other obvious abnormality. She complained of occasional urinary incontinence. On examination, straight leg raising to 80 degrees on the right caused radiating leg pain, but the bowstring test was negative. There was dense hypalgesia over the lateral aspect of the right foot and calf, absent right ankle reflex, and slight weakness of plantar flexion of the right ankle. Antineuralgic and antiinflammatory medication was ineffective. An epidural nerve root block at S1 produced anesthesia over the lateral right ankle and calf and seemed to give near total pain relief. A series of three epidural corticosteroid injections at S1 gave relief lasting only a few weeks following each injection. She then elected phenol chemical sensory rhizotomy rather than open surgical sensory rhizotomy. In August 1980, intrathecal injection of phenol in anhydrous glycerol was performed. This allowed her to discontinue opiates and become ambulatory, although she continued to complain of leg pain a year later.

Spinal and Lateral Recess Stenosis

Classically, *lumbar spinal stenosis* gives a picture of bilateral leg pains that are specifically aggravated by walking more than bending—so-called *neurogenic claudication*.[23] Spinal stenosis results most commonly from degenerative hypertrophy of ligamentum flavum, facets and their synovia and posterior annulus, often becoming symptomatic in patients with congenitally small spinal canals. An iatrogenic etiology was discussed earlier (page 25). Progressive hypertrophic degeneration can develop following resection of a disc rupture if the degenerative process that underlies many disc ruptures continues to worsen. The picture on myelogram and CT scan should be definitive for this syndrome. Unfortunately, some early or marginal forms of spinal stenosis may cause unilateral radiating leg pain in the presence of unilateral bone spurs or small disc bulges. Removal of the disc bulge alone, without performing an adequate decompressive laminectomy, may fail to relieve the preexisting nerve root pain.

A specific variant of lumbar spinal stenosis is the syndrome of *lateral recess stenosis* or *lateral canal stenosis*, in which a single nerve root may be entrapped laterally by hypertrophic bony changes as it curves around the facet (Figs. 3.9 and 3.10). Failure to extend the laminectomy far enough laterally or failure to add a foramenotomy may explain the relentless leg pain following discectomy alone for this condition.

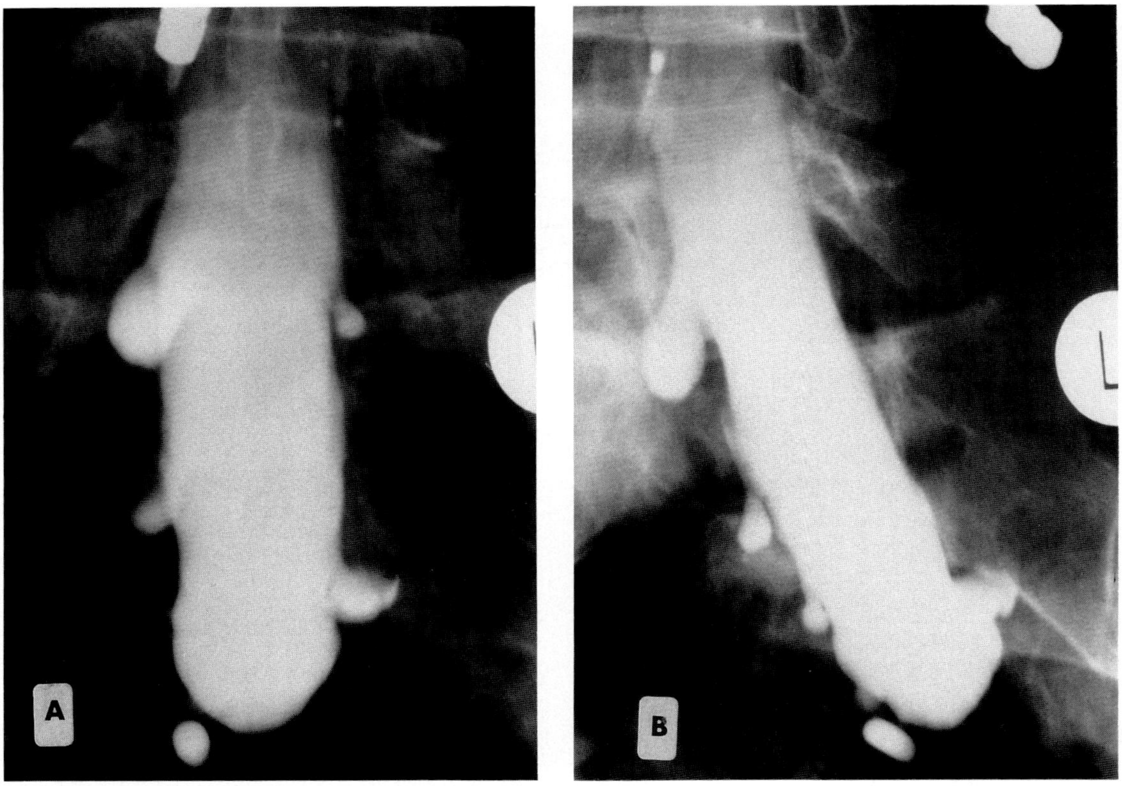

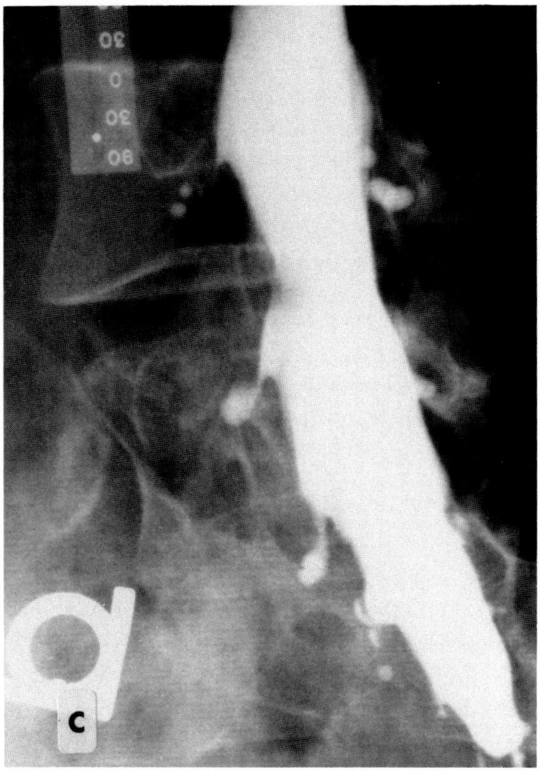

FIGURE 3.8. Myelogram films (**A and B**) demonstrate the lumbosacral nerve root cysts (Tarlov cysts) documented in the woman discussed as Case 2, prior to her first surgical intervention. The large cyst on the S1 nerve root was associated with an overlying area of apparent bony erosion. Operative plication/reduction of the cyst failed to relieve her persistent sciatica. The multiple small cysts seen in this patient and (**C**) in another patient are not uncommonly seen and rarely, if ever, are symptomatic.

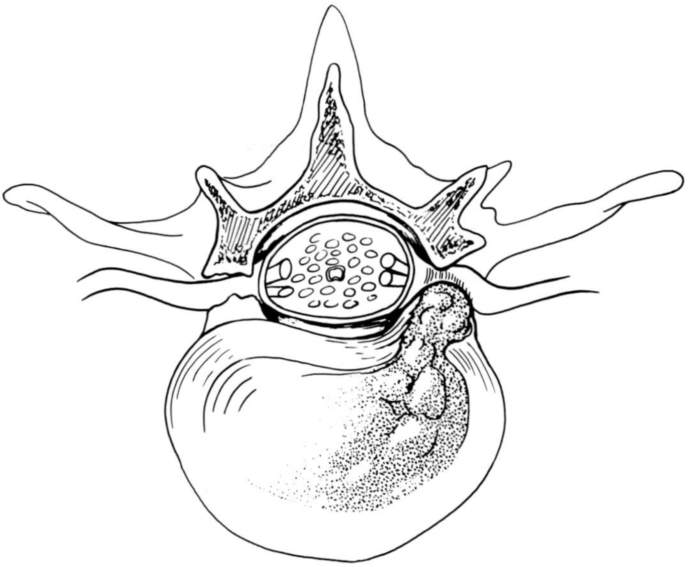

FIGURE 3.9. Two surgically correctable causes of sciatica usually go undetected on myelography. Lateral recess stenosis, secondary to degenerative arthritic changes **(left),** and far lateral disc ruptures **(right),** cause nerve root entrapment within the neuroforamen with little or no encroachment upon the thecal sac. A CT scan may be diagnostic, but surgical confirmation often requires careful exploration through an adequate bony exposure.

Facet Synovial Cysts

While the facet syndrome of painful degeneration or instability causes predominantly low back pain with posterior thigh radiation, cysts derived from *hypertrophied facet synovia* that project into the spinal canal cause focal nerve root compression. The symptoms produced closely resemble those of disc rupture, but, as with lateral recess stenosis, the nerve root may not be entrapped, and nerve root tension signs may be absent. CT and MRI scans showing a dorsal and lateral rounded mass adjacent to a facet joint are usually diagnostic. If sciatic symptoms are not sufficiently controlled by other means, surgical excision usually provides prompt relief. Not uncommonly, these cysts occur in association with a facet syndrome or painful spinal instability, so cyst removal may be combined with interbody-facet fusion and wiring or other forms of spinal stabilization.

Postoperative Arachnoidal Cysts

Leg pain that develops following back surgery may also develop from postoperative *arachnoidal cysts.* These CSF-filled cystic outpouchings are similar in etiology to, but less extensive than, pseudomeningoceles (see page 18). Whereas pseudomeningoceles cause pain more severe in the lower back than in the legs, arachnoidal cysts are likely to cause sciatica with relatively little lower back pain. The development of a postoperative arachnoidal cyst is initiated at the time of surgery when a small dural tear occurs and is not corrected. The arachnoid, which herniates through this dural tear, forms the primary cyst, although over time this may become reinforced by an outer wall of fibrous scar tissue. Fluid pulsations within the cystic outpouching can slowly enlarge the dural opening somewhat, but usually the ostium remains no more than a few millimeters in diameter. A nerve root can herniate through this ostium and become stretched within the sac, and at times can even become entrapped in the sac and cause a chronic sciatic irritation. Because these cysts usually arise from the dorsal half of the thecal sac, the dorsally situated sensory roots are more likely to herniate than the ventrally situated motor roots. The resulting clinical picture is one of intense, burning sciatic pain that may be constant and is usually sharply aggravated by activity or motion.

Psychogenic Factors

The intertwining of psychogenic and somatic factors in the failed disc syndrome is one of the most challenging and frustrating aspects of the management of this disorder.[26,27] Patients who are chronically in pain and are incapable of performing the activities that they feel they need to do or want to do are quite likely to become *depressed* or *anxious.* Conversely, patients who are depressed because of

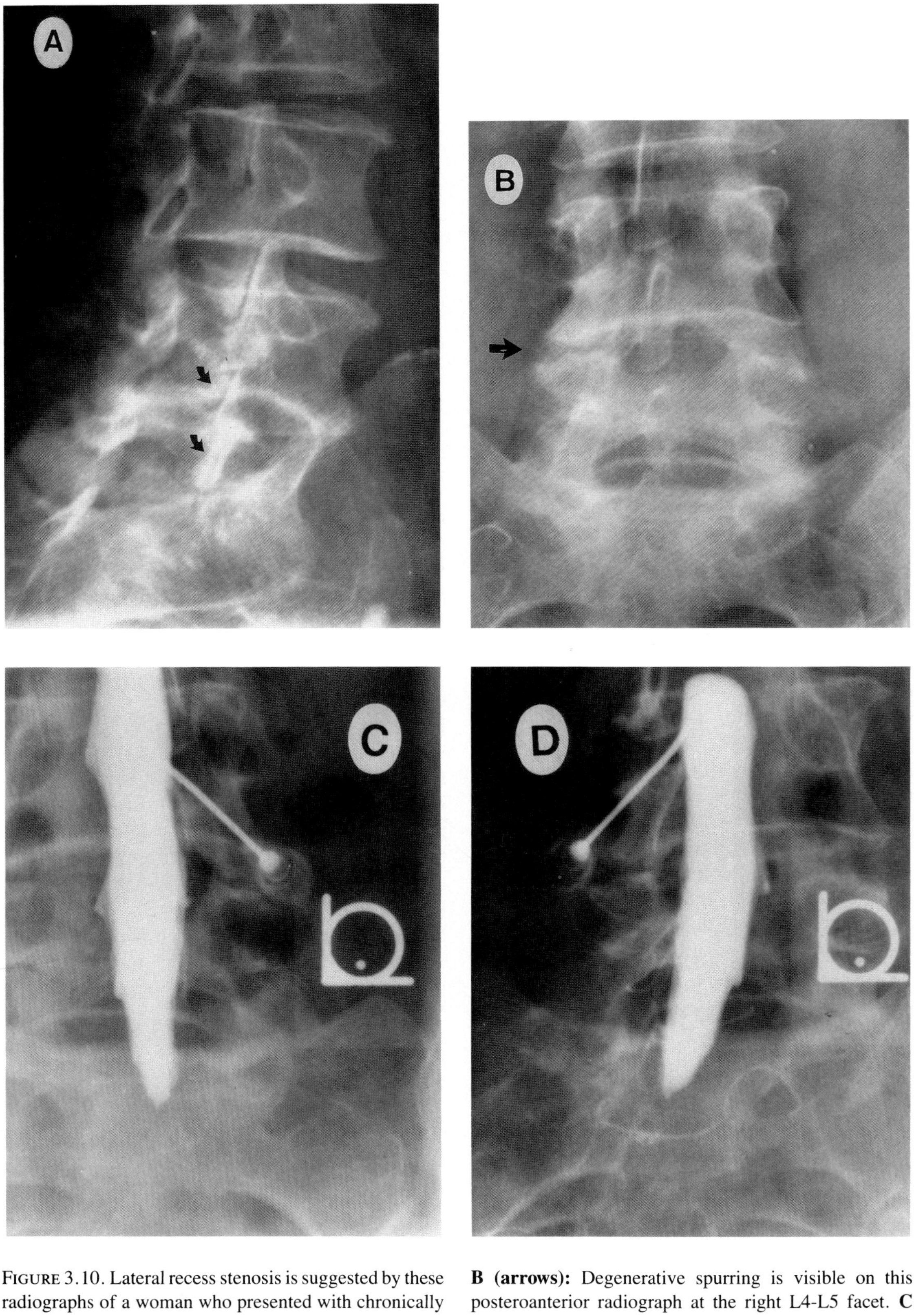

FIGURE 3.10. Lateral recess stenosis is suggested by these radiographs of a woman who presented with chronically progressive sciatica. **A (arrows):** Sclerosis and narrowing of the facets are best seen on oblique radiographs. **B (arrows):** Degenerative spurring is visible on this posteroanterior radiograph at the right L4-L5 facet. **C and D:** Myelography was normal but pain was relieved by surgical decompression of the lateral spinal recess.

family problems, job stresses, or other problems will certainly be *more conscious of, and more disabled by, somatic pain*. When depression coexists with somatic pain and disability, successfully treating one aspect of the problem will usually have a beneficial result on the other. Instituting primary psychiatric treatment may prove difficult unless the patient can first be convinced of its relevance to his situation and the potential benefit to him. It is frustrating for a surgeon to receive a report from a consulting psychiatrist to the effect that "after you've cured his pain, I'll help him with his depression," since the surgeon frequently needs the psychiatrist's help in order to be able to relieve the patient's pain.

Every physician who deals with failed back syndrome patients should make at least a brief attempt at assessing the potential *role of psychologic factors* in the overall disease process. Obtaining a history of other family members with back disease suggests a hereditary weakness of the patient's back. However, if these other family members have been severely disabled or chronically afflicted by their back problems, this should raise concerns about the risk of prominent psychologic factors in this patient's problem. Additional factors of importance include patients who are dependent on manual labor for their livelihood, patients with low intelligence, and patients with a developmental or family history of excessive punishment and parental violence. Intercurrent social stresses, such as divorce or loss of a loved one, may also predispose a patient to the development of chronic pain.

The physician should suspect that psychologic factors may be etiologically important in patients who exhibit *denial* or *hostility* as they deal with their present problems; in patients who seem to be *preoccupied by their illnesses* to the point that they lose all productivity, even for hobbies and other outside interests; in patients who show *obvious signs of depression, anxiety,* or *repression of normal affect;* and in patients who show evidence of *significant invalidism* through dramatic recounting of their problems or seemingly excessive dependence on others. Patients are most likely to develop chronic pain conditions if they give a prior history of excessively compulsive work addiction with limited outside interests and limited ability to react emotionally with others. A history of *sleep disturbance* should be carefully noted. Normal sleep patterns may be disrupted by pain, anxiety, or depression. On the other hand, the patient who claims to have severe, chronic pain, yet who denies difficulty sleeping, should be suspected of a problem in which psychologic difficulties or overt malingering plays a prominent role.

It is even more important to obtain *corroborating history* from the spouse or other family members in dealing with problems that have a strong psychologic component than in dealing with problems that involve tissue injury in a patient who reacts effectively psychologically. A discrepancy in the recounting of the impact of pain upon a patient's life between that given by the patient and the report given by the spouse or relatives may provide an important clue to the patient's excessive use of denial or symptom amplification. Descriptions by the spouse or other family members of the impact of the patient's pain upon his life-style and of the patient's reaction to his pain may be extremely helpful in quantitating the seriousness of apparent psychologic maladaptations to pain. The office nurse may be particularly helpful by talking formally or informally with other family members in the waiting room either while the patient is present or while the patient is in the examining room.

Evaluating the degree of emotional overlay is not always easy and various *testing devices* have been proposed.[28–31] One device is a depression rating scale in which the patient checks off his responses on a list of phrases or questions and his "depression score" is totaled. Another device is a printed body outline on which the patient is asked to draw specified symbols showing the location, quality, and intensity of his pain. Pains that are diffuse in area and quality, especially if they are graded at maximum severity, are more likely to be associated with depression—although one may question whether the depression is primary or secondary.

If depression is allowed to remain untreated and if no satisfactory relief of chronic pain is forthcoming, *suicide* becomes a distinct possibility. This is one of the clearly recognized complications of the failed back syndrome—a complication that, unfortunately, is not rare. Patients who express suicidal ideation, even if mentioned in apparent jest or by oblique reference, should be taken quite seriously in the hopes of preventing this "final solution" to chronic pain. Such patients should be challenged directly with the questions, "Are you planning to end your life? How do you plan to do it?" A person who answers affirmatively and has a specific plan in mind should be considered to be in a suicidal crisis and in urgent need of emotional support and psychiatric aid.

One type of psychologic problem encountered in failed back syndrome patients is potentially preventable. *Iatrogenic anxiety* or *anxiety-depression* is rarely discussed, but may occur at some perceivable level in many patients. Iatrogenic psychologic problems refer to psychologic problems that are initiated or aggravated by the patient's physician or other therapists. *Three major forms of iatrogenic psychologic disturbance* may be recognized in the management of the failed back syndrome.

In the first form of iatrogenic psychologic disturbance, the patient develops increasing anxiety or anxiety-depression because of an increasing fear of his painful and disabling disease. This process may begin preoperatively if effective surgical therapy is available but is withheld from a patient for an unduly long period of time in an effort to pursue what is self-righteously termed a "conservative" course. I define *medical conservatism* as a course of treatment likely to effect a satisfactory or useful result with the least investment of effort and risk. Simply prolonging ineffective therapy is not conservative treatment if effective alternative therapies are available. If nonoperative therapies prove inadequate, it may be that the quickest and safest therapy, entailing the least effort and medical cost, is surgical intervention. This is not an endorsement of a cavalier approach to surgery on the spine, but instead represents a plea to each health care practitioner involved with chronic failed back syndrome sufferers to be constantly mindful of the full gamut of nonoperative and operative therapies available.

In the second form of iatrogenic psychologic disturbance, a patient's anxious fear of pain may be further heightened in the early postoperative period by overly zealous *withholding of effective analgesic medications*. The past decades have witnessed, especially among young physicians, a vigorous reaction to the drug-abusing excesses of recent years and a laudable sensitivity to and fear of the danger of narcotic addiction. The risk of narcotics taken for pleasure is different from that of narcotics taken for the control of pain in a situation of finite duration. Patients who undergo surgery with reasonable expectation of a significant lessening of their pain within one or two weeks are far less likely to develop narcotic addiction than are the casual street users of narcotics. Although it is still wise to discontinue narcotics prior to hospital discharge, withholding adequate narcotic therapy in the early postoperative period guarantees the patient severe pain and forces him into the position of dreadful anticipation of the return of pain. This frequently results in a prolongation of and an increase in the patient's requirement for narcotics. As pain diminishes, narcotics can be withdrawn gradually, substituting nonnarcotic analgesics in a progressive fashion. I find it valuable to allow a period of several days of overlap during which the patient principally receives nonnarcotic medications, but understands that he may request narcotics when necessary. This is useful, since early ambulation and return to the activities of daily living may briefly leave patients with more pain than their nonnarcotic medication will adequately control.

The third form in which iatrogenic psychological disturbance may be encountered is a *fear of pain or rejection* in the long-term care of failed back syndrome sufferers. Pain is by definition a nociceptive phenomenon, implying a physical threat or danger to the organism. Thus, continued pain is inherently capable of inducing anxiety. Despite the intended overall optimism of this book, many failed back patients cannot be relieved of their pain or, at least, not all of their pain. These patients must learn to cope with their discomfort and must learn to function in spite of it. For them, heightened anxiety may be extremely destructive. To be rejected by their physicians or other health care providers engenders a feeling of aloneness and helplessness that is likewise anxiety generating. Dr. Eugene Stead, former Professor of Medicine at Duke Medical School, has observed: "A doctor often cannot solve the problem or cure a patient. Therefore he, along with the patient, must learn to live with it."[32] For these patients it can be beneficial to be reassured through careful medical attention that their conditions are not dangerous and are not likely to be progressive. Even if one is not able to offer total relief of pain, one can often succeed to some degree in reducing the patient's discomfort and disability. At the same time, if one can lessen the patient's anxiety, his functional and emotional status may be distinctly improved. Carefully listening to the patient's history and medical complaints, carefully examining him at each visit, and recommending useful diagnostic tests when these become advisable will do much to ameliorate the patient's anxiety. It is, however, necessary for the physician to go beyond the mechanics of medical care and to convey convincingly to the patient not only an interest in him as a person, but the rationale for the plan of medical care and the thoroughness with which it has been created. It is always more reassuring to persuade a patient that "nothing needs to be done" than to simply tell him that "nothing can be done."

Not all psychogenic factors in patients suffering from the failed back syndrome are iatrogenic. The intervention of *workers' compensation coverage* or other *third-party financial or legal interests* is always an important factor. Nearly every study that has examined the role of workers' compensation coverage or other adversarial or potentially adversarial third-party intervention has confirmed that a sizable percentage of patients in this category achieve a less satisfactory outcome than patients with similar back problems but without such third-party involvement. The potential availability of third-party funds raises the possibility of secondary gain in terms of financial reward or longer time off from work, which at times can lead to malingering. A more common cause of delayed or impaired recovery is not overtly fraudulent. An interest in seeking one's due in terms of money or time off or in punishing the company is often actively pursued by back-injured workers within the limits of the system and quite often may be covertly or overtly supported by a patient's fellow workers. In this situation, a failure to return to work may be perceived by a patient's fellow workers as a successful exploitation of the system and can actually be subverted into an improved standing with one's peers. On the other hand, patients who receive painful and disabling injuries at work may justifiably fear the prospect of returning to that same work. This is especially likely to be true if the work was unpleasant, and such fear is likely to be quite severe if the worker was already finding it increasingly difficult to keep up his work performance, because of either age or decreasing physical capability. Dr. Dietrich Blumer, Professor of Psychiatry at the Henry Ford Hospital, has described in detail the personality profile most commonly seen in chronic pain sufferers.[33,34] The patient he describes is often a "hyperachiever" who has throughout his life been overly industrious and usually quite restricted in outside interests beyond his job or source of livelihood. Patients with this personality structure are likely to be seriously shaken by the prospect of having to return to work in an impaired physical condition. For them the prospect of returning to work at a slowed pace or of returning to a modified work situation where they must be given special support and assistance may be psychologically intolerable. Interestingly, this phenomenon is rarely seen in physicians, a group almost universally composed of hyperachievers and work addicts. The distinguishing feature may well include both a consideration of personality differences and the fact that most professional people have neither the financial support of workers' compensation nor the peer support that tolerates or even condones disability.

Adhesive Arachnoiditis

Lumbar adhesive arachnoiditis is one of the more unpleasant causes of the failed back syndrome.[35,36] The etiology of this condition is poorly understood, and the existence of the disease has all too often been ignored, overlooked, or questioned in the past. Adhesive arachnoiditis may vary in severity from small adhesions around individual nerve roots to massive, multisegmental total obliteration of the subarachnoid space. When encountered following lumbar disc surgery it is more likely to be found at one or two segmental levels, almost always corresponding to the level of previous disc disease. At this level, the adhesive changes may be one of three types: *Type I*, unilateral involvement centered at the root exit zone; *Type II*, or circumferential involvement of nerve roots with an open, CSF-filled central communication; or *Type III*, total transverse obliteration of the subarachnoid space.

The *clinical manifestations* of arachnoiditis likewise vary greatly. Many patients remain asymptomatic despite incidental demonstration of significant lumbar adhesive arachnoiditis. In some patients, relatively minor myelographic changes may be associated with severe monoradicular pain or neurologic deficit (Fig. 3.11). In its extreme form, arachnoiditis can cause a progressive cauda equina syndrome with multisegmental pain, bilateral sciatic neuropathy, and progressive loss of bladder and bowel control. Always bear in mind that arachnoiditis may be completely asymptomatic, yet may mask underlying treatable conditions such as recurrent disc rupture, lateral recess bony entrapment of nerves, or spinal stenosis.

Although arachnoiditis has been associated with a variety of clinical disorders, in modern experience over 90% of cases in the lumbar region *occur in association with lumbar disc disease* (Fig. 3.12). Nonetheless, the *precise etiology remains unclear.*

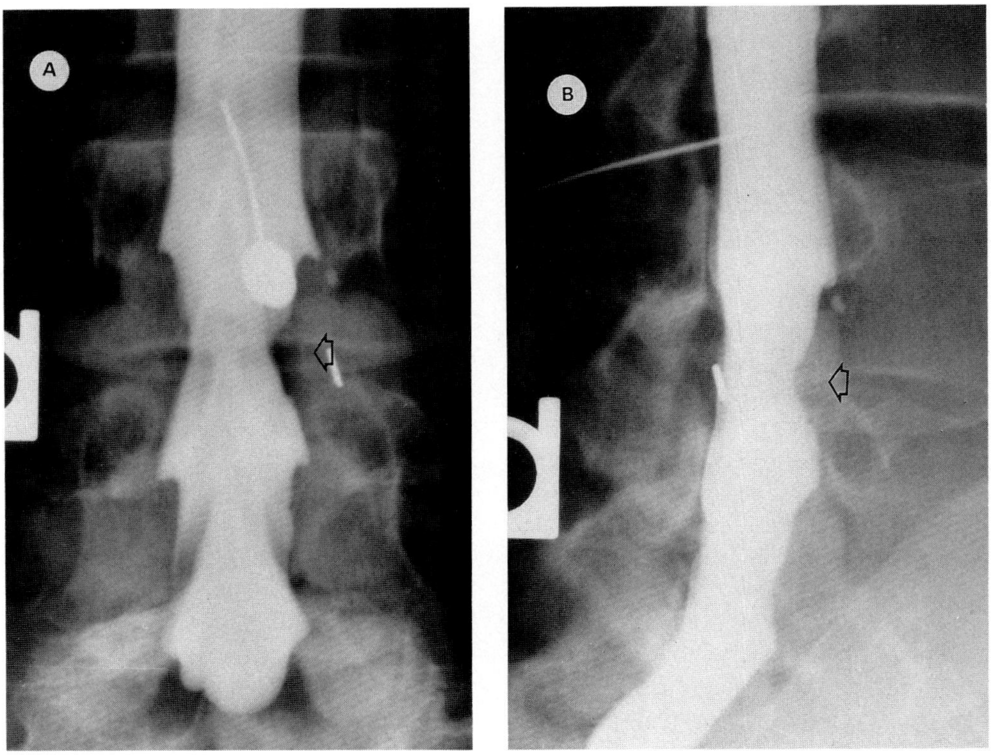

FIGURE 3.11. Lumbar adhesive arachnoiditis: localized type (Type I). These PA (**A**) and oblique (**B**) myelogram films demonstrate a focal anterolateral defect centered at the nerve root exit pouch adjacent to the intervertebral disc space. The patient presented with gradual onset of sciatica and sciatic neuropathy. Lumbar disc rupture was initially suspected clinically. Operative exposure failed to disclose a disc rupture or to alter the myelographic picture. The ragged outline of this defect should be contrasted with the smoother outline that is more typical of lumbar disc rupture, as depicted in Figure 4.15.

In every series, a small number of patients are described in whom arachnoiditis presents as their primary disease, without prior history of disc rupture, myelography, surgery, or other spinal instrumentation. At least one family has been described in which several members suffered from a spontaneous and apparently inherited form of the disease. Myelography has been implicated as a causative factor, yet lumbar arachnoiditis is rarely seen following myelography performed for cervical or thoracic disease. Mayfield has stated that he has never seen lumbar arachnoiditis following cervical myelography in a personal series of 3,000 cases.[37] If iophendylate (Pantopaque) or another myelographic contrast medium is the major causative factor, one would expect to find maximum adhesions forming at the tip of the caudal sac where any residual contrast material would be likely to lodge. However, this does not occur, and instead the adhesive process is most often confined to the site of previous disc disease.

Because arachnoiditis may clearly occur as a *spontaneous disease,* it is uncertain how many patients who are subsequently diagnosed as having arachnoiditis in fact have been initially misdiagnosed as having lumbar disc ruptures. In my personal series nearly all of the patients who subsequently required surgery for adhesive lumbar arachnoiditis were noted to have had atypical myelographic changes on their original myelograms, initially diagnosed as lumbar disc ruptures.[38] These defects took the form of bilateral or multisegmental abnormalities that were not consistent with the typical sharply localized anterolateral defect seen with a herniated nucleus pulposus. Patients with such myelographic atypicalities that are, in reality, caused

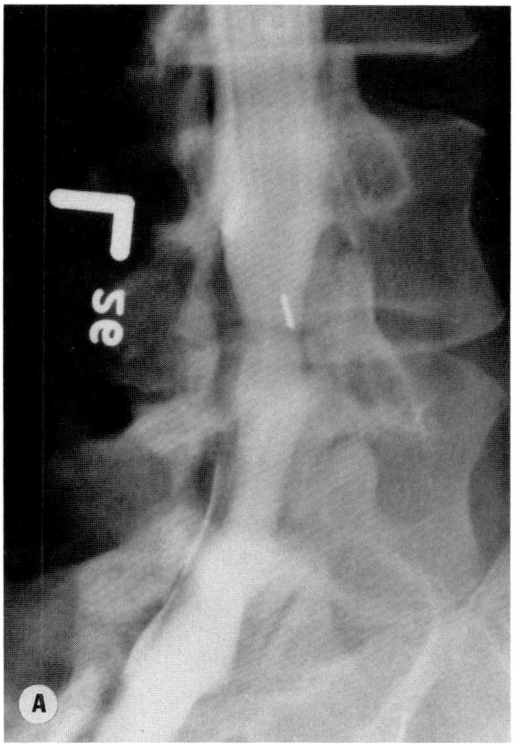

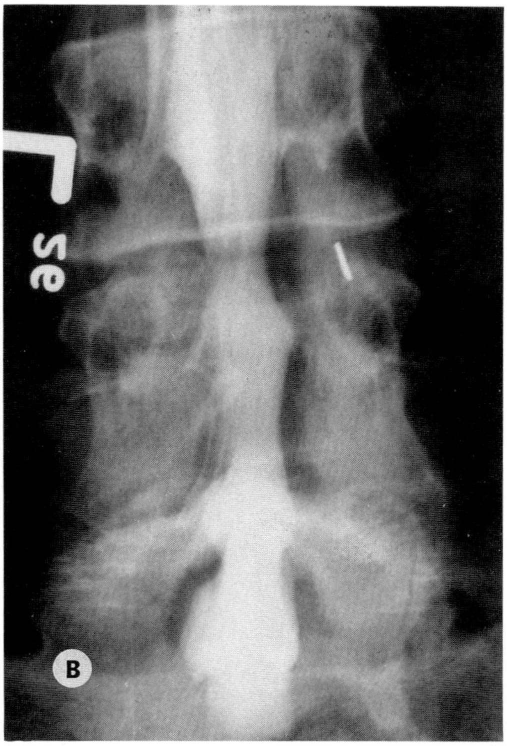

FIGURE 3.12. Lumbar adhesive arachnoiditis: annular or circumferential type (Type II). These myelogram films, taken in right oblique **(A)**, PA **(B)**, and left oblique **(C)** projections, document a more advanced stage of arachnoiditis in a patient who presented with bilateral but asymmetric leg pain, diffuse sensory loss, and mild weakness. At operative exploration, nerve roots were found to be bound to the outer walls of the thecal sac by dense white fibrous tissue with a persistent open central lumen filled with spinal fluid.

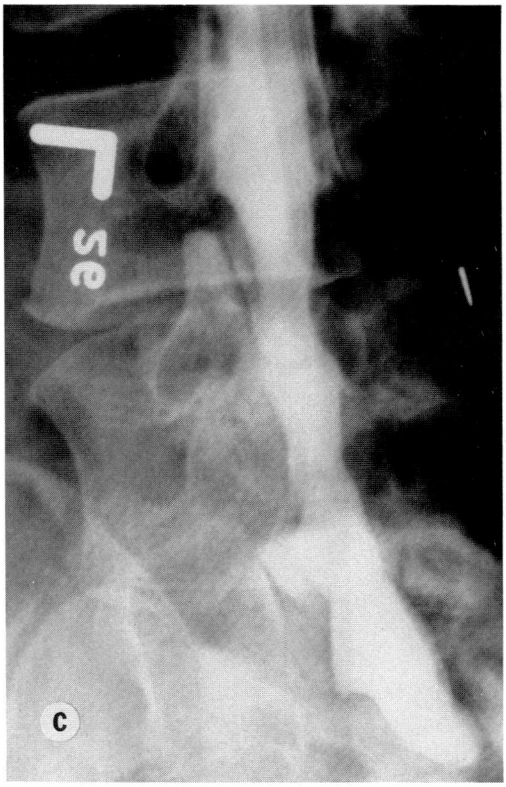

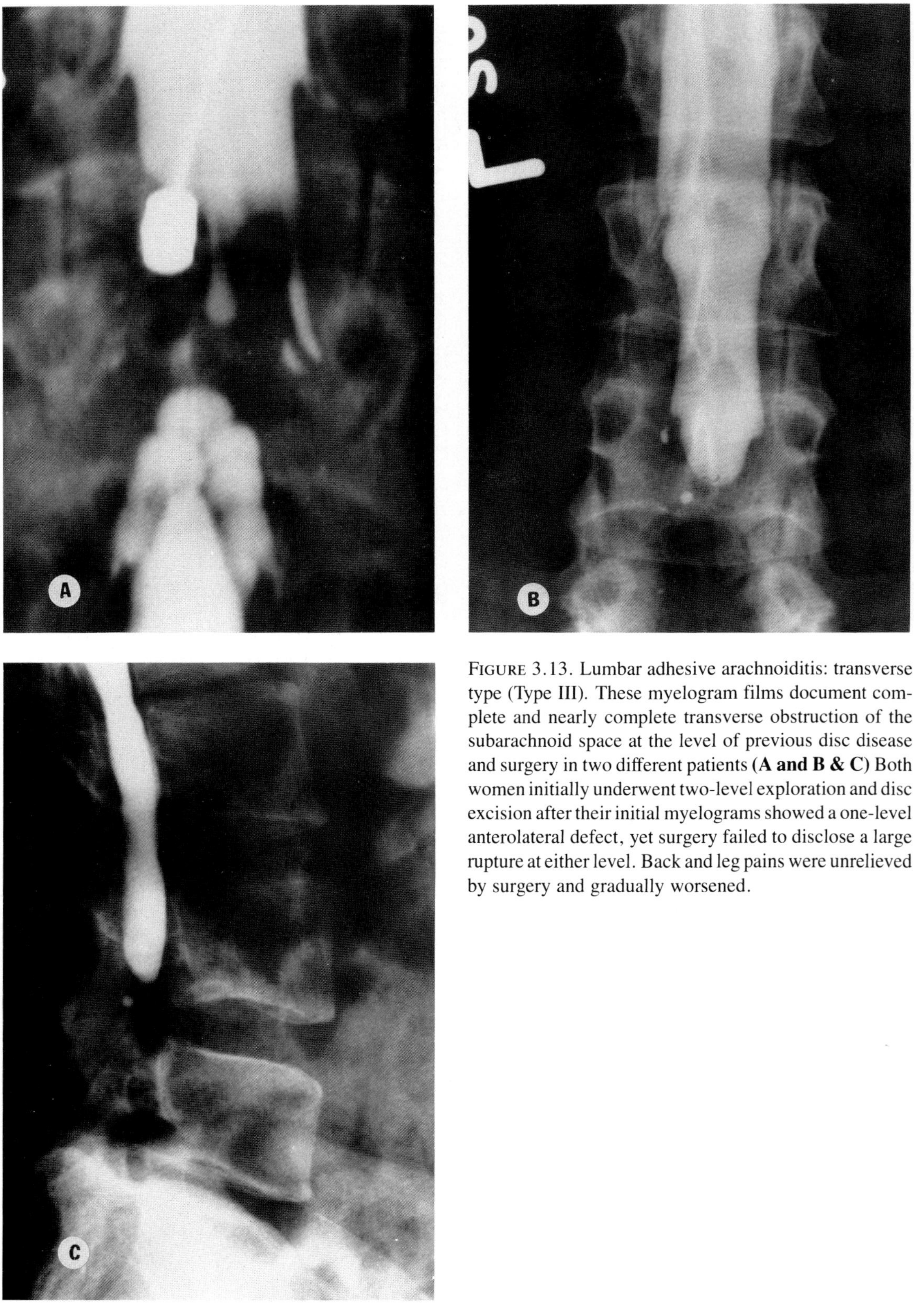

FIGURE 3.13. Lumbar adhesive arachnoiditis: transverse type (Type III). These myelogram films document complete and nearly complete transverse obstruction of the subarachnoid space at the level of previous disc disease and surgery in two different patients **(A and B & C)** Both women initially underwent two-level exploration and disc excision after their initial myelograms showed a one-level anterolateral defect, yet surgery failed to disclose a large rupture at either level. Back and leg pains were unrelieved by surgery and gradually worsened.

by arachnoiditis rather than disc rupture will remain severely symptomatic following disc excision, with or without spinal fusion.

Perhaps in the future, neurosurgeons will be more wary of such atypical myelograms and will be prepared to perform intradural inspection when extradural inspection fails to reveal an appropriately large disc rupture. With the current trend toward diagnosing lumbar disc ruptures with CT or MRI scans and eschewing myelography, it is unclear what will happen to those patients with primary arachnoiditis—which cannot be diagnosed with CT scans without intrathecal contrast, and which can be diagnosed with MRI scans only if the disorder is extensive. The discovery of extensive epidural adhesions at the time of primary disc surgery should always alert the surgeon to a considerably increased risk of intradural arachnoiditis.

Lumbar spinal surgery has also been implicated as an *etiologic factor* in the development of lumbar adhesive arachnoiditis (Fig. 3.13). It has been suggested that a more extensive laminotomy, exposing a greater surface of dura mater, may predispose to extradural and intradural adhesions. Many neurosurgeons, however, feel that a failure to perform a sufficiently large laminotomy is more likely to lead to nerve root trauma and thus increase the incidence of nerve root fibrosis and adhesive arachnoiditis. In any event, the use of epidural fat grafts at the conclusion of laminectomy seems to reduce the frequency of both of these complications, even when adequately large laminotomies have been performed. It has been suggested that multiple-level or bilateral laminectomy increases the risk of subsequent development of adhesive arachnoiditis. In my series of 17 patients requiring subsequent lysis of severely symptomatic lumbar arachnoiditis, two thirds of the patients had undergone an average of 2.5 operations each prior to their surgery for arachnoiditis, suggesting an increased likelihood of arachnoiditis following multiple operations.[38] On the other hand, those patients operated on initially by me had undergone an average of 1.25 operations per patient—a frequency of surgery almost identical to that encountered by me in a series of over 800 patients operated on for lumbar disc disease.

Thus, it remains unclear whether lumbar adhesive arachnoiditis develops as a result of disc rupture or whether it is in any way etiologically associated with myelography or disc surgery. It may be that a large percentage of cases, in fact, arise as a spontaneous disease and are simply misdiagnosed as lumbar disc ruptures. For these patients, of course, a failed back syndrome is the expected result if discectomy without intradural lysis is performed for a minimally bulging disc in the face of a large and atypical myelographic defect caused by primary arachnoiditis.

4

Precise Diagnosis of Specific Syndromes

Patients with the failed back syndrome should usually be treated initially with nonspecific and generally safer therapies. When simpler therapies fail, continued successful therapy must be based on a *precise understanding of the disorder* to permit an appropriate choice of specific therapy. As our knowledge of the complexity of the disorders that may cause the failed back syndrome increases, it becomes more apparent that the "wastebasket diagnoses" of *postoperative back, chronic lumbar derangement,* or even the all-encompassing term *failed back syndrome* are not sufficiently precise to permit accurate therapy for many patients. Attempts at diagnosing precise causes of the failed back syndrome should be undertaken in a systematic fashion. A carefully taken *history* is vitally important in all aspects of medicine, and this dictum holds true in understanding the causes of the failed back syndrome. The *physical examination* is equally fundamental, but in diagnosing the causes of the failed back syndrome many of the specific steps in testing that should be undertaken may not be familiar to all practitioners who deal with these patients. The available *laboratory* and *radiographic diagnostic procedures* can be categorized as either *invasive* or *noninvasive;* generally the noninvasive studies are undertaken prior to subjecting the patient to the more unpleasant and potentially dangerous invasive tests.

Not every patient requires extensive tests. Since 80% of all American workers will lose some work time during their careers due to low back pain, this should be considered a "symptom" and not a "disease," even a "normal" part of the human condition.[39] Extensive testing is not only expensive, but it can also reinforce the concept of "disease," with destructive psychological consequences. For many patients, history taking and physical examination will prove sufficiently confirmatory of a specific diagnosis to permit institution of appropriate nonspecific or specific therapies. If these therapies achieve the desired improvement in the patient, it may not be necessary to advise further diagnostic tests. It is often sufficient to be satisfied with a successful outcome even in the face of some residual uncertainty about the specific etiology of the patient's problem. Sparing the patient expensive, uncomfortable, and potentially dangerous tests is most commendable if the patient can be satisfactorily improved through therapy based on available information. This does not imply that specific testing should be withheld for an inordinately long period of time to permit extensive conservative therapy when this therapy proves ineffective. In my opinion, conservative therapy becomes radical when it is ineffective and is unduly prolonged.

History

General Considerations

For maximum effectiveness, history taking must be both a *passive* and an *active* process. By this I mean that one must be both receptive and directive in history taking. It is necessary to be sufficiently receptive to permit the patient to state his symptoms and perceptions of the impact of his illness upon his life, although rambling, repetitive, and nondirected narratives must be disciplined by the interviewer.

Dr. Eugene Stead, former Professor of Medicine at Duke Medical School, placed great emphasis on the history-taking process.[32]

> The history can never be a mere mechanical recording of data. Each statement must be scrutinized for its possible bearing on the present status of the patient and, more particularly, for any light it may shed on the symptoms of which he now complains. The mind of a physician must be constantly alert to the possibility that any event related by the patient, any symptoms, however trivial or remote, may yet hold the key to the solution of the medical problem.
>
> . . . It is the taking of the history and in the analysis and interpretation of the data contained therein that the skill, knowledge and experience of the physician are most frequently and rigorously tested.

If allowed to tell their stories, patients frequently recount symptoms that may seem minor to them but that may significantly alter the interpretation of their clinical stories. On the other hand, patients are not medically trained, and symptoms that are not present may be as significant as symptoms that are present. These symptoms must be *inquired after* by the interviewer.

Once an adequate outline of the patient's perception of his illness has been obtained, the interviewer must actively direct the history-taking process in an effort to uncover further symptoms, both present and absent, that may materially alter the clinical interpretation. Active intervention is also useful in attempting to establish the severity of symptoms and the impact they have on the patient's physical functioning, sense of well-being, functional capacity in job and at home, and overall happiness or emotional status. Although an assessment of the presence or absence of specific symptoms is the chief ingredient in interpreting the specific etiology of the patient's failed back syndrome, assessment of the severity or significance of symptoms is more often the chief determinant of the type of therapy to be offered. Symptoms that are of mild severity and have little disruptive impact on the patient's life usually call for a more cautious and low-risk approach to therapy. On the other hand, symptoms of major severity that have a major impact on the patient's life may justify more aggressive therapeutic intervention, especially if more limited therapies have failed. One of the major quandaries of the practice of medicine, one that stresses to the fullest the experience and philosophy of the physician or surgeon, is the frequently encountered clinical situation in which patients present with symptoms of seemingly limited severity that are poorly tolerated and fail to respond to carefully tailored and well-applied low risk or nonaggressive therapy. Is one justified in proceeding to more aggressive, more involved, and more risky therapy in these patients?

Historical information obtained from failed back syndrome sufferers falls into three major categories: symptoms that suggest a *"mechanical" etiology* of the patient's pain, symptoms that suggest *neurologic or neuralgic difficulties,* and a *miscellaneous group* of symptoms that suggest conditions other than lumbar disc disease or neuralgia. For each of these symptom categories it is important not only to assess the presence or absence of specific symptoms but also to attempt to assess the *severity* of the symptoms. Ascertaining factors that ameliorate or exacerbate symptoms is especially valuable in assessing the severity of symptoms, but may also be helpful in defining the symptoms etiologically. Similarly, information about the *duration* and *time course* of symptoms is likely to be of value in assessing the impact of symptoms on the patient's life, but may also be materially helpful in identifying the etiology of the symptoms. Symptoms that are of recent, rapid onset or that are progressively increasing in severity demand more urgent treatment for the underlying condition, even though the condition may be essentially the same as that which in another patient causes a static, long-standing, and low level of symptomatology. If long-standing low-level symptoms change for the worse, one is then obligated to explore the reason for this change. If symptoms increase because of the superimposition of a second disorder, altered therapy tailored to the new condition may be indicated. If the basic disorder remains the same with only an increased level of symptomatology, the factors responsible for this increased symptomatology must be identified to permit both an extension of therapy and institution of preventive measures in an effort to ward off future relapses.

There is a strong correlation between the *anatomical localization* of symptoms and a *categorization of symptoms by etiologic type*. Symptoms suggesting mechanical etiologies are most commonly associated with back pain, although this pain may radiate to the buttocks and posterior thighs. Symptoms suggesting neurologic or neuralgic difficulties in the failed back syndrome patient are most commonly associated with sciatic radiation of pain into the lower leg. Pains of mechanical etiology are characteristically aggravated by posture or activity, usually with an increase in back pain. Sciatic neuralgic pain may be aggravated by posture or activity in conditions such as arachnoid cysts and epidural adhesions beneath a pseudarthrosis or when the nerve is entrapped by disc rupture or scar, but neuralgic pains are usually more constant than the pains of mechanical etiologies and are usually incompletely relieved by rest.

Mechanical Etiologies

Symptoms suggestive of mechanical etiologies generally involve weight bearing, body position, or activity. The term *mechanical symptoms* generally refers to *symptoms that derive from bones, joints, ligaments, or intervertebral discs.* Weight bearing on the lower back, through sitting or standing, causes axial loading on *lumbar discs* and will result in pain if the annulus is incompetent and the posterior longitudinal ligament is stretched or distorted by protruding disc material. Pain will also occur if the disc space is inflamed or irritated, as seen in painfully arthritic or degenerated but not ruptured discs or in inflammatory discitis. *Sacroiliac joints* are stressed both by weight bearing and by lateral and rotational stresses on the pelvis caused by walking, upper body movement and by specific pelvic stresses involved in pregnancy and sexual coupling. *Facet joints* also may become painful under axial loading if they are inflamed or if their normal relationship has been distorted by collapse of an interspace. For patients with disc ruptures, painful degenerations, or symptomatic facet syndromes, bed rest is usually beneficial. These patients retire to bed to obtain relief and are likely to be most comfortable on awakening. The pain of inflammatory discitis is also improved by bed rest, but usually not as rapidly or completely as in the other conditions just mentioned. Patients with discitis frequently continue to experience significant back pain even after being in bed for several days.

Merely maintaining an erect posture may elicit pain from *tender or inflamed tissues* in the lumbar thecal sac. With erect posture, the water-column effect of the spinal fluid transmits a maximum pressure to the lumbar thecal sac, causing local distention and distortion. This effect is sharply aggravated if the patient coughs, sneezes, or strains while erect. Patients with severe *meningeal inflammation* or *spinal stenosis* may experience increased back pain while erect. Patients with lumbar spinal stenosis often find the fully erect posture to be painful and adopt a posture of partial forward flexion at the waist, since the fully erect posture stresses degenerated facets and increases the infolding of hypertrophied ligamentum flavum and facet joint capsules against nerve roots. Patients with *lumbar pseudomeningoceles* are likely to experience both mechanical back pain and sciatic leg pain when they attempt to maintain an erect posture (Fig. 4.1). Patients with large and acutely inflamed *disc ruptures or nerve root fibrosis* are likely to experience predominantly sciatic pain, although mechanical back pain may also be significant.

Sitting provides another postural type of mechanical stress in patients with low back disorders that many find to be particularly uncomfortable. Sitting may be poorly tolerated because of its mechanical effect on joints, bones, and ligaments or because of the presence of areas of local tenderness. Sitting

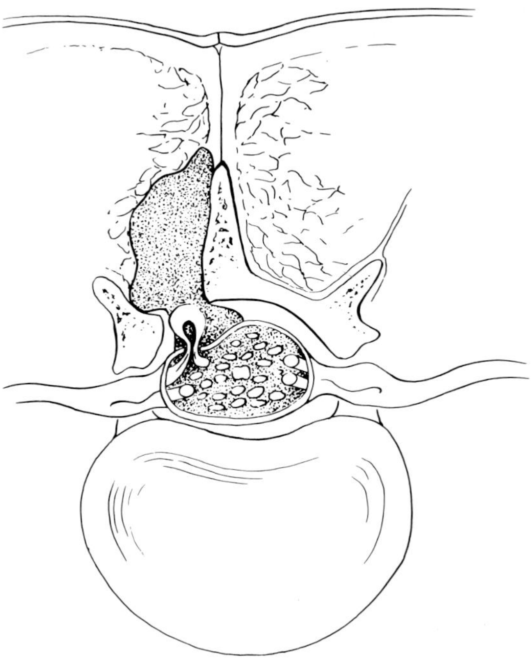

FIGURE 4.1. Lumbar pseudomeningoceles can develop when surgical tears in the dura and arachnoid go unrepaired. Spinal fluid accumulation in soft tissues of the back leads to formation of a pseudomembrane and clinically causes severe back pain aggravated by standing or straining. Herniation of a dorsal sensory root through the narrow mouth or ostium of the pseudomeningocele can cause sciatica, in addition to low back pain.

Tu 13

January 2004

s	m	t	w	t	f	s
				1	2	3
4	5	6	7	8	9	10
11	12	13	14	15	16	17
18	19	20	21	22	23	24
25	26	27	28	29	30	31

February 2004

s	m	t	w	t	f	s
1	2	3	4	5	6	7
8	9	10	11	12	13	14
15	16	17	18	19	20	21
22	23	24	25	26	27	28
29						

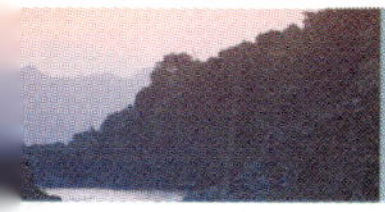

Appointment Schedule

✔ Task Completed
→ Planned Forward
✗ Task Deleted
G✔ Delegated Task
• In Process

↓ ABC Prioritized Daily Task List

Framingham office
Mitchy - assistant
508 - 879 - 9889

10:00 am on
May 26.
463 Worcester Rd (Rte 9)
Framingham.

[illegible]

6
7
8
9
10
11
12
1
2
3
4
5
6
7
8
9
10

The leader releases energy, unites energies, and all with the object of not only carrying out a purpose, but of creating further and larger purposes.
—Mary Parker Follett

Monday, January 12, 2004

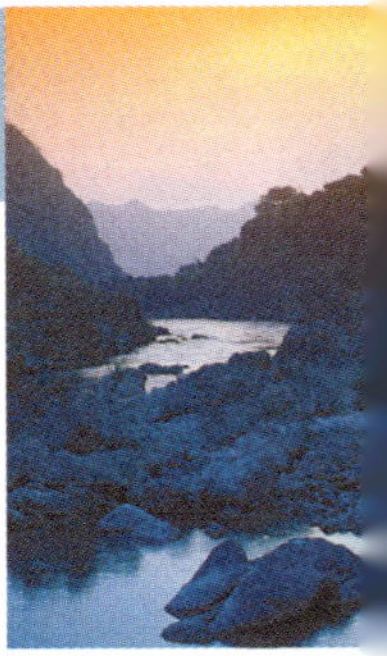

Daily Record of Events

involves partial *flattening of the normal lumbar lordotic curve,* since full forward flexion of the hips to 90 degrees causes some pelvic rotation. When this is done with persistent weight bearing on the lumbar spine, pain may be generated from sacroiliac joints or lower back structures, including discs that are still painful from surgery, inflammatory discitis, facet syndrome, arthritis, or spinal fractures. The persistent vertical posture also causes persistent *distention of the lumbar thecal sac,* which may cause pain (as discussed above). Lumbar trigger points at the posterior iliac crest may cause pain when compressed by the chair back or when they are simply stretched by the bending plus weight bearing entailed in sitting. Coccydynia, ischiogluteal bursitis, and inflamed sciatic nerves may cause pain through direct compression against the chair bottom. Sitting while riding in a motor vehicle is usually particularly troublesome for those who suffer from the failed back syndrome. In this circumstance, not only is the back placed in a weakened position, but vibratory stress is added through the motion of the vehicle; this is apt to be more severe when traveling over rough pavement or ground. Similarly, the discomfort brought on by sitting may be aggravated when sitting is continued for prolonged periods of time or when sitting is coupled with upper extremity activity. Upper trunk and upper extremity activities of necessity require tightening of supporting lower trunk musculature and invariably cause some motion in the lower back as the body's center of gravity shifts and as the upper extremities pull the trunk in different directions. This is often particularly troublesome for failed back syndrome sufferers who attempt to return to work. These patients may find that they can tolerate sitting quietly at home long enough to enjoy meals or watch television, but that pain limits their ability to sit for prolonged periods at their jobs or to undertake upper extremity activities while seated at work.

An *aggravation of pain by activity* is also typical of mechanical pain. Bending the lower back places horizontal or rotational stresses on intervertebral discs, facet joints, back muscles, and ligaments. Bending in any direction is frequently painful, but *hyperextension* may be dramatically more painful than other back movements in patients with *facet syndromes* or *kissing pseudarthrosis* following spinal fusion (Fig. 4.2). In these patients, hyperextension maximally impacts on painful facet joints and maximally compresses together the painful bony components of the pseudarthrosis. *Forward bending* elicits pain from a variety of lower back musculoskeletal disorders, with the pain in each of them tending to be maximum in the lower back but commonly with radiation into one or both buttocks and posterior thighs. This pain characteristically does not radiate below the knee; such radiation would suggest a sciatic nerve origin of pain. Bending pain originating from the intervertebral disc (discogenic rather than radiculopathic), from facet joints, or from sacroiliac joints in each instance is maximal in the lower back. The buttock and posterior thigh radiating component is more likely to be unilateral with the latter two conditions than with primary discogenic pain, although bilateral facet or sacroiliac joint involvement is certainly not uncommon. Back pain from bending caused by paraspinal muscle spasm *or* ligamentous strains is less likely to cause radiation of pain into the buttocks and posterior thighs. The pain from muscle spasm, in fact, may more often radiate into the thoracic area or groin. Patients with epidural scarring rarely experience only back, buttock, and posterior thigh pain on bending; a radiculopathic component of pain radiating below the knees is commonly present also. With severe meningeal inflammation and severe paraspinal muscle spasms, back pain may be reproduced simply by *forward neck flexion,* which causes stretching of the thecal sac and lumbodorsal muscle mass.

Neurologic Etiologies

Symptoms of neurologic involvement are likely to involve complaints of *pain* or *loss of neurologic function.* One form of pain that patients may complain of is *neuralgic pain,* which derives from injured or irritated nerves. This pain is generally felt in the distribution of one or more adjacent nerve roots. With lumbar problems the area of distribution usually conforms to the territory of the sciatic nerve. Patterns of pain referral, however, may be confusing at times, so that it is not uncommon to hear complaints of pain radiating into the groin, scrotum, or genitalia in association with more typical buttock and leg pain. A pain may usually be identified historically as being neuralgic in type by a description of the quality of the pain. Neuralgic pains are most often described as burning, tingling, itching, oı numb. Neuralgic pain is more likely to

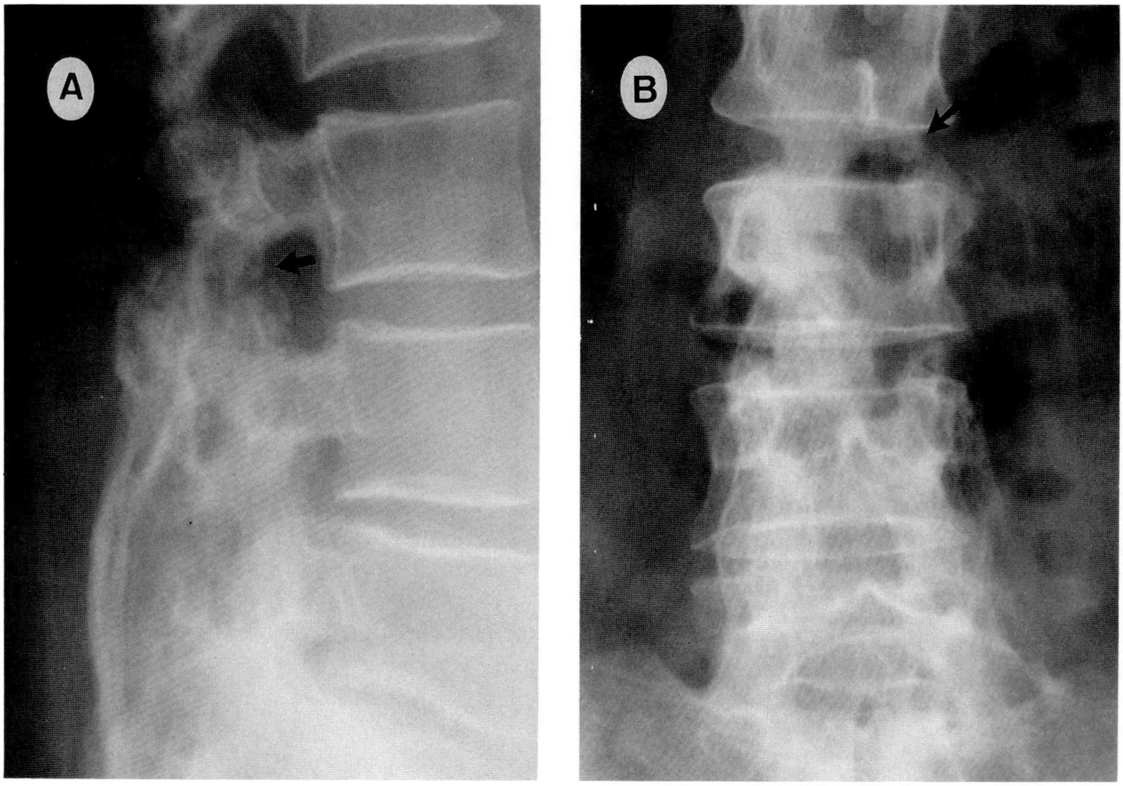

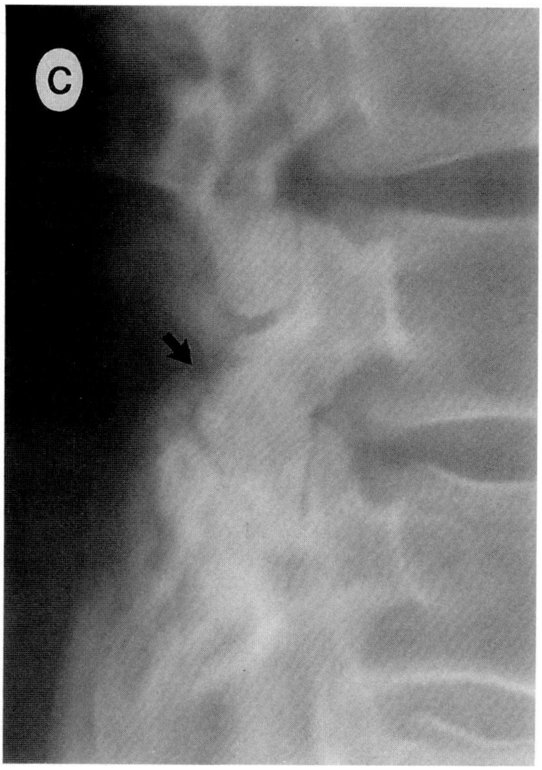

FIGURE 4.2. **A and B:** Plain radiographs document a kissing pseudarthrosis **(arrows)** in a woman who had previously undergone three lumbar laminectomies with fusions. Back pain became severe following trauma six years after her latest fusion, with a major component of pain on attempted hyperextension of her back. **C (arrow):** Surgical exploration for reduction/excision of the kissing pseudarthrosis also confirmed an unstable transverse pseudarthrosis that could not be positively identified on tomography or CT scan, but was suspected clinically and on the basis of a positive uptake on isotope scan.

be relatively constant. Although it may be aggravated by activity or pressure, it is rarely completely relieved by inactivity or rest. Occasionally, a patient will experience a sudden "jangling," "blasting," or "lightning bolt" pain into the lower extremity. Symptoms suggesting *nerve tenderness* are less often recounted. A description of local tenderness on sitting without sciatic radiation does not imply pain of nerve origin, since this is more suggestive of ischiogluteal bursitis or some other etiology. Local tenderness at sites such as fusion bone donor sites may derive from specific nerve involvement if painful neuromata are present.

The pain that derives from *nerve entrapment* characteristically has a strong relationship to activity and is considerably improved by bed rest, proper positioning, or inactivity. If a nerve root is entrapped by a disc rupture or scar tissue, activities and positions that cause stretching of that nerve root will elicit radiating pain into the extremity supplied by that nerve root. The patient will usually comment that forward bending, lifting the leg, or walking causes a sharp or strongly aching pain into the buttock and lower extremity. Coughing, sneezing, straining at stool, or prolonged standing causes distention of the lumbar thecal sac and may also bring on sciatic pain. Once such a pain develops, the patient will usually report that he obtains significant relief by recumbency, frequently with the knee and hip slightly flexed—a maneuver that relaxes the nerve roots.

One specific form of *root compression, spinal stenosis,* can usually be suspected by its characteristic history of pain.[23] Spinal stenosis causes a compression of the entire intraspinal nervous tissue, but it is usually a compression of low grade without entrapment of the nerve (Fig. 4.3). Nerve roots in the area of compression usually slide freely so that bending or leg elevation rarely elicits sciatic pain. The pain is usually worse on standing, which distends the thecal sac, and especially standing fully erect, which impacts hypertrophied facets and posterior ligaments into the spinal canal, compressing nerve roots. On the other hand, sustained activity, especially walking, causes metabolic hyperactivity and slight swelling of the nerve roots. When nerve roots swell within the limited confines of the spinal space, this sharply aggravates the compression and causes the patient to complain of aching pain in both lower extremities or lower back, a pain that mimics vascular claudication. Like the pain of vascular origin, this neurogenic claudication pain is usually rapidly improved by cessation of walking.

Lateral recess stenosis—that is, maximal hypertrophic stenosis laterally in the spinal canal and compressing nerve roots more than thecal sac—likewise causes nerve root compression without entrapment or fixation of the nerve to surrounding structures.[40] As is true with spinal stenosis, patients with lateral recess stenosis are usually less bothered by bending or leg elevation than they are by prolonged standing or walking—although the symp-

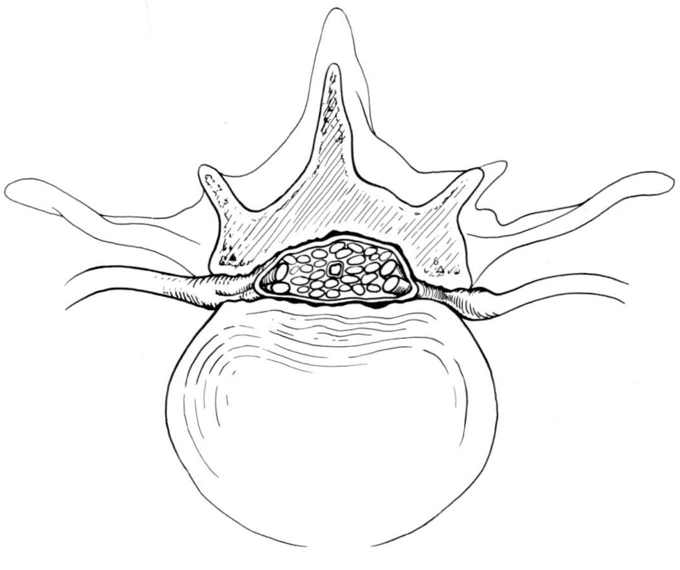

FIGURE 4.3. Lumbar spinal stenosis usually becomes symptomatic due to the superimposition of hypertrophic degenerative changes on a congenitally narrow spinal canal. Nerve roots that are already crowded together in the narrow canal become diffusely compressed by arthritic degenerative bars, a compression that is acutely worse when the nerve roots and lumbar veins are engorged by the activity entailed in ambulation. Because nerve roots are compressed, but not actually entrapped, the straight leg raising test usually fails to produce sciatica.

toms that do develop tend to be more circumscribed and are chiefly referable to a single involved nerve root.

Pain deriving from the autonomic nervous system, *causalgic pain,* is difficult to confirm, and its frequency is not clearly known. The patient classically complains of a diffuse burning throughout the affected limb with an associated dramatic hypersensitivity to even light touch. He may note bluish discoloration or blanching of the limb either constantly or in association with pain, activity, or changes in ambient temperature. On examination, these patients often exhibit *trophic changes* of the extremity. They may comment on their dry and shiny skin during history taking. Unfortunately, this classical constellation of symptoms is not always present; many patients seem to complain of more nonspecific or vague pain without trophic changes, and the *dysautonomic basis* of their pain may be difficult to confirm or may not even be suspected by the examiner.

The symptoms of neurologic loss include *weakness, sensory loss, and autonomic involvement.* Complaints of generalized weakness or asthenia do not ordinarily imply specific neurologic loss. Although such symptoms can be seen with generalized peripheral neuropathies, these conditions are usually not painful. *Focal weakness* of a single muscle group is much more important, and a complaint of a dragging toe or difficulty climbing stairs is much more suggestive of a specific neurologic loss. Patients with significant pain will frequently complain that their legs "suddenly give way." This phenomenon probably represents a reflex response to pain rather than specific motor weakness—as discussed on page 51.

Sensory loss is often overlooked by the patient unless it becomes severe. This is especially true if there is little or no pain in the affected extremity. Complaints of *diffuse numbness* throughout an extremity are likely to represent a reverse acupuncture effect, as discussed on page 52. When the sensory loss is due to specific nerve injury, a more *focal cutaneous sensory loss* is usually reported. In failed back syndrome patients, this focal loss generally involves a specific portion of the calf or foot, often with extension into the posterior thigh, buttocks, groin, or even the genitalia (Fig. 4.4).

Autonomic loss is more rarely encountered and, like causalgic pain, autonomic loss in the lower extremities is more difficult to confirm. A complaint of *impotence* more often than not reflects a psychologic impairment secondary to pain, discomfort, or distress. If a complaint of difficulty in *initiating urination or urinary incontinence* is obtained, it is necessary to consider the possibility of a severe involvement in the lumbosacral region; this should bring to mind diagnoses such as arachnoiditis, complete disc prolapse, or spinal tumor. Medications taken for pain relief or pain itself, especially pain aggravated by straining to void, can also interfere with micturition, but the new emergence or rapid development of urinary difficulty is strongly suggestive of a major neurologic abnormality, which could become permanent if not treated promptly and appropriately. *Incontinence of stool* is less frequently encountered, even with severe autonomic loss, but is of equal significance and dire import. Constipation is rarely secondary to autonomic involvement in the lumbar region, even though it is frequently encountered in failed back syndrome sufferers as a result of inactivity, poor diet, and narcotic medications.

Miscellaneous Etiologies

Other symptoms obtained from failed back syndrome sufferers suggest a miscellaneous group of etiologies. Pain referred to the back from *intrapelvic* or *intraabdominal diseases* is most commonly overshadowed by abdominal or genital pain and is usually associated with gastrointestinal, urinary tract, or menstrual symptoms. A rarely encountered form of sciatic neuralgia is caused by pelvic retroperitoneal perineural *endometriosis.* Women who suffer this disorder classically describe a periodic form of sciatica that is exacerbated during menstruation and usually becomes progressively more severe with each menstrual cycle. Intrapelvic or retroperitoneal endometriosis can also cause pain predominantly in the back rather than in the leg. This pain likewise exhibits a characteristic cycling crescendo. An aggravation of back pain and sciatica in the perimenstrual period without a crescendo increase from cycle to cycle usually does not indicate the pain of endometriosis. The significant hormonal changes and characteristic fluid retention that occur at the time of menstruation may aggravate mechanical or sciatic pain of almost any etiology. Also, pregnancy may severely aggravate back pain because of hormonal changes and, in later stages of pregnancy, because of the added weight and mechanical distortion of the back secondary to the patient's altered center of gravity.

Pain secondary to arthritis or arthritis-like conditions exhibits a characteristic temporal *double peak*. The characteristic pattern is one of aching stiffness upon arising in the morning, with improvement following initial activity and ambulation. With the passage of hours, pain in the back or other joints gradually increases in severity and may become disabling by afternoon or evening. This form of pain is improved by resting and by local applications of heat. This pattern of pain is to be expected in patients suffering from diffuse degenerative or inflammatory arthritis, but is also typical of the pain seen with a lumbar facet syndrome and discogenic back derangement, which might be better termed *arthropathy of the intervertebral disc*.

In the failed back syndrome patient, lower extremity *claudication pain* is not always neurogenic. Younger patients who develop claudication-like symptoms in one or both lower extremities following laminectomy should certainly be suspected of suffering from neurogenic claudication secondary to iatrogenic spinal stenosis or lateral recess stenosis. However, one of the potential complications of lumbar disc excision is injury of iliac vessels. This usually results in massive intraoperative bleeding or early postoperative retroperitoneal hemorrhage. These complications are readily apparent. Occasionally, the vascular damage may be less extreme and may simply lead to thrombosis. This can then induce a unilateral leg ischemia, and true vascular claudication may result. The following case report documents this potential complication.

Case 3

This 53-year-old woman was referred to me three months after having undergone lumbar laminectomy and disc excision by an orthopedic surgeon. Postoperatively, right leg pain persisted and repeat myelography continued to show a small defect at the L4-L5 operative site. I was asked to recommend therapy for her persistent sciatica.

During questioning, the patient stated emphatically that her present pain was decidedly different from her preoperative pain. The preoperative pain was sharply circumscribed to anterior shin and foot, was aggravated by bending more than by activity, and was associated with focal numbness of her foot. In contradistinction, her present pain was diffusely aching in character, seemed unaffected by bending, was severely aggravated after walking 100 feet, and was associated with a global feeling of vague numbness throughout the leg. On examination, straight leg raising to 75 degrees caused "tightness" only and no pain. Motor and sensory examination was normal. The right foot felt slightly cooler than the left. Dorsalis pedis and popliteal pulses were strikingly absent on the right and boundingly present on the left. Referral to a vascular surgeon resulted in arteriographic confirmation of iliac artery obstruction just ventral to the L4-L5 interspace. This was surgically corrected, with prompt improvement in claudication symptoms.

Muscle spasm pain usually occurs as episodes of cramping discomfort in the extremities or back. The classic gastrocnemius charley horse is well-known to athletes and would-be athletes. This form of acute muscle cramping and the related anterior compartment, or tibialis anterior, cramping are particularly prone to occur following activity or exercise. They frequently occur at night when the foot is allowed to relax into partial ankle extension. *Acute muscle spasms* of this type produce visible, tender tumescence in the muscle body and appropriate tonic deflection of ankle or toes. These pains are improved by stretching the affected muscle, by limited exercise, and by application of heat. Acute muscle spasms of this type rarely persist for more than a few minutes or a few hours, but they may leave behind a residue of local tenderness and aching. They may reappear repetitively and, for many patients, predictably with activity or sleep. Failed back syndrome sufferers may also develop acute muscle spasms in lumbar paraspinal muscles or glutei. These spasms may follow activity or exercise, but may also occur with little apparent provocation as an acute worsening of chronic backache. A typical story is that of a patient who recounts: "I was leaning over the sink to brush my teeth when suddenly a severe pain grabbed my back and caused me to fall to the floor." The pain that these spasms produce is typically back pain, but it may radiate into the thoracic area, into one or both buttocks, and less commonly into posterior thighs. Visible and palpable tender tumescence is usually detectable. Relief is sometimes obtained by lying flat or by flexing the hips, often aided by local applications of heat and liniments.

Not uncommonly, back muscle spasms may enter the chronic phase of a *"fixed muscle spasm."* These fixed spasms cause an intense form of back pain that may persist for days or even weeks if appropriate therapy is not instituted. Even with effective therapy a residue of deep aching in the back often persists for one or two weeks after relaxation of the muscle spasm. The pain that these spasms cause is some of the most intense suffered by victims of the failed back syndrome. Its characteristic abrupt onset or progressive buildup, its localization to the back, and the findings of local muscle tightness and tenderness are usually diagnostic.

Muscle spasms are frequently implicated as a cause of chronic persistent back discomfort. Although muscle spasms can occur repetitively and muscle pain is a part of the *"flabby back syndrome"* (see page 18), actual muscle spasm lasting chronically for months or years probably occurs extremely infrequently, if at all. As a result, it is rarely logical to treat patients who suffer chronic back pain for long periods with muscle relaxing medications only, although these medications may be helpful as prophylaxis against acute spasms or may be helpful because of their tranquilizing or antineuralgic properties. In the flabby back syndrome, the combination of chronic overweight and underactivity so commonly seen in our affluent society leads to chronic weakness of muscles and laxness of ligaments and tendons. Patients with this syndrome frequently develop diffuse, aching back pains and may be subject to frequent muscle spasms. However, their underlying chronic pain is usually not that of true muscle spasm but rather results from the use of underprepared muscles.

Physical Examination

Neurologic Examination

The neurologic examination of the patient with a failed back syndrome has two major parts: tests for nerve tenderness or irritability and tests for nerve function.

Limitation of *straight leg raising* is one of the cardinal, well-known features of lumbar disc ruptures.[41–44] This can be an important indicator of nerve root irritation or tenderness secondary to entrapment of the nerve or fixation to surrounding structures by a disc rupture, epidural scar, arachnoiditis, tumor, or traumatic postoperative neuroma. Conditions that cause nerve root compression without entrapment characteristically do not produce nerve root pain on straight leg raising. This distinction is an important finding in the diagnosis of spinal stenosis and lateral recess stenosis, both of which involve nerve root compression without entrapment. Simply eliciting pain on straight leg raising is not enough to confirm nerve root involvement. If the pain that is elicited arises from a sciatic root the pain will be experienced as true *sciatica*—that is, a pain radiating down the leg into the calf and foot. Distorting the pelvis by straight leg raising may cause pain that is felt only in the back or posterior thigh. This form of pain is *mechanical or discogenic* in origin or originates from painful facets, sacroiliac joints, paraspinal muscles, or ligaments. Straight leg raising may also elicit pain from an *abnormal hip joint* that may radiate into the posterior thigh and lower back. Characteristically, of course, hip pains are elicited by a variety of other movements that stress the hip joint only, such as rotation, abduction, adduction, and hip joint impaction (Fig. 4.4).

Straight leg raising should be done not only with the *hip flexed,* but also with the *hip hyperextended.* Forward flexion straight leg raising is done with the patient standing or supine. Backward hyperextension straight leg raising may be done with the patient standing, prone, or on his side. Forward straight leg raising is especially effective in stretching L5 and S1 roots, which enter the lower portion of the lumbosacral plexus and are therefore relatively fixed in position near the sciatic notch. Backward straight leg raising is especially effective in stretching L3 and L4 roots, since they enter the upper portion of the plexus. As a result, they may curve away from the pelvic wall during forward flexion and be stretched less than the more caudal roots. During backward hyperextension, the lumbosacral plexus is flattened against the back of the pelvic wall, and the L3 and L4 roots that may have escaped painful stretching during forward straight leg raising are forcefully stretched, causing sciatic pain if the root is entrapped or inflamed. This form of straight leg raising is particularly useful and important to include in the physical examination of patients suspected of having L3-L4 disc disease or with a history of prior back surgery at L3-L4 or higher in the lumbar area.

A variety of *modifications of the straight leg raising test* have been described, all eliciting or preventing stretch of the sciatic nerve roots with induction of pain in a sciatic distribution. A variety of eponyms have been given to these various tests, but I

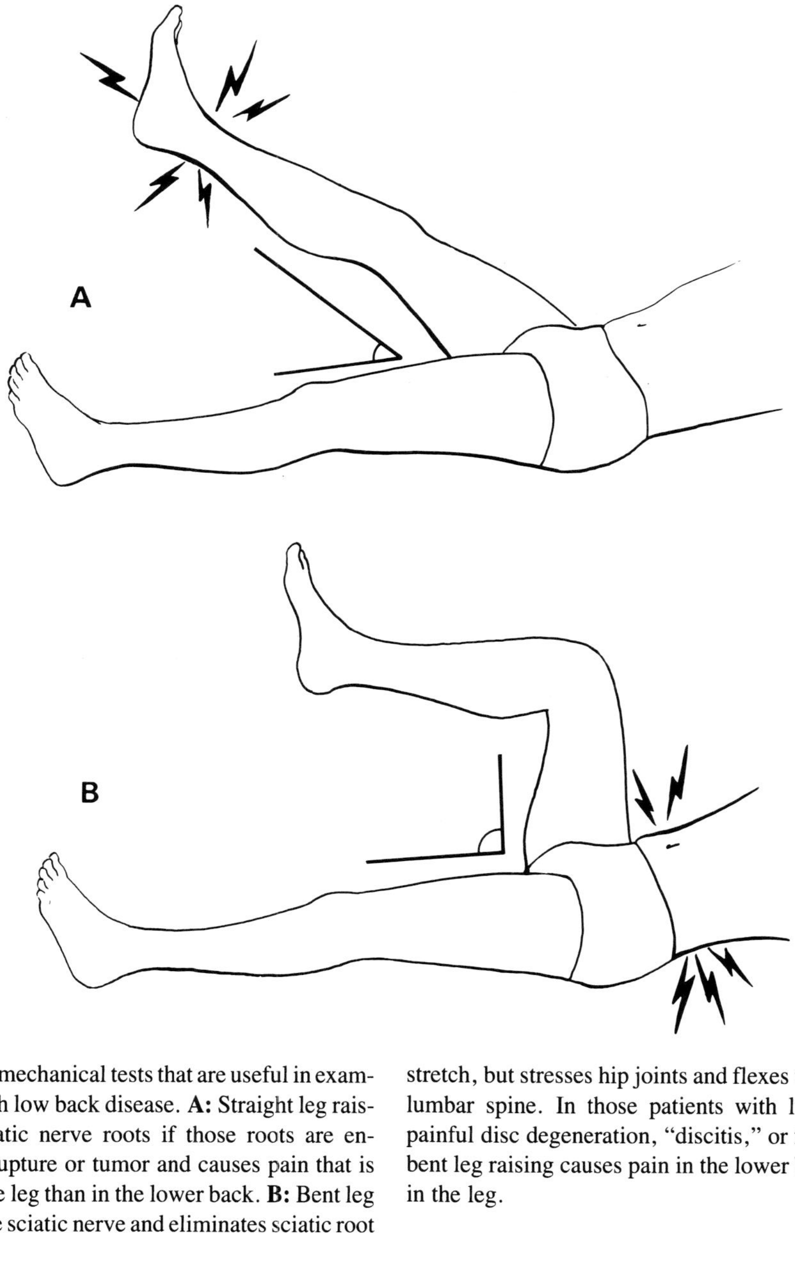

FIGURE 4.4. Two mechanical tests that are useful in examining patients with low back disease. **A:** Straight leg raising stretches sciatic nerve roots if those roots are entrapped by disc rupture or tumor and causes pain that is more severe in the leg than in the lower back. **B:** Bent leg raising relaxes the sciatic nerve and eliminates sciatic root stretch, but stresses hip joints and flexes the pelvis on the lumbar spine. In those patients with lumbar arthritis, painful disc degeneration, "discitis," or facet syndrome, bent leg raising causes pain in the lower back, more than in the leg.

find this a confusing practice that I do not recommend. Lasegue described six versions of his test that cover almost all of the other eponymically identified testing procedures.[42] All of these tests are based on the principle that simultaneous flexion of a hip and extension of the ipsilateral knee will put traction on the sciatic nerve and will elicit sciatic pain if the nerve root is entrapped within the spinal canal or at the pyriformis muscle. In contrast, flexion of the hip with knee flexed does not put traction on the sciatic nerve roots even at a point where hip flexion is sufficient to cause pelvic rocking and distortion of painful structures in the back. The various eponymically differentiated techniques of straight leg and bent leg raising involve dynamically moving from one basic position to the other. With all these tests, the severity of entrapment can be estimated by quantitating the angle of leg elevation at which sciatic radiation of pain becomes obvious to the patient.

The leg pain that results from straight leg raising can be further confirmed as originating from sciatic root entrapment by eliciting radiating pain by one or more of *three other tests that involve stretching the nerve*. The addition of forced ankle plantar flexion, then ankle dorsiflexion while the affected leg is elevated to the point where leg symptoms become obvious to the patient can be useful, especially in patients who have difficulty describing the pain that straight leg raising induces. Forced plantar flexion of the ankle adds to the relaxation of the sciatic nerve, while *forced dorsiflexion* adds to the nerve stretch and therefore should specifically and acutely aggravate the sciatic component of pain. I have found forced ankle dorsiflexion to be more valuable than elicitation of the *bowstring sign*. In this test, the patient sits or lies with hip and knee flexed and the examiner compresses the sciatic nerve by manual pressure in the popliteal fossa. When this maneuver elicits radiating leg pain to the foot, it is indeed strongly confirmatory of nerve root compression, but I have found the test to be positive only in patients with flagrant root entrapment. The third method of eliciting sciatic pain by stretching is the *crossed well-leg raising test* (of Fajerstajn).[43,44] This test is performed by having the patient lie or stand with the affected leg straight, then performing straight leg raising on the contralateral leg. To be positive, the test must elicit sciatic radiation in the straightened leg, not in the leg that is being elevated. In these patients, straight leg raising on the affected or abnormal side should always elicit ipsilateral sciatica at a lower angle of elevation than that necessary to achieve contralateral pain from the crossed well-leg raising test. This test elicits contralateral pain by stretching the sciatic nerve roots sufficiently to cause distortion of the entire lumbar theca with transmitted distortion across the spinal sac to the contralateral nerve roots. This test is said to be highly specific for nerve root entrapment, usually by a disc rupture (Fig. 4.5).

The origin of pain from the sciatic nerve can also be confirmed by documenting *nerve tenderness* by direct palpation over the sciatic notch. A sciatic

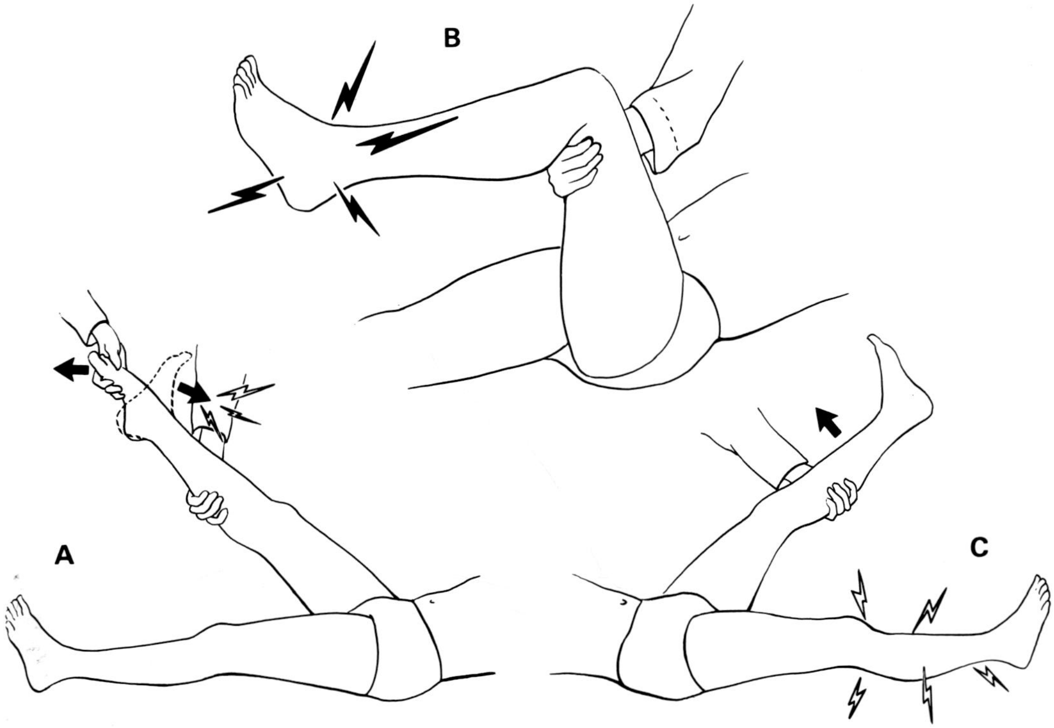

FIGURE 4.5. Supplementary tests for lumbosacral nerve root entrapment. **A:** Once straight leg raising has been carried to the point of discomfort, forced ankle dorsiflexion causes further painful sciatic stretching, and forced ankle plantar flexion relaxes sciatic roots and relieves radiating leg pain. **B:** Bent leg raising relaxes the sciatic nerve, but the bowstring test selectively stretches the sciatic nerve by compression within the popliteal fossa. **C:** The crossed well leg raising test causes sciatic radiation of pain in the opposite leg by stretching asymptomatic nerve roots so far that they cause distortion of the contralateral entrapped roots.

nerve origin of pain will also be suggested by observing the *"one cheek sign."* This sign is frequently observed in patients with lumbar disc disease but is not specific, since it can be observed in patients with sciatic irritation of other causes, ischiogluteal bursitis, or a painful fasciitis or trigger point. This sign is elicited by watching the patient sit and is most pronounced if the patient sits in an armchair. It will be observed that the patient consistently maintains weight bearing on one ischial tuberosity or buttock cheek, even at the expense of some twisting of his back and frequently with the added support of an elbow on the arm of the chair. The basis of this distinctive sitting posture is an effort by the patient to avoid compression of a tender sciatic nerve or ischial tuberosity or to avoid stretching or stressing a painful fasciitis or trigger point.

The other signs of neurologic involvement in patients with the failed back syndrome are related to the functional status of the involved sciatic nerve or root. *Neurologic dysfunction* may be expressed as weakness, sensory loss, reflex loss, or autonomic or causalgic changes. The specific patterns of neurologic impairment seen with lumbosacral nerve root dysfunction are summarized in Figure 2.3 in Chapter 2.

The true extent, or even the existence, of *motor power impairment* may be difficult or impossible to determine accurately in the face of significant pain and tenderness. Patients will often recount that their painful extremity suddenly "gave way," resulting in a fall. This phenomenon seems to be related to the primitive *nociceptive withdrawal reflex,* in which a painful stimulus to the foot causes an abrupt and involuntary withdrawal of that extremity. Of course, if this occurs while the patient is standing, the result will be a sudden loss of support, with a tendency to fall. In patients with the failed back syndrome, the nociceptive stimulus may originate internally rather than from an externally applied stimulus, causing the patient to fall without encountering any external stimulus. This same phenomenon also becomes a consideration in the physical examination of motor power. If the patient attempts to perform a motor movement that elicits pain from muscles, joints, or other structures, he may not only consciously suppress or limit the motion but may also find his motor efforts actively inhibited by this withdrawal reflex.

In the absence of significant pain on exertion, *specific weakness* of one or more muscle groups should be sought. Muscle strength may be graded numerically (0 to 4+, 5+, or 10+ power; or 0 to 4+, 5+, or 10+ weakness) or verbally (poor to excellent power; severe to no weakness), but the numerical scale used should be declared to avoid confusion. It is frustrating to read in a medical report "gastrocnemius—3+." This may mean anything from "3+ weakness on a scale of 4+" to "3+ power on a scale of 10+." It is always helpful to be able to confirm apparent weakness. Watching for evidence of weakness when the patient is not being specifically muscle tested is useful; so is asking distracting questions, such as: "Does it hurt your back when you walk on your toes? Your heels?" Obviously, significant weakness should impair the motor activity even if no pain is produced. A muscle weakened by nerve root injury should lose its deep tendon reflex, and long-standing weakness should leave visible, palpable, or measurable atrophy.

A careful and reliable *sensory examination* is essential in the diagnosis and management of failed back syndrome patients. The basic essentials of the sensory examination should be quite familiar to all physicians and surgeons, but performing an accurate and reliable examination may at times tax the skill and concentration of the examiner. From a systems analysis point of view, the sensory examination entails three parts: input, output, and interpretation. The examiner is solely responsible for the input portion of the examination. He must decide which neurologic testing technique is indicated and how extensively to pursue this technique. The examiner must also perform the testing in a reproducible fashion that is presented clearly enough to the patient so that the patient can provide an accurate output of information. In the output segment of the examination, the patient must detect, transmit, and consciously perceive the applied stimulus, interpret the stimulus, and formulate a response. The response may be reflex, mechanical, or verbal, the latter being especially important during sensory examination. Once this output has been generated, the examiner must not only listen for a verbal response but must also observe carefully for nonverbal responses or nonverbal concomitants to verbal responses. The examiner must then formulate an interpretation of the response that is entered in the medical record as the result of the sensory examination. The complexity and importance of a careful sensory examination are obvious to physicians and usually rapidly become obvious to patients who are carefully examined at intervals by their attendant surgeons during the course of the management of a lumbar disc problem. I am indebted to a former patient of mine, Mr. Melvin Levinson, for his witty but perceptive observations on this point:

Thoughts While Convalescing
or
Ode To A Neurosurgeon

The doctor-patient relationship which is established at the initial contact is of paramount importance to the successful conduct of the patient's illness.

Certain specialists of the medical profession are magnificently equipped with imposing tools and equipment which properly impress the patient with the compass of the physician's knowledge and technique.

The stethoscope of the GP
The saws and chisels of the Orthopedist
The x-ray machines of the Radiologist
The lenses and chart of the Ophthalmologist

But . . . towering above these symbols of scientific and medical progress stands the Neurosurgeon admirably equipped with his collection of . . . safety pins!!!

Cutaneous pain perception may be seriously impaired by the underlying spontaneous pain. The classic teaching in neurology is that a *stocking* or *glove sensory loss* usually represents a *hysterical* sensory loss. This phenomenon is characterized by sensory loss usually involving all modalities in a distal extremity with a circumferential upper border not following segmental patterns of innervation. There is no doubt that hysterical sensory loss does exist, but it is my impression that such loss is apt to be more extensive than simple *antalgic sensory loss*. Hysterical sensory loss more commonly involves the trunk, if not the entire side of the body, with arm, leg, and face included. On the other hand, antalgic sensory loss is usually confined to the painful extremity, with an upper border that may vary from mid calf to upper thigh. My assumption is that this form of sensory loss can be likened to "*reverse acupuncture*." It is reasonably well accepted now that acupuncture and transcutaneous neurostimulation (TNS) induce pain relief and some sensory loss by competitive inhibition within the central neuraxis. The *"double-gate" theory* of pain postulated by Wall and Melzak explains the pain relief and hypalgesia generated by acupuncture or TNS as being caused by a competitive inhibition of the central ascending reticular nociceptive pathways.[45–48] This is brought about by large-volume stimulation of the long-fiber touch-transmitting pathways that synapse competitively with long-fiber pain pathways into the reticular ascending system. When the reticular system is flooded by touch signals, pain signals are not able to pass through, and noxious stimuli are perceived without their nociceptive quality. In antalgic analgesia I assume that a similar process works in reverse—that is, the long-fiber pain pathways are firing actively and actively flooding the reticular pathway. When additional nociceptive stimuli attempt to feed into this system they are blocked as effectively as they might be if the reticular system were overloaded with collateral input from the touch pathways. The result is a loss of ability to perceive painful stimuli that does not follow normal segmental patterns but is likely to involve the entire extremity.

Disturbance of functioning of *individual roots of the sciatic nerve* results in specific patterns of neurologic abnormality (see Fig. 2.3). As discussed in Chapter 2, some variability exists from person to person about the level of exit of these individual nerve roots, as well as the recognized variability in the neurologic functions subserved by a given nerve root. A classic example is the discrepancy shown on different sensory charts of the cutaneous representation of various nerve roots (see Fig. 4.6). Some charts show bands of sensory loss extending up the leg from the foot to the buttock, while others show the corresponding sensory loss confined to the distal lower extremity only. In practice, the situation is usually even more complex than that because of the considerable overlap that takes place between peripheral nerves in nearly every part of the body. To completely denervate any one given segmental area of skin usually requires interruption of a minimum of five sensory nerve roots, two above and two below the major sensory root. This can be amply demonstrated in patients who have undergone lumbar sensory rhizotomies for pain relief. Sectioning a single nerve root may leave little or no easily detectable cutaneous sensory loss, and sectioning two adjacent roots may induce hypalgesia but rarely, if ever, induces anesthesia. Nonetheless, the pattern of neurologic abnormality caused by disordered functioning of the sciatic nerve roots is sufficiently constant to be extremely useful clinically. The most commonly encountered patterns of *sensory* loss, usually hypalgesia with or without hypesthesia, are:

L4 root (usually an L3-L4 disc rupture)—medial knee and upper medial calf.
L5 root (usually an L4-L5 disc rupture)—shin and dorsal medial foot, including great toe.
S1 root (usually an L5-S1 disc rupture)—lateral calf and lateral foot, including small toe and lateral half of plantar surface of foot.

Muscle weakness is most often encountered in the following patterns:

L4 root—weakness of knee extension.
L5 root—weakness of dorsiflexion of ankle and especially of great toe. Testing the latter is all too often not included in the routine physical or neurological examination.
S1 root—weakness of plantar flexion or ankle.

Weakness of ankle movement can be tested nicely by asking the patient to walk first on the toes, then on the heels. If the patient's attention is distracted by the physician asking whether or not this elicits back pain, one often discovers that the patient is able to perform these two functions even though on objective testing he seems incapable of dorsiflexing or plantar flexing that ankle. Obviously, if the patient can carry his entire weight during the process of toe walking or heel walking, motor weakness must not be profound, and an alternative explanation for apparent severe weakness on direct testing must be sought.

Impairments of *deep tendon reflexes* also form a part of the neurologic picture seen with sciatic root abnormalities. The knee reflex is most commonly lost with L4 radiculopathy, and the ankle reflex is most commonly lost with S1 radiculopathy. L5 radiculopathy rarely results in a detectable loss of deep tendon reflex because the tibialis anterior reflex, which is disturbed by L5 radiculopathy, is difficult to elicit in normal persons. Thus, it is both possible and not uncommon for a patient to exhibit a significant sciatic radiculopathy with no detectable reflex loss—even though a prominent orthopedist testified that the contrary was true in a much publicized malpractice trial.

Even the examination of *deep tendon reflexes* must be done carefully because the patient's state of muscle tension and relaxation may either augment or impede induced reflex responses. Many patients

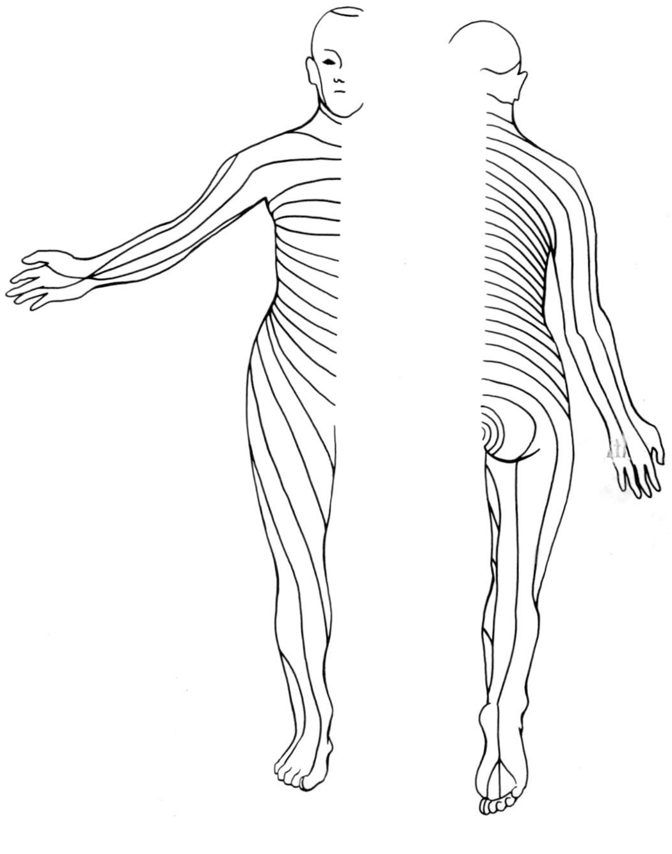

FIGURE 4.6. Approximate cutaneous representation of dermatomally arranged segmental spinal nerve roots. Not all such sensory charts depict cutaneous representation of lower lumbar and upper sacral nerve roots over the posterior thigh and buttock, but this chart is more consistent with what I observe in most patients.

with a failed back syndrome take muscle relaxing medications, so that bilaterally hypoactive reflexes may be drug induced and therefore carry little or no localizing information. In these instances, reinforcing maneuvers, such as the *Jendrassik maneuver,* may be quite helpful in identifying reflex asymmetries. To do this maneuver, the patient is asked to hook together the fingers of both hands. Reflex testing is done repeatedly at perhaps five-second intervals, beginning with the patient's arms relaxed. While repetitive reflex testing continues, the patient is asked to pull strongly against himself and then moments later is told once again to relax. The reflex being tested should be augmented by this maneuver, especially just as the patient begins to pull.

Autonomic changes in lower extremities are less commonly seen in the failed back syndrome than are loss of sensory or motor function, but *reflex sympathetic dystrophy* or *causalgia* may occasionally accompany or follow painful conditions, usually those that include sciatica. In these patients, trophic changes may be identified in the extremity under question, consisting of dryness, thinning, and skin discoloration. One other autonomic phenomenon may be sought in patients with apparent severe sensory loss in whom segmental loss is suspected, even if this occurs in association with a more global and antalgic analgesia. If there is severe interruption of the nerve root, the *wheal and flare response* to a skin scratch in the affected area may be lost. Scratching the affected area with a sharp object will cause a linear wheal to appear, but no erythematous flaring will accompany this response. In contrast, scratching other cutaneous areas that retain their innervation, even if analgesia is present in these areas on an antalgic basis, causes both a wheal and flare to appear.

Mechanical Examination

The *mechanical examination* of the back is the second important part of the physical examination of patients with the failed back syndrome. The term *mechanical examination* has been maligned for its imprecision and inelegance, but it is a convenient term for an examination that emphasizes bones, joints, and ligaments.

The back should first be *visually inspected* for evidence of spinal curvature laterally (scoliosis) or exaggerated forward bowing (lordosis). Abnormal sharp forward angulation (kyphosis) is less often encountered in patients with the failed back syndrome, since this is usually related to spinal tuberculosis, extensive vertebral fractures, or extensive vertebral collapse secondary to metastatic carcinoma. A visible scoliosis is quite frequently the result of unilateral paraspinal muscle spasm, which frequently occurs with no underlying bony abnormality. On the other hand, an exaggerated lordosis, and occasionally scoliosis, may indicate chronic poor posture, with the resultant ligamentous relaxation and stretching being the cause of the patient's persistent back pain. *Pelvic tilt,* or elevation of one iliac crest higher than the other, may also be the result of either muscle spasms or poor posture. Pelvic tilt, however, should alert the physician to measure the lower extremities, since a difference in leg length greater than a centimeter or two may result in sufficient distortion of back mechanics to result in chronic back pain. Pelvic tilt should also alert the physician to examine the hips, since *hip disease* can cause local muscle spasms or even bony deformity and can cause pain in the buttock, thigh, and lower back that may confuse the assessment of a failed back syndrome.

Manual *manipulation* of the lumbar spine can yield helpful information. With the patient supine, the examiner's forceful lifting of each vertebral segment in turn with his fingers may trigger pain in areas that are not tender to palpation or even to percussion. Focal movements of degenerated or damaged facets or discs will produce localized pain if those joints are painfully arthropathic. Pain on manipulation is less frequently encountered with spinal sepsis or metastatic cancer.

Because the mechanical structures in the back are concerned with *weight bearing* and *bending,* examination of these functions occupies a preeminent portion of the mechanical examination of the back. Valuable information can be obtained by simply observing patients as they walk into the office or examining room, stand, sit, or rise from sitting. This information is even more valuable if it is obtained during the course of initial contact or history taking rather than as a formal part of the examination. It is, however, sometimes useful to repeat this portion of the examination to look for exaggerated responses in patients who realize that they are being examined. Such exaggerated responses suggest the possibility of conscious attempts to alter the examination, but may reflect only nervousness, anxiety, or even a well-intentioned but overdone attempt to cooperate with the physician.

Standing posture should be observed for associated spinal curvature and for symmetry of hip and lower extremities. Does the patient bear weight evenly an equal amount of time on both legs, or does he avoid full or repetitive weight bearing on one extremity? *Bending tests* of the back and hip obviously overlap considerably with the neurologic tests of nerve stretching (see page 48), but the differences are worth emphasizing. I have found that many practicing physicians (especially those who are neither neurosurgeons nor orthopedists) seem to have a very limited understanding of this aspect of the physical examination. The basic differentiation is that bending that causes stretching of entrapped sciatic nerve roots will elicit distal radiating leg pain if the root entrapment (as in a lumbar disc rupture) is the cause of the patient's pain. On the other hand, movements of the back and hip that do not cause nerve stretching, but that still cause pain in the back, buttock, or upper thigh, indicate a mechanical cause for the patient's pain.

Mechanical *mobility testing* for the failed back syndrome concentrates principally on back motions. These are done with the patient standing and include testing of motion in several directions. The patient is asked to forward bend, backward bend, lateral bend, and rotate the back, with the first two of these motions being the most important. The range of motion in each direction is quantitated, and an effort is made to ascertain whether restriction in motion is due to pain or merely due to stiffness or tightness of joints and ligaments. Quantitation of motion is usually given as degrees of angulation or rotation of the back. The amount of forward bending may alternatively be quantitated in terms of how far down the patient's leg he is able to touch (e.g., "patient is able to forward bend to touch three inches below his knees"). Other tests of mobility include bent leg raising and straight leg raising, as discussed in the section on the neurologic examination. Internal and external rotation of the hips and upward impaction of the hip joint by sharp and forceful compression of the sole of the foot with the leg extended help to exclude the possibility of hip disease masquerading as low back disease.

Miscellaneous Examination

Several features of the physical examination suggest etiologies of pain other than mechanical or neurologic problems. *Visual inspection* of the back may reveal *pilonidal sinus openings* or *midline nevi,* which increases the suspicion of an underlying lipoma or other congenital neoplasm. Visually inspecting the back, especially with the patient prone, may reveal evidence of paraspinal muscle spasm, with unilateral tumescence and scoliosis concave to that side. This is confirmed by palpating a firm and exquisitely tender muscle mass that does not relax when surrounding muscles relax.

Palpation of the lower back, coccyx, pelvis, hips, and leg bones frequently elicits other areas of *local tenderness* without visible changes in the skin or underlying tissues. The more focal this tenderness, the more suggestive it is of a precise etiology that may respond nicely to locally directed, usually nonoperative therapy, and that may even be aggravated by laminectomy (see page 145). In contrast, *diffuse tenderness* is a more nonspecific manifestation of a variety of painful conditions, especially fibromyalgia, diffuse arthritis, the flabby back syndrome (see page 18), or psychologically painful states. The chief causes of marked *focal tenderness,* other than muscle spasm, are painful trigger points or fasciitis, bone donor sites, coccydynia, and ischiogluteal bursitis. Painful sacroiliac joints, facet joints, or interspinous or sacroiliac ligaments, or pain at the site of a pseudarthrosis, are other common sources of local tenderness, although the tenderness is less likely to be severe on palpation, but more so on percussion (see page 23). Pseudomeningocele (see page 18) and spinal infection (see page 19) characteristically cause local tenderness, but neither condition is commonly encountered. Fat herniations through the fascial aponeurosis in the lumbosacral paraspinal area (see page 22) may also cause back pain and local tenderness. Although such herniations are claimed by some to be common, in my experience local tenderness is far more common over the periosteal and muscular edge of the iliac crest than over the aponeurosis covering lumbosacral paraspinal muscles.

In my experience, painful *periosteal trigger points* are by far most commonly encountered over the posterior iliac spines, with 69% of trigger points occurring at these sites in my personal series[49] (see page 21). It is especially important to palpate for trigger points, since they occur frequently, can be discovered only by palpation, are often not diagnosed, and usually respond well only to specific therapy (frequently local injection) (see page 99). Palpation at these sites frequently elicits not only local pain but also pain radiating into the posterior or posterolateral thigh or even into the region of the ipsilateral knee. Periosteal trigger points may also be elicited from other locations along the posterior iliac crests, from the tips of spinous processes, or from interspinous ligaments. *Muscular trigger points* occur over muscle bellies, away from sites of periosteal insertion, and are frequently multiple. The distinctions among periosteal and muscular trigger points, fasciitis, and ligamentous tenderness are vague and ill-defined, so that tenderness over interspinous ligaments or sacroiliac ligaments may be variously termed ligamentous tenderness, trigger points, or fasciitis. In all of these conditions, histologic examination of the painful area (which is rarely possible clinically) is usually unrewarding, because ordinarily there are no obvious histologic changes and no cellular evidence of inflammation. Local tenderness over a *bone donor site* may reflect a similarly nonspecific histology, but histologic examination will occasionally reveal one or more local neuromata. Despite this difference in histology, the pain elicited on palpation is quite similar to that from other local painful sources (i.e., local tenderness with frequent radiation into buttock or posterolateral thigh).

Ischiogluteal bursitis also causes marked focal tenderness and pain. The location is diagnostic (see page 22) and, like periosteal trigger points, ischiogluteal bursitis can be diagnosed only by palpation, is frequently not diagnosed, and usually responds best to specific therapy. This condition has been termed "the classical pain in the arse."[22] Pain is usually maximum in the buttock rather than the lower back, and point tenderness can be elicited from the ischiogluteal bursa overlying the point of the ischial tuberosity. The area of maximum tenderness may be palpated in the erect or prone patient by thrusting upward from the gluteal fold. The derivation of the tenderness from the ischiogluteal bursa is usually easily confirmed by palpating the ischial tuberosity with the patient seated or in the lateral decubitus position with hips flexed. In this position, gluteal muscles move aside to uncover the ischial tuberosity, thus sparing these muscles from prolonged compression during sitting.

Tenderness is less frequently elicited from *facet joints*, but when it is elicited it differs from that elicited from trigger points, fasciitis, or painful ligaments in that the pain is usually more obvious on firm pressure or percussion than on light palpation (see page 19). The tenderness is usually less severe than that elicited from trigger points, but quality and radiation of pain are usually quite similar. Likewise, the pain elicited from palpation over a *pseudarthrosis* is more obvious with firm or deep palpation or percussion than with superficial palpation (see page 20). The pain that is elicited usually remains local, but may be associated with radicular pain secondary to transmission of pressure through the pseudarthrosis to underlying nerve roots tethered by epidural scar. Palpation over an *inflamed sacroiliac joint* evokes local pain that frequently radiates in similar fashion to that evoked from trigger points, fasciitis, and tender ligaments, although the distinguishing feature is the location of the tender point over the sacroiliac joint.

Examination by *percussion,* gently using a fist or a rubber hammer, supplements examination by palpation and manual manipulation. Percussion transmits a wave of tissue motion below superficial structures and can elicit pain when palpation or even manipulation is painless. The condition in which percussion most reliably elicits pain is metastatic vertebral cancer, but percussion pain may also be elicited in spinal sepsis, aseptic discitis, pseudomeningocele, and painful arthropathy of degenerated or injured discs, facets, or sacroiliac joints.

Coccydynia is most commonly seen following local trauma to the coccyx, but is occasionally encountered as a minor or major component of the failed back syndrome. These patients complain of pain on sitting, defecation, and intromission during sexual intercourse. Examination shows marked local tenderness over the coccyx and severe pain is elicited when the coccyx is manually manipulated with one finger in the rectum (Fig. 4.7).

When one encounters patients with local tender areas, the history of localized pain and tenderness may often be confirmed by visual inspection, *if the patient has used local heat extensively.* At the area of maximum heat application, brownish discoloration of the skin will often be seen and, of course, blistering may result from injudicious heat application.

Laboratory Studies

Hematologic studies are usually normal in patients with the failed back syndrome. Patients who present within days after surgery with excruciatingly severe back pain and tenderness, with or without radiating leg pains or increasing neurologic deficits, may suffer from a bacterial wound infection. If so, the hemogram will usually show an elevated white blood count (WBC) with polymorphonuclear predominance. Within the first several days following back surgery, especially if spinal fusion is included, an elevation of WBC with polymorphonuclear predominance is often seen in association with the *"bone fever"* that results from the trauma of surgery without bacterial infection. The patient with a wound infection will show persistent temperature elevation, as well as a persistent and usually increasing elevation of WBC. Sciatic neuritis caused by, or at least temporally related to, systemic viral infections or herpetic infections usually presents after postoperative temperature elevations have returned to normal. WBC will be normal or low, and a lymphocytic predominance will be encountered.

The *erythrocyte sedimentation rate* (ESR) will be elevated in the presence of bacterial wound infection, but may also be selectively elevated even though the WBC is normal. This picture is typical of acute inflammatory arthritis or *inflammatory discitis;* the latter sometimes called *aseptic interspace necrosis*. Inflammatory discitis is an extremely painful condition in which bacteria cannot be cultured from the interspace, but it is likely to represent a form of acute autoimmune disorder triggered by the hematogenous release of antigenic substances from the disc space at the time of surgery. The progress of the disease can be charted by serial determinations of sedimentation rate, with a falling sedimentation rate usually correlating with improved pain and clinical recovery.

Acute rheumatoid arthritis, ankylosing spondylitis, and Reiter's syndrome are all forms of *inflammatory arthritis* that may cause the failed back syndrome. These conditions may have been present prior to back surgery and may have been improperly diagnosed or, less frequently, they may have developed postoperatively. All will characteristically cause an elevation of the sedimentation rate. Patients with acute rheumatoid arthritis will also have elevations in their rheumatoid agglutinins, and patients with ankylosing spondylitis will most likely have an HLA-B27 serotype.[9,10] Degenerative osteoarthritis is much more commonly encountered in patients with the failed back syndrome, but hematologic or serologic tests are not confirmatory, because this is a degenerative rather than an inflammatory disorder.

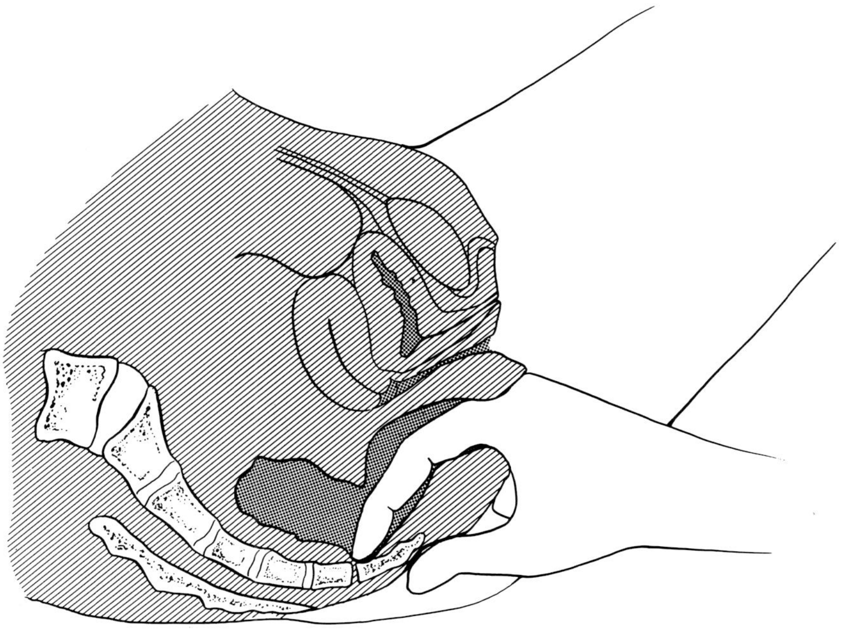

FIGURE 4.7. Coccydynia may cause lumbar or sacrococcygeal pain and tenderness on sitting, defecation, or intromission. Its presence is confirmed by digital compression and manipulation of the sacrococcygeal joint during rectal examination.

Additional laboratory tests may be helpful in distinguishing other specific conditions important in the differential diagnosis of the failed back syndrome. *Gouty arthritis* occurs with a frequency that surprises many clinicians and may occasionally present with a significant spinal involvement. An elevated serum uric acid is highly suggestive of gout. Kidney stones, pyelonephritis, or other *urologic disorders* can occasionally cause back pain that is sufficiently severe and isolated to require differential diagnosis from the failed back syndrome, or at least from an exacerbation of that disorder. Urine analysis in these conditions becomes important, with inspection for microscopic hematuria, white blood cells, or casts.

Electrodiagnostic Studies

The usefulness of electrodiagnostic studies in the diagnosis of virgin lumbar disc disease remains controversial and of uncertain value. Clearly severe pain can occur in the absence of neurologic damage. The usefulness of these techniques in patients with failed back syndrome is even more uncertain, especially since lumbar surgery itself causes electrical abnormalities of paraspinal muscles.

Electrical *nerve conduction studies* can unquestionably be of value in patients in whom the differential diagnosis includes primary neuropathy, such as painful diabetic mononeuropathy. Electrical demonstration of slowed nerve conduction in one or more peripheral nerves can be most helpful in the differential diagnosis of weakness or sensory loss in the lower extremity, especially when these symptoms are combined with spontaneous pain. Lumbar disc ruptures and other abnormal conditions that damage the nerve roots rather than the peripheral nerves usually do not cause a slowing of peripheral nerve conduction. Focal nerve compression may result from *pyriformis entrapment syndrome,* but this condition is difficult to diagnose by nerve conduction tests because of its proximal location. Confirmation of slowed conduction at the pyriformis muscle requires placement of one set of needle electrodes in the paraspinal region, a technique that is usually not included in routine nerve conduction studies.

Electromyography (EMG) can detect muscle reinnervation several months prior to the reappearance of sufficient muscle strength to be detectable by physical examination. Similarly, areas of muscle denervation caused by nerve root injury may be apparent electromyographically while weakness is still undetectable on physical examination. This is particularly suggestive of nerve root injury if denervation potentials are detected in paraspinal muscles, as well as in muscles of the lower extremity. Unfortunately, once patients have sustained nerve root injury it is difficult, if not impossible, for EMG to differentiate the time of onset of that injury. For the patient who presents with a failed back syndrome, denervation potentials from the lower extremity may exist for many months even after the nerve root has been adequately decompressed. Paraspinal muscles will of course yield abnormal denervation potentials once they have been disrupted during the performance of a laminectomy. This electrical abnormality may persist for many months, perhaps even for years. Many patients will experience severe sciatic pain and irritation without developing peripheral denervation, and in these patients, a normal EMG will be recorded despite the presence of painful nerve root entrapment. EMG may be beneficial to the failed back syndrome sufferer if an electromyographic study is abnormal and if a previous study obtained since the original surgery was either normal or unequivocally showed a less severe or less widespread abnormality. Simply documenting an abnormal EMG in a failed back syndrome sufferer does not confirm whether new damage has occurred or whether the recorded electrical changes are merely the residue of a previously decompressed nerve root injury. Similarly, the recording of a normal EMG does not preclude the presence of a painful disorder of nerve roots, and patients should not be denied appropriate nonsurgical or surgical therapy solely on the basis of a negative EMG.

Noninvasive Radiologic Studies

Plain Radiographs

Radiographs or x-ray pictures of the back are an indispensable but often frustratingly unhelpful part of the diagnosis of the failed back syndrome. By definition, all of these patients have undergone previous back surgery, perhaps at the hands of another surgeon. Radiographs may give valuable information about the previous operation. The *laminotomy defect,* a term used to describe the "window" through the lamina created by a unilateral partial hemilaminectomy, will help to localize the level of previous disc surgery and may reveal whether more than one level was explored operatively (Fig. 4.8). If the interlaminal space is large or if the surgeon performed microsurgery, however, the laminotomy may have included relatively little bone removal and may be difficult or impossible to visualize on plain radiographs. If the surgeon has left a *metallic marker,* often a metal hemostasis clip, at the operative site, confirmation of the previous operative level can be made unequivocally. This may be extremely important if myelographic abnormalities or clinical features of the patient's failed back syndrome suggest symptomatic pathology at a level different from that initially operated on, or if the initial operation was thought by the surgeon to have been performed at a level different from that confirmed by the radiograph. Intervertebral disc space narrowing is not confirmatory of the site of previous disc surgery, since disc space narrowing is often seen as part of the pathology of disc degeneration and rupture, as one element of degenerative arthritic changes of the spine, and even as a normal variant.

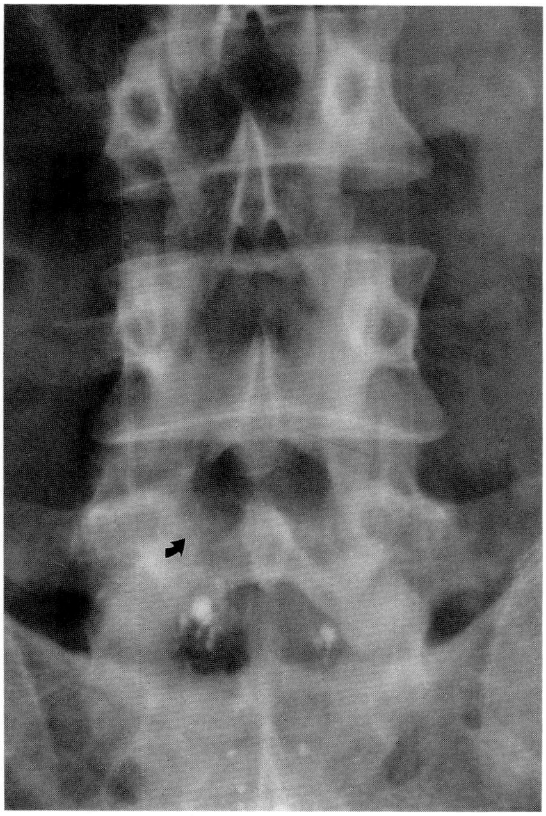

FIGURE 4.8. The laminotomy bony defect left by this woman's previous discectomy is difficult to visualize on a postoperative radiograph **(arrow).** A microsurgical approach with even more limited bone removal would make identification even more difficult, unless a metal marking clip had been placed at the time of surgery. Localization of the previous operative level may be important in excluding the possibility of surgery at an incorrect level as one cause of a failed back syndrome.

Plain radiographs may disclose causes of the failed back syndrome that were overlooked prior to the first surgery or that developed subsequently. A number of back patients develop their original symptoms following *trauma,* and in rare instances a *fracture* of the lumbar spine, especially a fracture of a transverse process, may be overlooked preoperatively. Furthermore, small, simple linear fractures may become more obvious with the passage of time as osteogenic sclerosis develops during healing or around a pseudarthrosis.[18] Even ligamentous tears may become obvious as calcification develops in the area of damage many months following the time of original injury. Lumbar or lumbothoracic *tumors* can at some stage of their development mimic, with disturbing accuracy, the symptomatology of lumbar disc disease. Initial preoperative radiographs may have failed to include the lower thoracic spine, where intradural benign tumors may affect individual lumbar or sacral nerve roots. This form of tumor rarely causes significant bony erosion or expansion of the canal until multiple nerve roots have been compressed, although late in the stage of a failed back syndrome this feature might surface in a patient with an otherwise confusing picture of increasing disability of poorly understood etiology. *Metastatic carcinomas* may also be overlooked if initial films are not carefully reviewed, or if bony changes are late in development. Occasionally, severe back and leg pain may be caused by a predominantly epidural metastasis in which plain radiographs and even radioisotope scans of the spine fail to show obvious abnormality.

Preexisting *congenital disorders* may also have been overlooked, or their significance underestimated, on initial films. *Spina bifida occulta* of L5 or S1 is a relatively common congenital variation and carries no pathologic or etiologic significance in its minor form. However, on occasion, widely bifid spines, especially if the process includes more than one vertebral level, may signify the presence of an underlying occult *meningocele* and *lipoma,* even if there is no obvious cutaneous evidence of this anomaly (Fig. 4.9). Even these lesions are commonly asymptomatic, but may occasionally cause low back pain or pains in the buttock or saddle regions. An anomaly of this type should be particularly suspected in the patient who presents with neurogenic bladder involvement. *Diastematomyelia* may also present as sciatic pain, with pain often preceding the development of objective neurologic deficits. Symptomatic diastematomyelia is most likely to be encountered in adolescents or young adults, but may occasionally be encountered in middle-aged persons. A careful review of plain radiographs will often show the characteristic bony midline intraspinal post or peg, usually in the lower thoracic region. Tomography or computerized tomography (CT) or magnetic resonance imaging (MRI) scans may be necessary for complete delineation of the nature of the disorder. A variation of the above two conditions that is occasionally referred to as a cause of low back and sacral or saddle area pain is the *filum terminale* syndrome, or tethered cord. In this syndrome, which is rare except in patients with myelomeningoceles or other spinal dysraphism, a foreshortened filum terminale is said to cause traction on the conus medullaris as the patient grows taller during youth and adolescence. Symptoms are aggravated by activity, and relief is said to follow sectioning of the filum terminale. Radiographs are generally normal in this condition, which may be associated with occult meningocele or other lumbar congenital defects, but CT scans with intrathecal contrast or MRI scans will usually disclose the thickened filum terminale and low-lying conus medullaris.

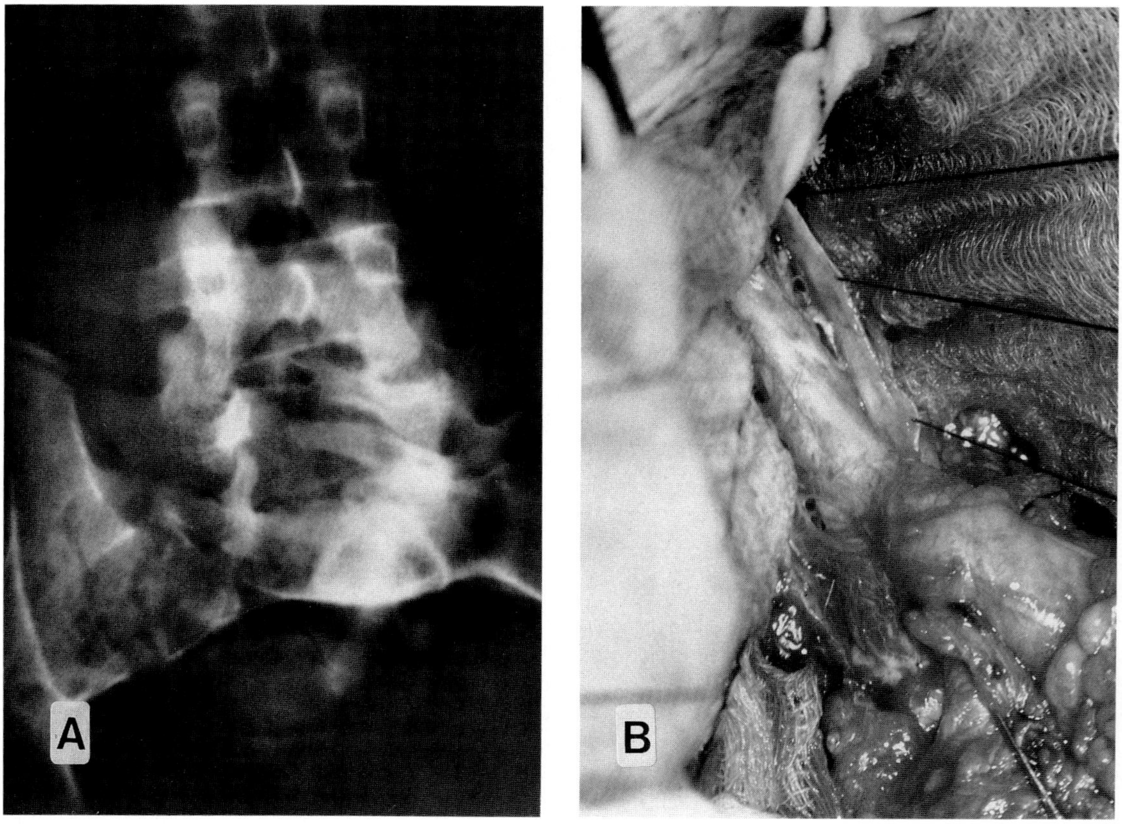

FIGURE 4.9. This 18-year-old girl was suspected of suffering from lumbar disc disease until she developed neurogenic bladder and advancing sensory loss down the medial aspect of both thighs. **A:** The significance of the abnormality on her plain radiograph had been underestimated, even though it demonstrates severe spina bifida occulta and interlaminar widening. **B:** Operation disclosed a lipomatous tumor that extended from the conus medullaris of the spinal cord intradurally through the dura and bony defect and into the subcutaneous tissues of the back.

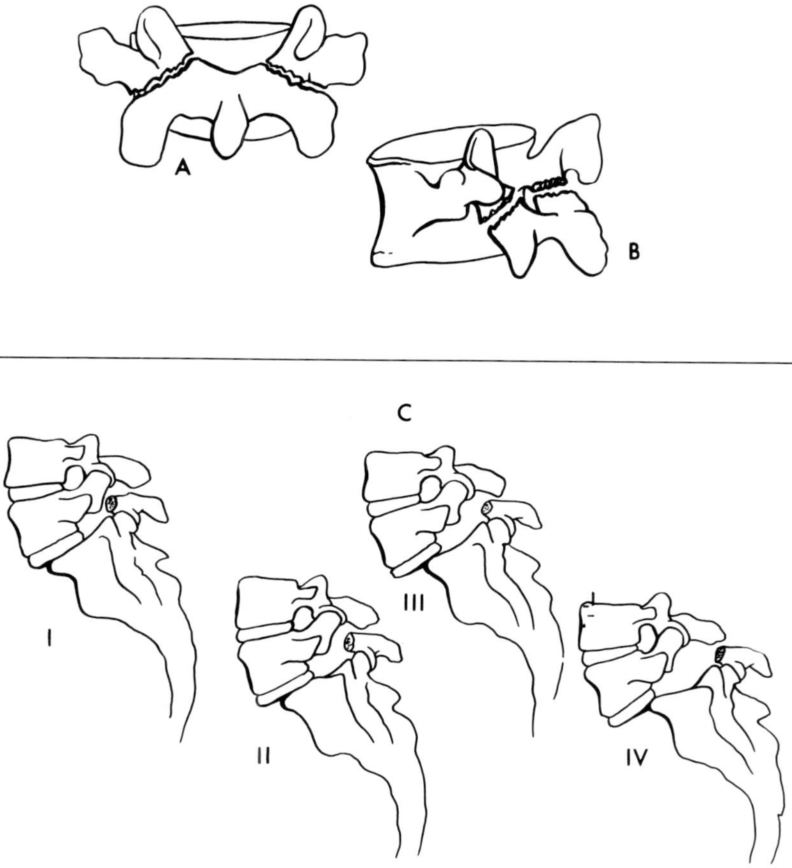

FIGURE 4.10. Spondylolysis may occur with or without spondylolisthesis. **A and B:** Depicted here are posterior and oblique views of a lumbar vertebra that demonstrate the congenital defect in the pars interarticularis which constitutes spondylolysis. If this bony defect results in separation and anterior displacement of the vertebral body, this dislocation is referred to as a spondylolisthesis. **C:** Increasingly severe stages of anterior dislocation are referred to as spondylolisthesis of Grades I to IV.

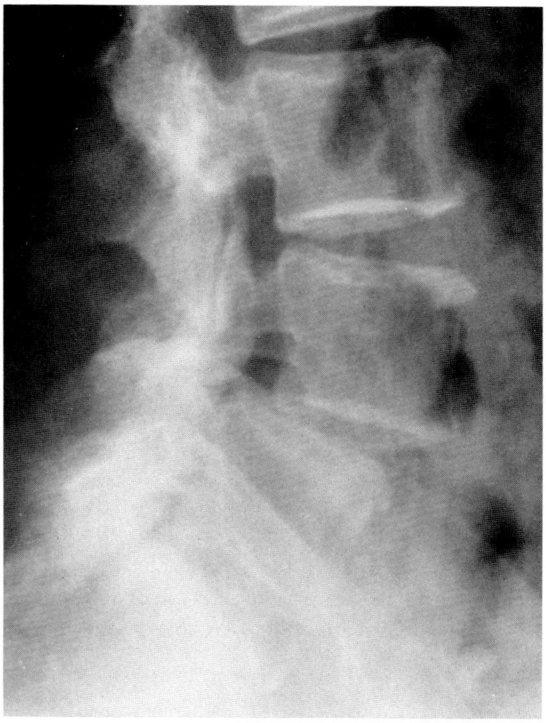

FIGURE 4.11. Spondylolisthesis may be aggravated following disc removal. This 38-year-old woman underwent disc excision without fusion at L4-L5 for sciatica greater than low back pain. Over the next few years, low back pain became progressively more severe. This radiograph disclosed progressive spondylolisthesis at the operative site with forward slipping of L4 on L5.

In contrast, an extremely common form of congenital anomaly is *spondylolysis with spondylolisthesis* (Fig. 4.10). A failure of spontaneous fusion of embryonic osteogenic centers can result in a failure of proper formation of the pars interarticularis of the lateral mass of the dorsal vertebral arch (spondylolysis) with progressive listhesis or slipping of one vertebral body over another (spondylolisthesis). Spondylolisthesis may have preceded simple disc excision, but its significance may have been underestimated. On the other hand, excision of disc material, along with some disruption of posterior bony elements, may aggravate spondylolisthesis and, therefore, may add to the patient's likelihood of developing persistent lower back pain (Fig. 4.11). This condition most frequently occurs at the lumbosacral junction and is said to be a common cause of persistent back pain in young persons. Spondylolysis may occur without spondylolisthesis, and in these instances careful oblique radiographs or CT scans are necessary to make the diagnosis—although it is uncertain whether spondylolysis without spondylolisthesis is ever symptomatic. Oblique radiographs reveal the characteristic "Scottie dog" appearance of the pedicle and facet, and the spondylolysis is evident as the "collar on the dog's neck." A numerical grading system is used to express the severity of anterior slippage in spondylolisthesis, with Grade I referring to minimal slippage and Grade IV referring to complete dislocation of the vertebral bodies.

Arthritis is a major component of many cases of the failed back syndrome, having been either overlooked or underestimated preoperatively or having developed postoperatively. Rheumatoid arthritis, ankylosing spondylitis, and Reiter's syndrome may become symptomatic before characteristic radiographic changes are present. With the passage of time, sclerotic changes should become visible in paraspinal ligaments or in the sacroiliac joint region of the pelvis. Osteoarthritis, on the other hand, is probably a normal accompaniment of the aging process and, therefore, is often symptomatic. Radiographs will delineate the extent of the abnormality, but the correlation between the severity of radiographic changes and the severity of symptoms is imperfect at best.

Plain radiographs may also be important postoperatively if they disclose evidence of a retained *foreign body.* It is unlikely that large steel instruments will inadvertently be left behind during the course of lumbar disc surgery, but I have encountered patients in whom radiographs have revealed the radiopaque markers of surgical cottonoids left at the laminectomy site and surgical sponges left at a bone donor site for spinal fusion. If such foreign bodies are discovered, they must be reported to the patient immediately, especially if the discovering surgeon was also the operating surgeon. The retained foreign body may continue to be a source of difficulty for the patient, causing mechanical nerve root compression or local irritation or acting as a source of sepsis. Accordingly, their recognition is extremely important, and their subsequent surgical removal is indicated except in special circumstances in which surgical removal of a small foreign body may do more harm than the foreign body is likely to do if left in place.

Previous spinal fusion should always be readily apparent on plain spine radiographs (Fig. 4.2). The fusion is usually quite easy to detect if it was performed posteriorly or laterally, but may occasionally be overlooked if an interbody fusion or modified interbody fusion was performed (Fig. 4.12). Occasionally, patients will spontaneously resorb most, if not all, of their fusion, and radiographic evidence of little or no persistent fusion bone may correlate with symptoms of persistent back distress. Fusion bone at times will overlap and contact or rub against adjacent bone, usually the next highest lamina or spinous process. These areas of so-called *kissing pseudarthrosis* may become quite symptomatic (see page 23). Their presence may be confirmed by radiographs or CT scans, but their symptomatic status cannot be. Many patients with close approximation of fusion bone to adjacent bone never develop symptoms at this site, so a confirmation of symptomatic kissing pseudarthrosis requires invasive testing with local anesthetization or surgical excision. Fusion bone may at times develop too exuberant a growth into the spinal canal, causing a form of *iatrogenic spinal stenosis.* This is difficult, if not impossible, to confirm by plain radiographs, but tomograms (laminograms) of the spine may be quite helpful. If this diagnosis is suspected clinically, CT scanning should be obtained to delineate the extent of bony proliferation.

Pseudarthrosis of a spinal fusion with failure to achieve stabilization is a frustrating condition for the radiologist as well as for the patient and his clinician. Spinal fusions are performed by placing fusion bone, often multiple small fragments, in con-

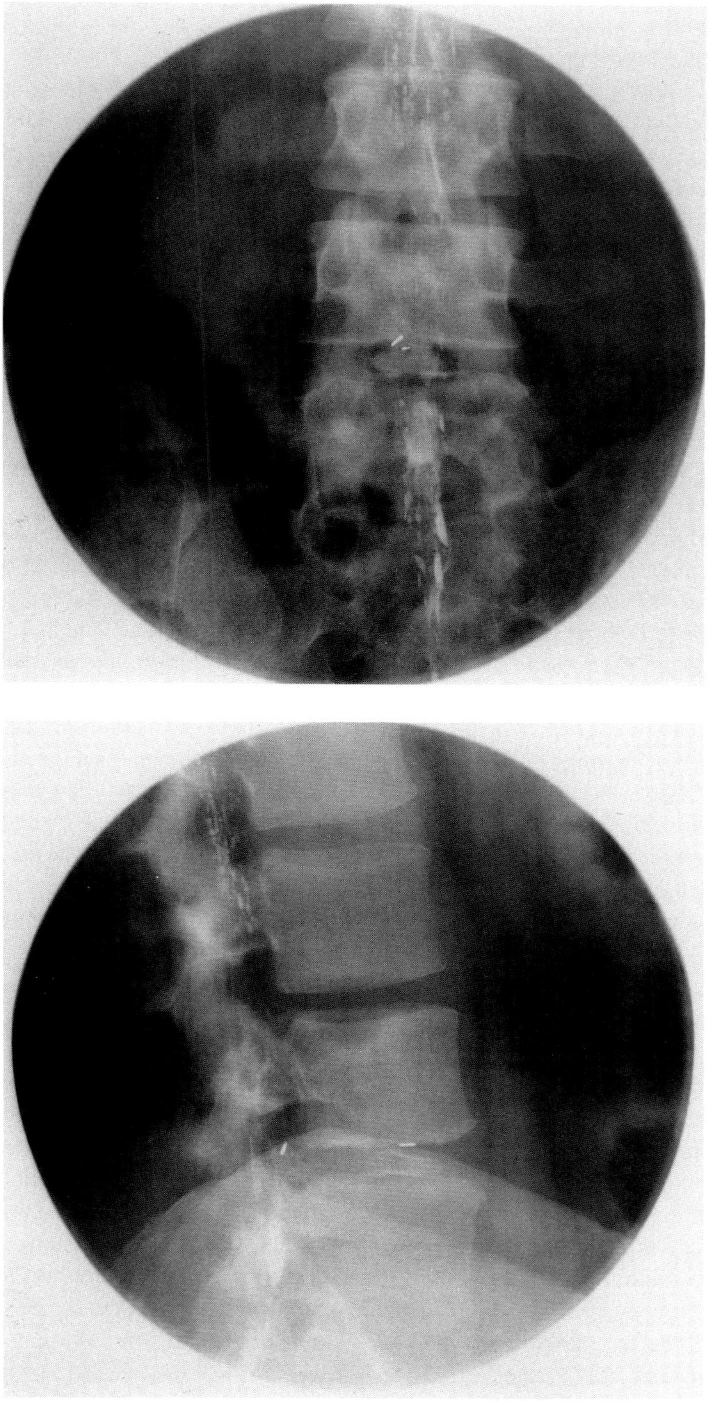

FIGURE 4.12. The Christoferson procedure of modified interbody bone fusion, not now in common use, was designed principally to limit interspace collapse and was not intended to guarantee spinal fusion. These AP **(top)** and lateral **(bottom)** radiographs demonstrate an interbody bone plug in place at L4-L5 in a patient who has been relieved of low back pain and sciatica following a large disc prolapse. The bone plug is marked at both ends with metal clips for x-ray identification. The wedge shape of the intervertebral disc space helps to prevent posterior dislocation of the plug. The posterior clip has migrated off the bone plug into the spinal canal.

tact with preexisting bony structures. Even if the majority of these small fragments grow and fuse together satisfactorily, a persistent line of nonunion and resulting mobility may develop, passing from one irregular bony fragment to the next. The resulting pseudarthrotic line is never straight and often meanders across the mass of fusion bone in serpentine fashion. A straight x-ray beam often cannot pass through the full length of the pseudarthrotic line, and on plain radiographs a pseudarthrosis is usually indistinguishable from the complex jungle and dense mass of a satisfactorily healing fusion site. X-ray tomography and CT scans give additional bony detail, but demonstration of defects in the fusion bone at one or even several nearby sites does not confirm that the fusion is unstable. In many instances, the fusion is deliberately left open in its center, and this intentional windowing must not be confused with instability or pseudarthrosis. Larger blocks or dowels of fusion bone may be in direct opposition with vertebral bone, but plain radiographs cannot confirm whether the two have grown together. Bony growth from one bony component into the other usually can be confirmed on the "bone window" settings of CT scans and may be sufficient to rule out pseudarthrosis.

Flexion and extension films are helpful if pseudarthrosis is extreme enough to permit at least several millimeters of motion. Considerably less motion than this, however, can result in severe symptoms, yet may be undetectable even on carefully reviewed flexion/extension films. Obtaining good flexion/extension radiographs can be a "Catch-22" situation: Flexion/extension radiographs are ordered for patients who experience severe back pain on back bending, but good radiographs to diagnose the cause of their limitations may not be obtainable because of the limitation of motion caused by the disease. Adequately premedicating the patients with anodynes, muscle relaxers, or both prior to attempting flexion/extension radiographs is important, since even the most stoic person may have trouble overcoming reactive muscle spasms to permit back flexion and extension sufficient to permit detectable movement of the pseudarthrosis. In patients with limited pseudarthrotic motion, the pain may arise from nerve endings at the pseudarthrotic site or from the hypertrophic scarring that frequently develops in the spinal canal beneath the pseudarthrosis. This soft-tissue scarring will not be visualized on plain radiographs. CT and MRI scans can detect scar within the spinal canal and can often detect scar within the fusion area, but they cannot detect whether this scar is likely to be symptomatic.

Radioisotope bone scans may be strongly positive in patients with symptomatic pseudarthrosis, but the physiologic postsurgical increased isotope uptake that persists for several months following surgery should not be misconstrued as proof of a symptomatic pseudarthrosis.

After years of frustration and subsequent surgical surprises in dealing with patients with fusion pseudarthroses, I can only conclude that there is no universally reliable radiographic method of detecting all symptomatic pseudarthroses, and even invasive diagnostic testing is not universally successful (see page 102).

In the past decade, the awareness of *facet joint syndromes* as a cause of back and upper leg pain has increased considerably (see the discussion of unnecessary surgery in Chapter 2).[50] Plain radiographs taken in right and left oblique views should visualize facet joints. Sclerotic and narrow joints, degenerative spurs at the margin of facet joints, slipping or subluxation of facets, and abnormal angulation of facets may all be demonstrated by such radiographs (Fig. 4.13). CT and MRI scans confirm that *degeneration in facet joints* commonly accompanies degeneration in the intervertebral discs, and facet degeneration is often documented on imaging studies in patients with back and leg pain. It must always be kept in mind that degenerative arthritis seems to be a concomitant of aging and that many patients develop degenerative changes in facet joints without becoming symptomatic. Nonetheless, imaging studies that demonstrate degenerative or other changes in facet joints in a patient with low back and leg pain should heighten one's clinical suspicion of a facet syndrome as the basis of the patient's pain. Flexion/extension views are also useful in demonstrating instability of the facet joints, but again, one must keep in mind that simply demonstrating forward slipping of a vertebra with flexion does not guarantee that this is the source of the patient's pain. When radioisotope bone and joint scans demonstrate a clearly focal abnormality at the site of one or more facet joints, the likelihood is greatly enhanced that this represents a significant source of the patient's pain. Invasive diagnostic studies are often helpful in supplementing anatomic imaging studies (see page 101).

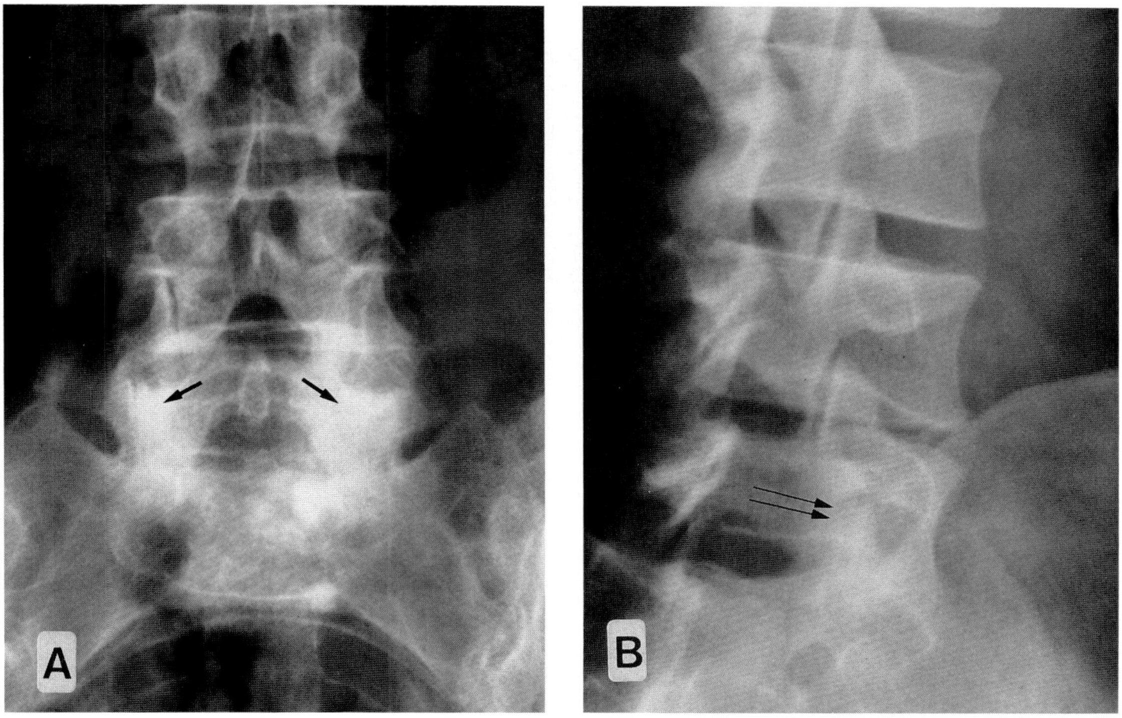

FIGURE 4.13. Lumbar facet abnormalities are being documented with greater frequency in patients with low back and leg pain. Demonstrated abnormalities (**A**) include degenerative and sclerotic changes (single arrows), and (**B**) abnormal facet angulation (double arrows). Clinical correlations with these abnormalities remain less certain, with some asymptomatic patients demonstrating severe abnormalities and some symptomatic patients demonstrating no radiographic abnormalities despite confirmed facet syndromes.

Plain radiographs are useful in diagnosing *postoperative wound infections* only if there is significant bony involvement. The majority of postoperative wound infections occur in the soft tissues, and neither these infections nor the more devastating intraspinal infections cause changes in the adjacent bone (Fig. 4.14). *Osteomyelitis* occurring in a fresh spinal fusion may be evidenced radiographically by progressive dissolution of the fusion bone. Osteomyelitis that occurs following discectomy is more likely to be secondary to bacterial infection of the disc space, with secondary involvement of the vertebral bodies adjacent to the interspace infection. The progressive destruction of vertebral bodies that occurs with sepsis contrasts markedly with the radiographic picture of aseptic *interspace inflammation or inflammatory discitis.* This nonseptic, autoimmune process causes initial sclerotic changes in the opposing surfaces of the vertebra across the interspace. Later, there is narrowing of the disc space, and in some patients eventual spontaneous fusion of the disc space occurs.

CT and MRI scans can document the presence of *intraspinal* and *extra-spinal collections,* which can help confirm the presence of spinal abscess. These scans also nicely delineate the extent of *bony destruction* or *lytic change,* and can be helpful in documenting disc space bacterial infection and in differentiating this from aseptic disc space inflammation. *Radioactive bone scans* also can be helpful—both bone and joint scans and white blood cell scans—as discussed later.

Computed Tomographs (CT) and Magnetic Resonance Imaging (MRI) Scans

CT scanning represents a technological revolution in radiographic imaging. This technique couples *radiographic imaging* and *computer reconstruction* of the resulting image. The area to be scanned is imaged with a thin beam of x-rays that passes across the area of interest at multiple angles of penetration.

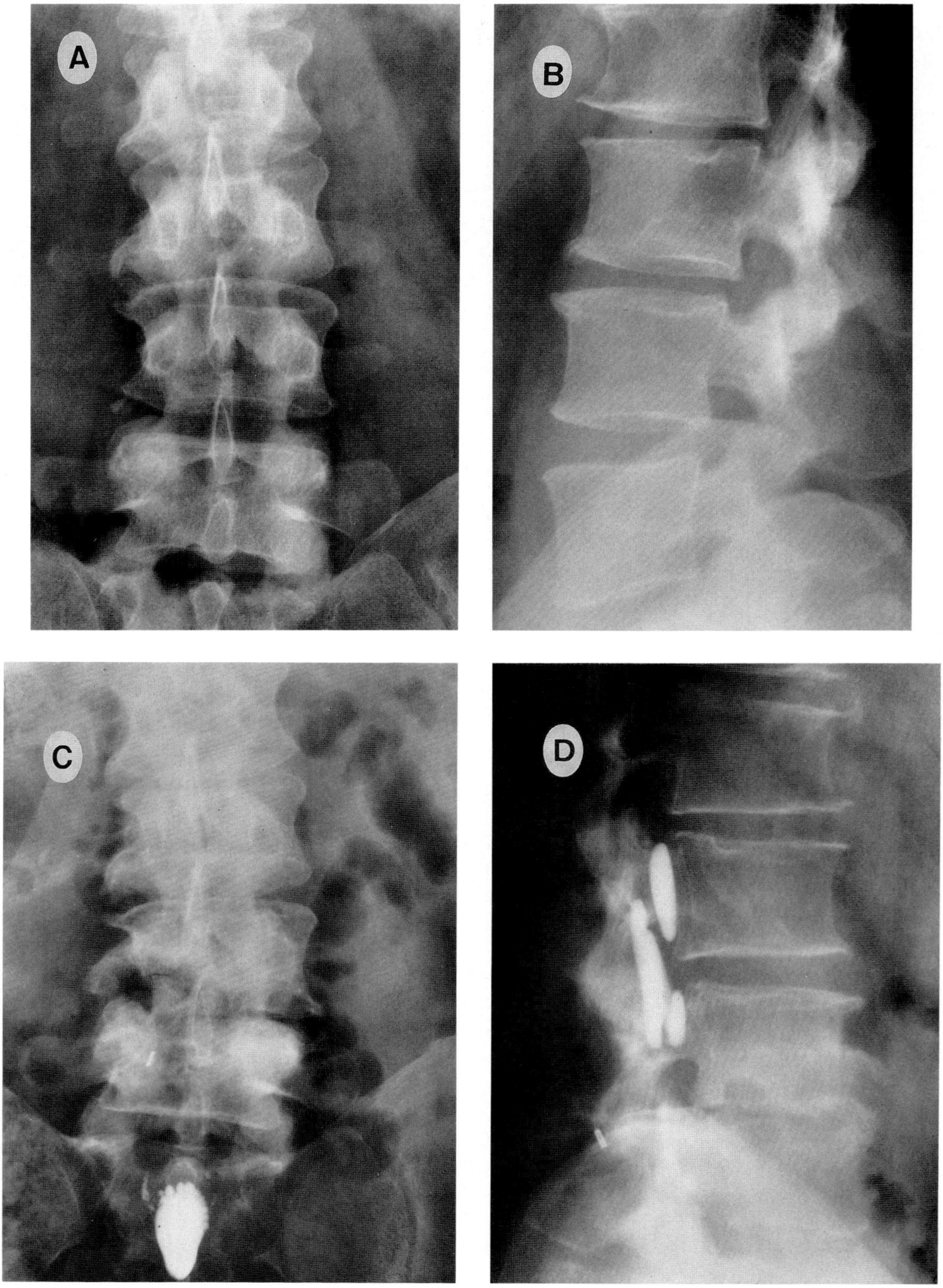

FIGURE 4.14. **A and B:** Postoperative infection of an intervertebral disc space may cause severe low back pain before radiographic changes become obvious. **C and D:** If untreated, pain, fever and leucocytosis increase as radiographically visible destruction of the disc space progresses.

The absorption of these x-rays is quantitated numerically, and sophisticated computer analysis yields a two-dimensional plot of numerical densities for volumes as small as one cubic millimeter. Three dimensional images can be constructed with special computer software. The computer element then displays these densities on a fluorescent screen, or transfers them to x-ray films, in the form of black-and-white or even color representations of different densities. The resulting picture resembles a photograph of a cross section of an anatomical specimen of the area being imaged (Fig. 4.15). The currently available third-generation CT scanners have a considerably improved resolving power over the earlier models. With these units, it is possible to visualize soft-tissue densities within the spinal canal, distinguishing between spinal fluid, epidural fat, and ruptured disc material (Fig. 4.15).[51] It is frequently impossible to distinguish between disc material and epidural scarring, but the presence of abnormal tissue at least can be documented.

MRI scanning represents another technologic revolution in anatomic imaging and does not employ ionizing radiation. The application of strong fixed and pulsed electromagnetic fields to body tissues induces a resonating response in the ions that compose those tissues, resulting in precise and ion-specific production of weak radio-frequency energy transmission from those ions. Detecting coils, coupled with special computers, can detect the origin of these transmissions with a three-dimensional spatial accuracy similar to that of a CT scan (Fig. 4.16). Furthermore, tuning the MRI scanner creates different images displaying the concentrations of different ions (commonly hydrogen, which is present in most body tissues) as different densities, producing light or dark spots on the image produced. Tuning to produce two or more different images greatly improves the sensitivity of MRI scanning in detecting anatomic variations between tissues and even in differentiating the composition of various tissues. Most MRI scans are obtained with images from at least two different machine settings.

CT and MRI scans have revolutionized the anatomic imaging of the lumbar spine. CT scanning produces transverse or axial tomographic computerized reconstructions of fine detail of the *absorption density* of materials to x-rays. The computerized analysis can be altered flexibly to produce "bone windows" or "soft-tissue windows"—machine settings that optimally display bony detail or soft-tissue detail. MRI scanning reconstructs in the axial, coronal, or sagittal plane finely detailed computerized reconstructions based on *chemical composition* of tissue. The detectors can be adjusted to produce several different types of images emphasizing different chemical composition—images labeled, for example, as spin echo, T1-weighted, or T2-weighted images. The T2-weighted image, for instance, emphasizes tissues containing water. Both techniques can be further enhanced by the administration of *intravenous contrast-enhancing agents:* iodinated compounds for CT scanning, and ferrous compounds for MRI scanning. In general, these compounds are valuable both while in the blood to highlight blood vessels and when they cross the blood-brain barrier of the central nervous system. They tend to concentrate in areas of increased vascularity such as tumors and infections. Contrast enhancement can also be obtained for CT scanning by the *subarachnoid injection* of low concentrations of iodinated myelographic contrast media to produce a *CT/myelogram* (Fig. 4.17). CT scans generally give better detail of bony anatomy than MRI scans, but MRI scans generally give better soft-tissue detail and have the major advantage of being available in all three dimensions; even though CT scan images can be reconstructed in sagittal or coronal planes, the reconstructions lack the precise detail of the initial axial images (Fig. 4.18).

CT and MRI scans detail the *anatomic changes* of *spinal degeneration,* but cannot detect the *physiologic significance* of those anatomic changes (Fig. 4.19). Hypertrophic changes or *spurs,* narrowing of disc or facet joints, irregularity and sclerosis of margins of discs or facets, and severe disc degeneration with replacement of disc material by nitrogen gas (the so-called vacuum phenomenon) are all precisely detailed on CT scans (Fig. 4.20). MRI scans likewise document hypertrophic changes and narrowing, but also document changes in signal intensity from desiccated and degenerated intervertebral discs and demonstrate altered signals from vertebral bodies adjacent to degenerated discs, which probably results from fatty infiltration (Fig. 4.21). Hypertrophic changes that cause narrowing of the spinal canal are excellently documented on axial images, but the sagittal images available on MRI scans can add a delineation of the rostrocaudal extent of the spinal stenosis. Lateral recess stenosis, with focal compression of nerve roots as they pass

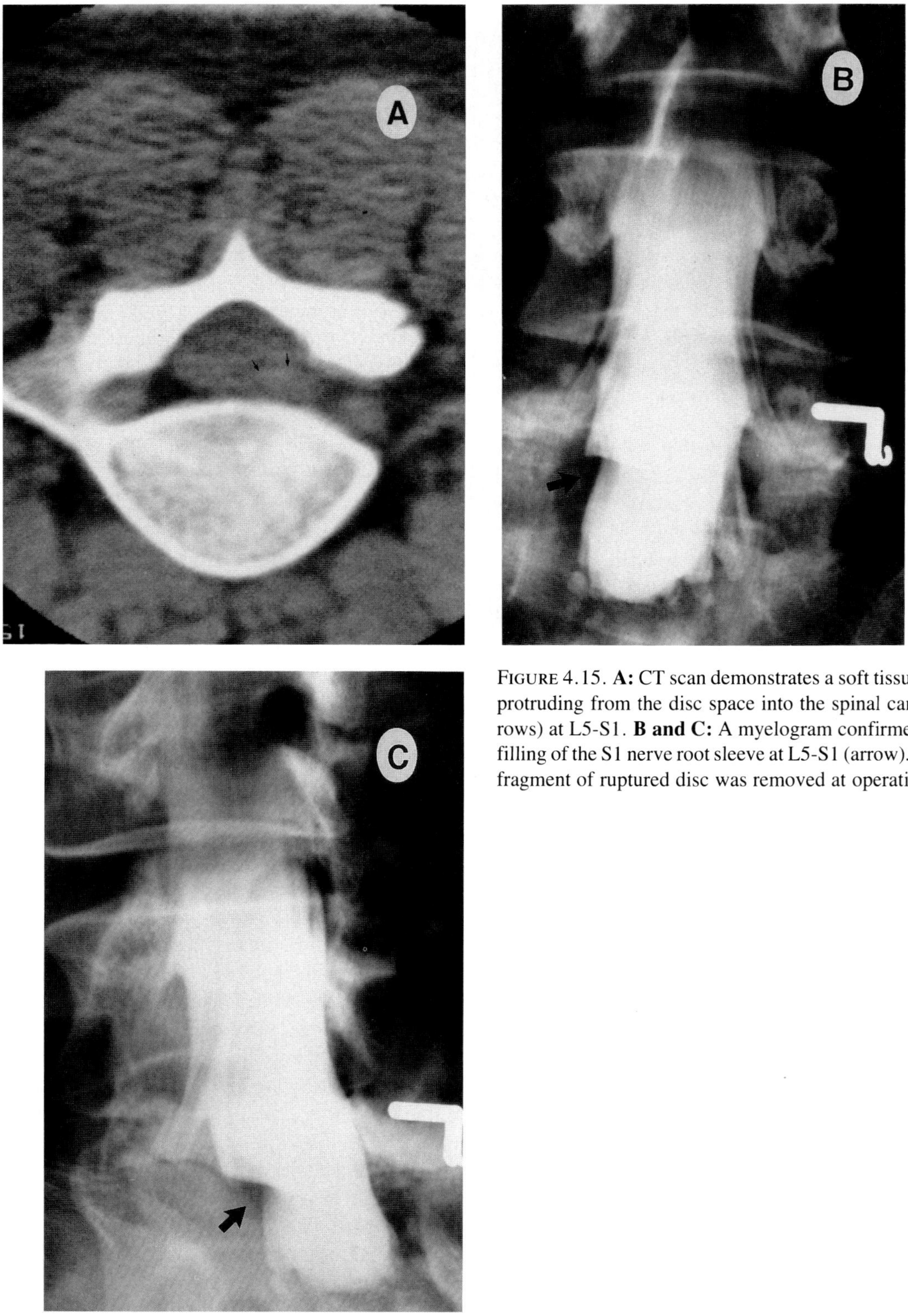

FIGURE 4.15. **A:** CT scan demonstrates a soft tissue mass protruding from the disc space into the spinal canal (arrows) at L5-S1. **B and C:** A myelogram confirmed nonfilling of the S1 nerve root sleeve at L5-S1 (arrow). A free fragment of ruptured disc was removed at operation.

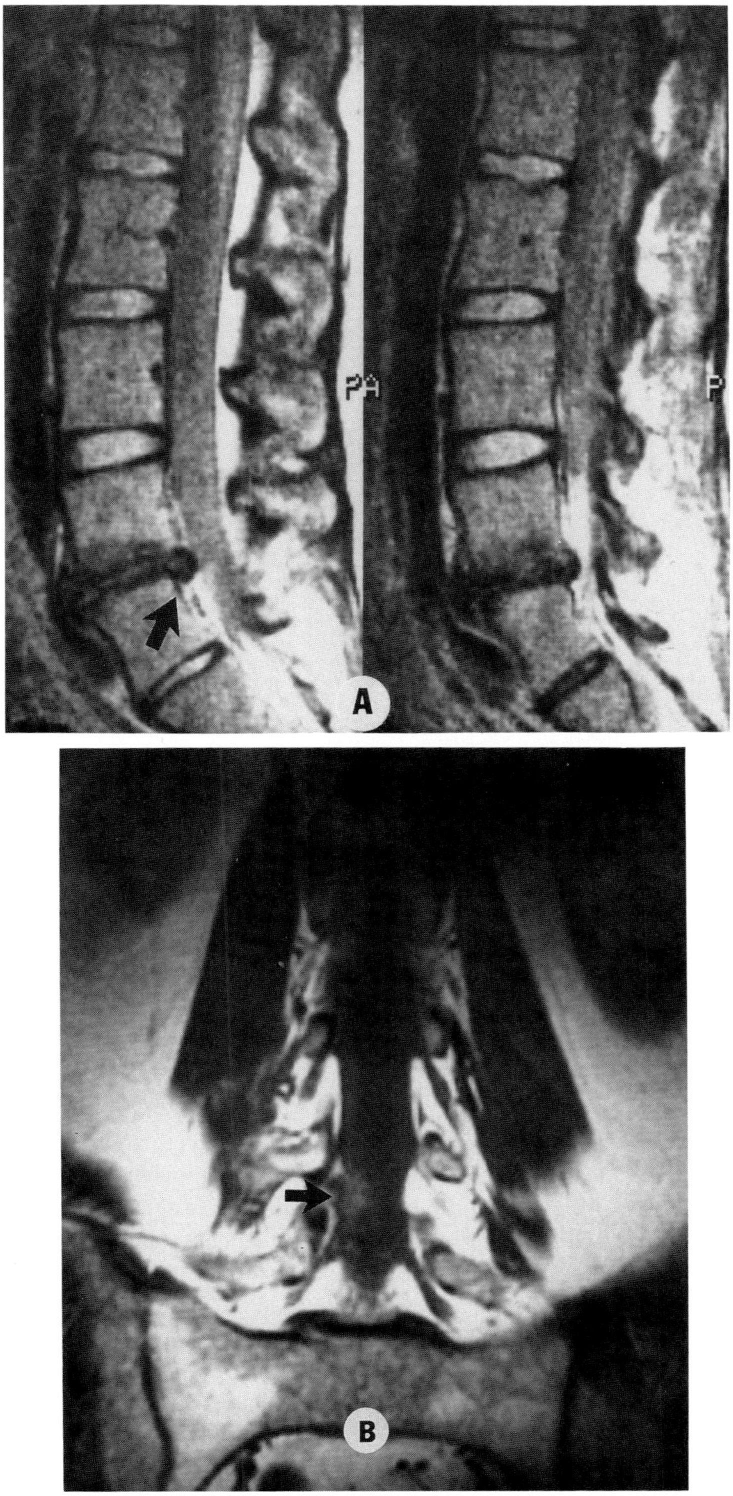

FIGURE 4.16. This MRI scan clearly shows a large disc herniation at L4-L5 and demonstrates this in sagittal (**A**), transverse (**B**), and (next page) coronal (**C**) planes. The displacement of theca and nerve roots is clearly obvious (arrows).

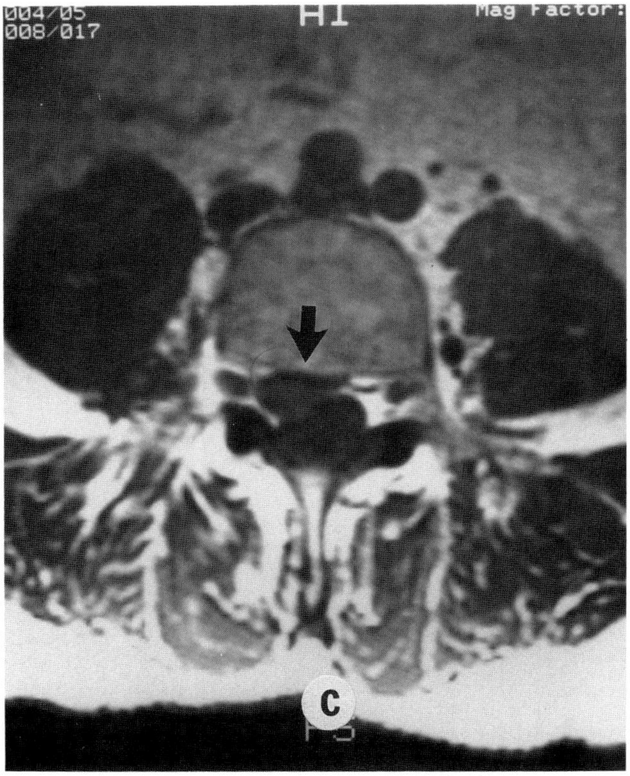

FIGURE 4.16 (continued). **C:** Coronal MRI showing large disc herniation at L4-L5.

around pedicles, can be beautifully demonstrated on CT scans and may be imaged on MRI scans of good quality (Figs. 4.22 and 4.23).

The detection of *disc ruptures* and distinguishing *recurrent disc ruptures* from *epidural scar* are areas of major importance for CT and MRI imaging (Figs. 4.24 and 4.25). The axial images can demonstrate not only disc ruptures within the spinal canal but also *far-lateral disc ruptures* occurring within or even lateral to the neural foramen (Fig. 4.26). Such far lateral disc ruptures were felt to be exceedingly rare prior to the advent of these imaging techniques, but now they are discovered more frequently and offer an explanation for some of the sciatic syndromes not detectable on plain radiography and myelography. MRI scans beautifully delineate soft-tissue changes in the spinal canal and can help distinguish physiologic bulging of discs, frank rupture of discs, and the presence of free disc fragments within the spinal canal. Even with CT or MR imaging, it is often difficult to distinguish when what a radiologist reports as a "bulging disc" is merely *physiologic* and a healthy sign of a flexible back and when this bulging becomes accentuated enough to raise the possibility of pathologic significance through stretching and distortion of annulus and spinal ligaments to cause back pain. Both MRI and CT scans can provide imaging evidence of when protrusions of the intervertebral disc into the spinal canal are large enough to cause distortion or apparent compression of nerve roots, and therefore are likely to be causative of sciatica.

The distinction between *postoperative scar* and *recurrent disc rupture* is now possible with fair, but imperfect, reliability through the use of *contrast-enhanced* CT and MRI scans. Without enhancement the scans merely document the anatomic presence of an extradural mass, but the addition of contrast enhancement causes an increased uptake in vascularized tissue (i.e., scar) and leaves unenhanced the avascular disc fragment.

Many surgeons are now accepting CT scan imaging of *disc ruptures* as definitively diagnostic and are forgoing myelography. Unfortunately, CT scans rarely include spinal levels above the mid lumbar area. Many patients have asymptomatic bulging of discs or bony spurring in the lumbar area, and spinal tumors that cause a sciatic syndrome clinically resembling that of lumbar disc sciatica may be overlooked. Even if CT scans are obtained through the

FIGURE 4.17. Myelography (**A**) was interpreted as showing "bilateral disc rupture" in this 40-year-old male with unilateral sciatica. CT scan (**B**) done immediately following the myelogram, a so-called "CT/Myelogram," failed to disclose a disc rupture but instead disclosed mild spinal canal stenosis with significant lateral or foraminal stenosis maximal on the right or symptomatic side. Subjecting this patient to disc removal without bony decompression would most likely have failed to relieve him of sciatica.

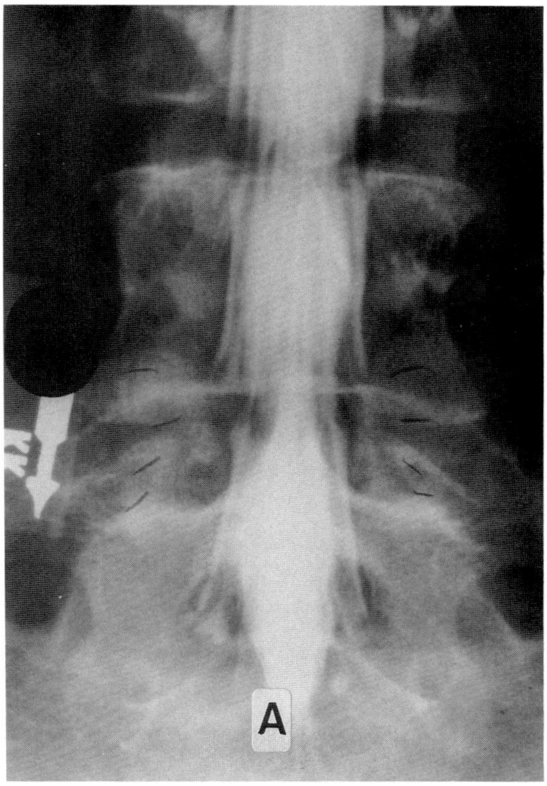

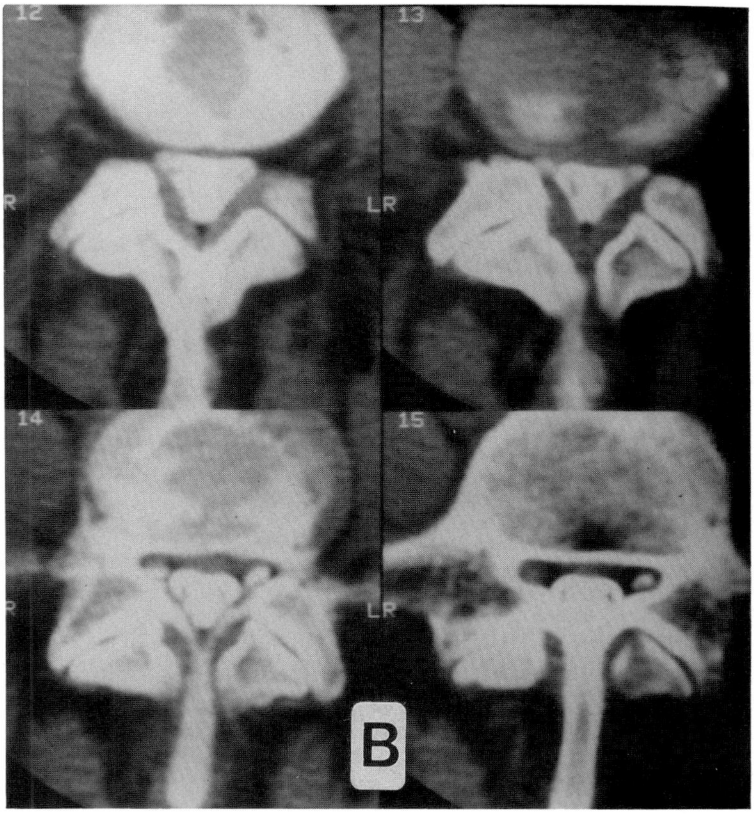

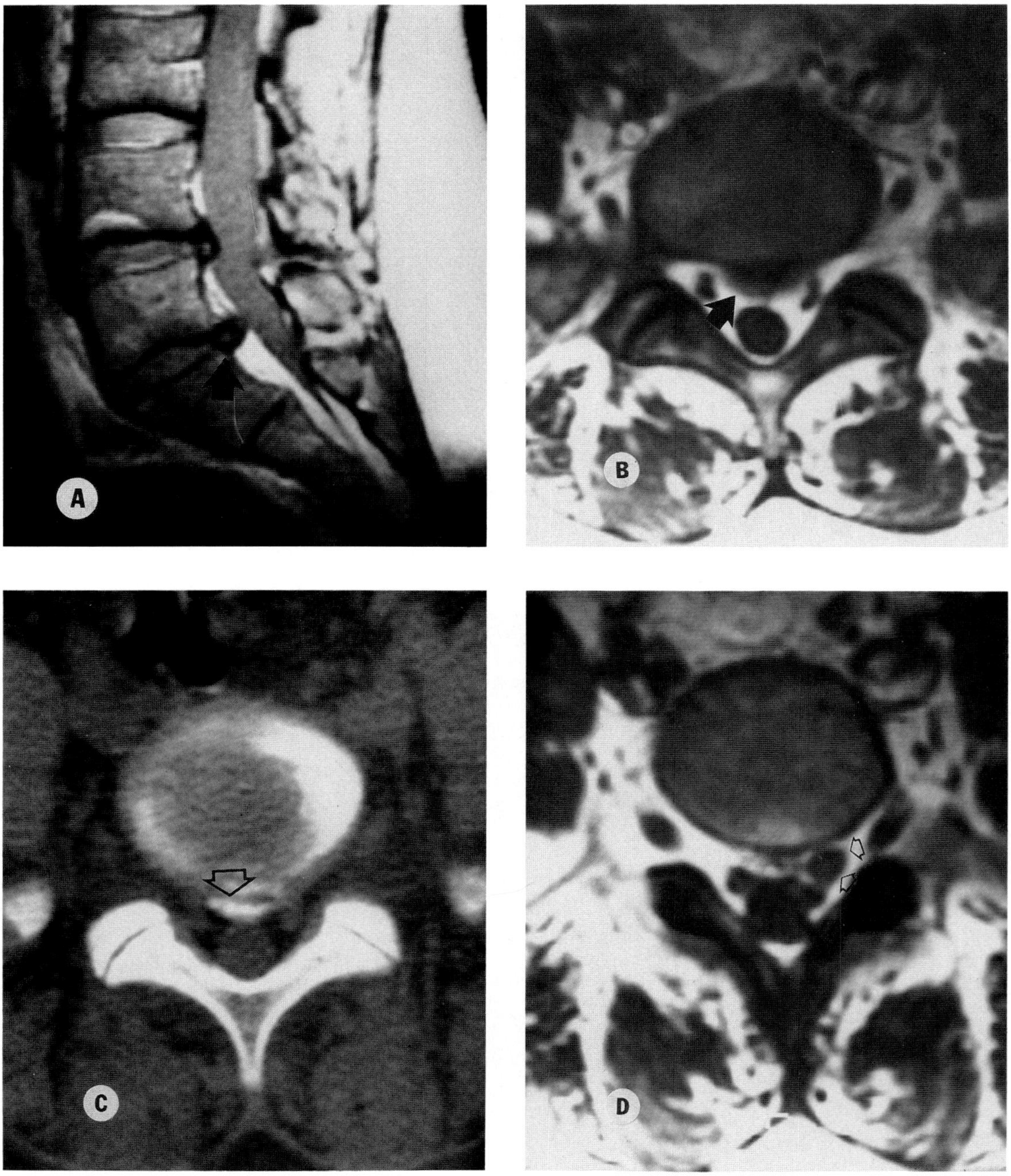

FIGURE 4.18. Sagittal and horizontal MRI images (**A and B**) show a sizeable abnormality behind the intervertebral disc at L5-S1 (arrows) in a lady who presented with unilateral sciatica. A CT scan (**C**) confirmed what was not evident on the MRI scan—i.e., that the protrusion was largely calcified. She initially improved with bed rest, then developed explosive sciatica with neurologic loss, and a repeat MRI scan (**D**) now showed a newly protruded free fragment of disc material (open arrows) overlying the vertebral body and severely compressing the nerve root. At surgery both a free disc fragment and a slipped epiphyseal ring were confirmed.

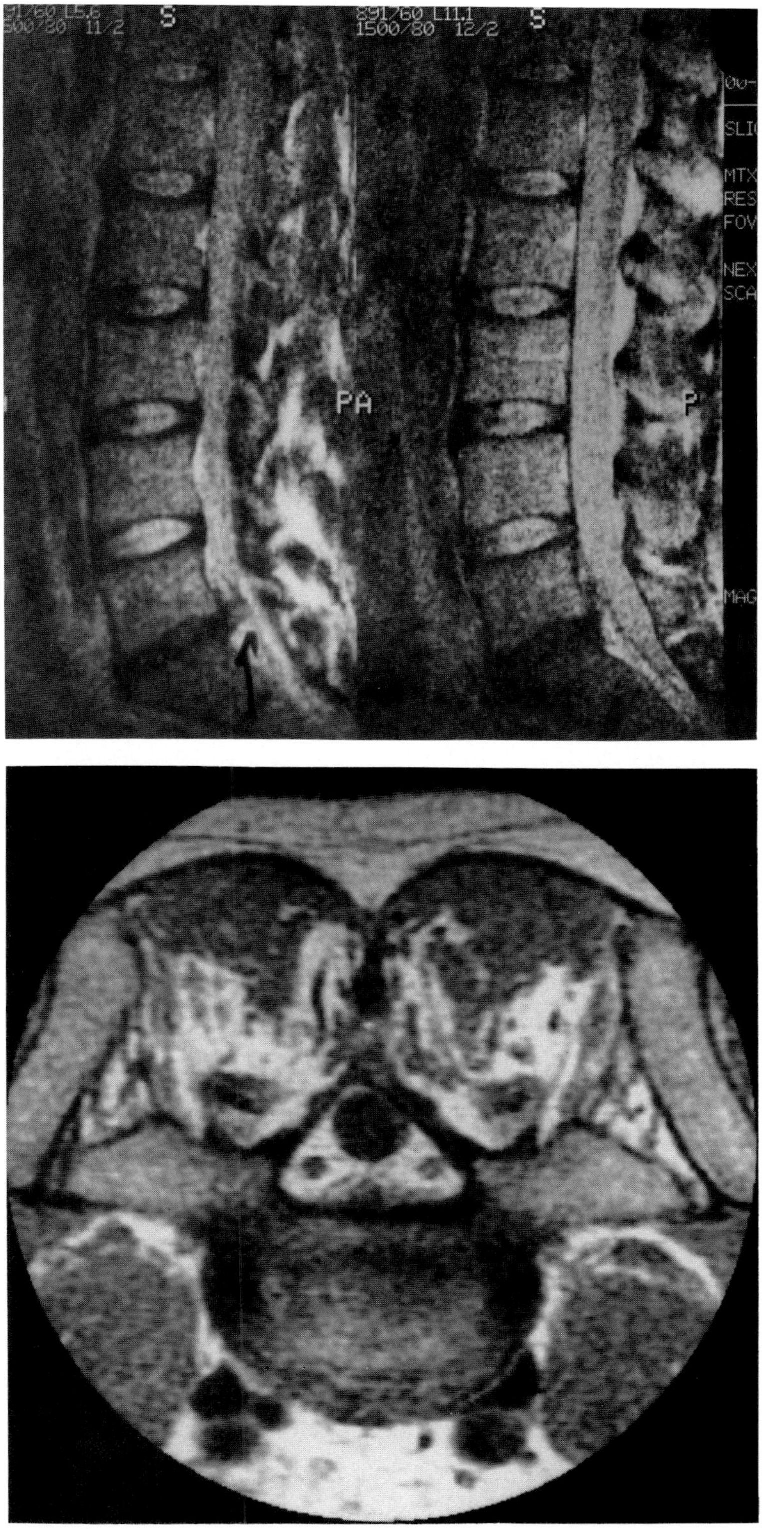

FIGURE 4.19. This MRI scan was interpreted by a radiologist as showing "a large disc rupture" on sagittal images **(top)** of a 34-year-old woman with chronic lumbago and no sciatica. The axial view **(bottom)** however shows that the abnormality lies in the midline of the canal, may be a bony degenerative change rather than herniated nuclear material, and is not in contact with nerve roots or theca. She ultimately responded well to nonsteroidal anti-inflammatory drugs and an exercise program without surgical intervention.

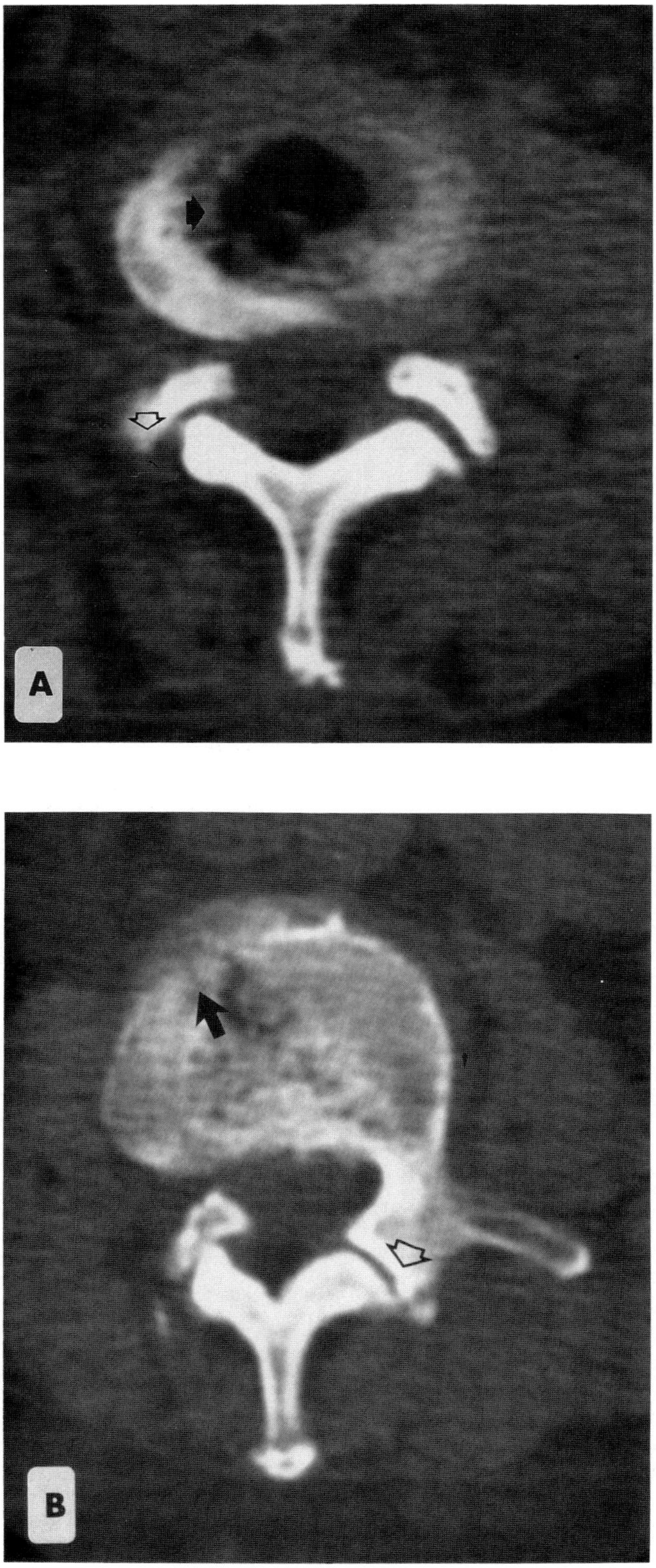
A
B

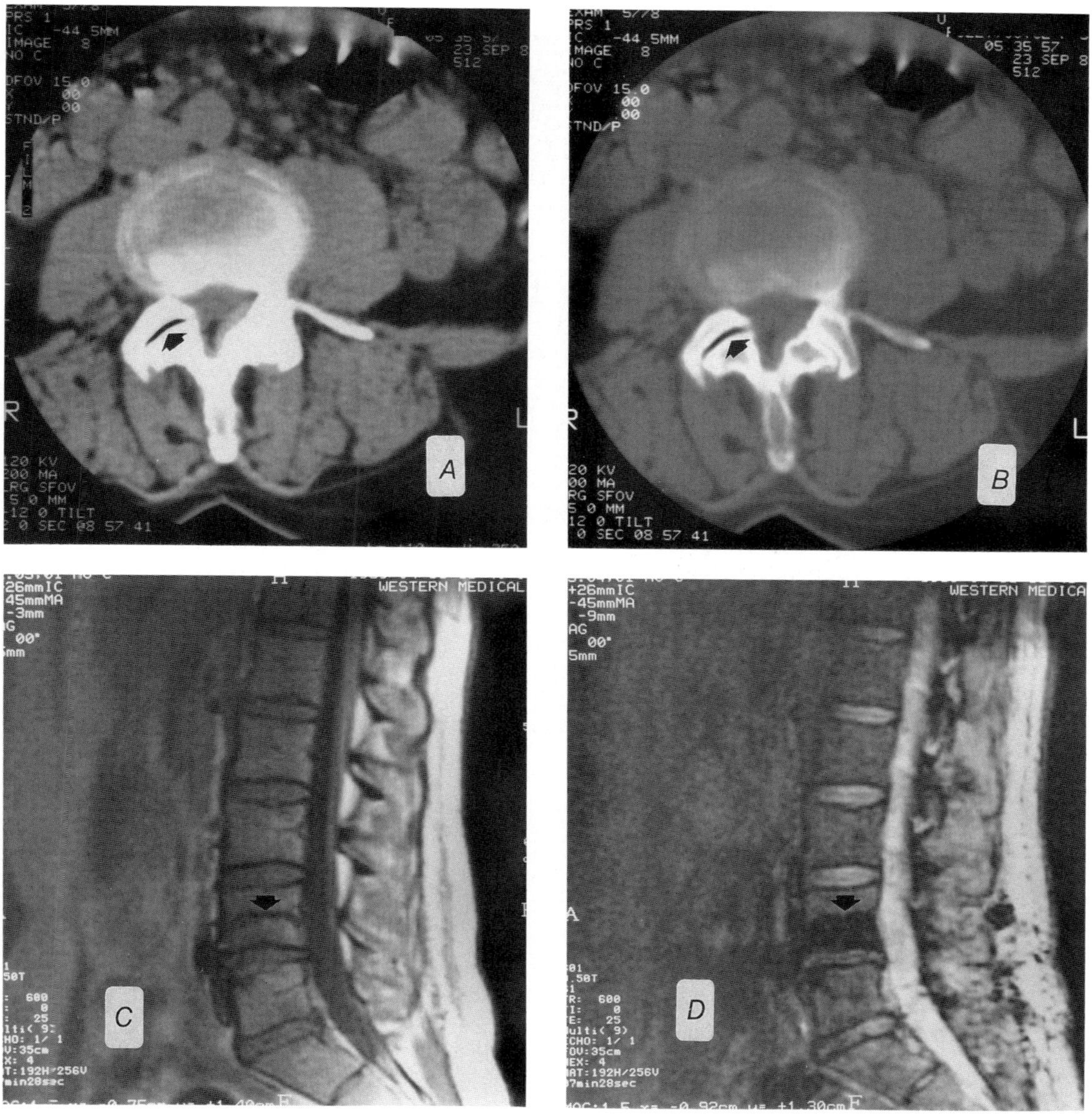

FIGURE 4.21. Severe spinal degeneration can be imaged both on CT and MRI scans, though CT scans generally show greater bone detail. Soft tissue **(A)** and bone **(B)** settings of this CT scan show a relatively healthy intervertebral disc but severe facet degeneration with "vacuum phenomenon" and hypertrophic spurring from the facet joint, suggesting this as a more likely source of the patient's pain than the disc. Sagittal, T1-weighted **(C)** and T2-weighted **(D)** MRI scans show loss of signal brightness from the L4-L5 disc with fatty infiltration of the L4 vertebral body (arrows)—signifying focal degeneration in a young woman with persistent lumbago despite resection of the L5-S1 disc.

FIGURE 4.20. CT scans give excellent depiction of spinal degenerative changes. **A:** Severe degeneration of the intervertebral disc often causes the "vacuum phenomenon" of intradiscal gas (arrow); also shown is degenerative spurring of the facet (arrowhead). **B:** Degenerative changes at disc space margins look like "spurs" on plain radiographs but are demonstrated on CT scan to be crescentic marginal lipping (arrow). Even more severe facet degeneration causes collapse of the joint space with more extensive marginal spurs (arrowhead). The apparent asymmetry from right to left resulted from degenerative scoliosis with lateral tilting of the vertebral body.

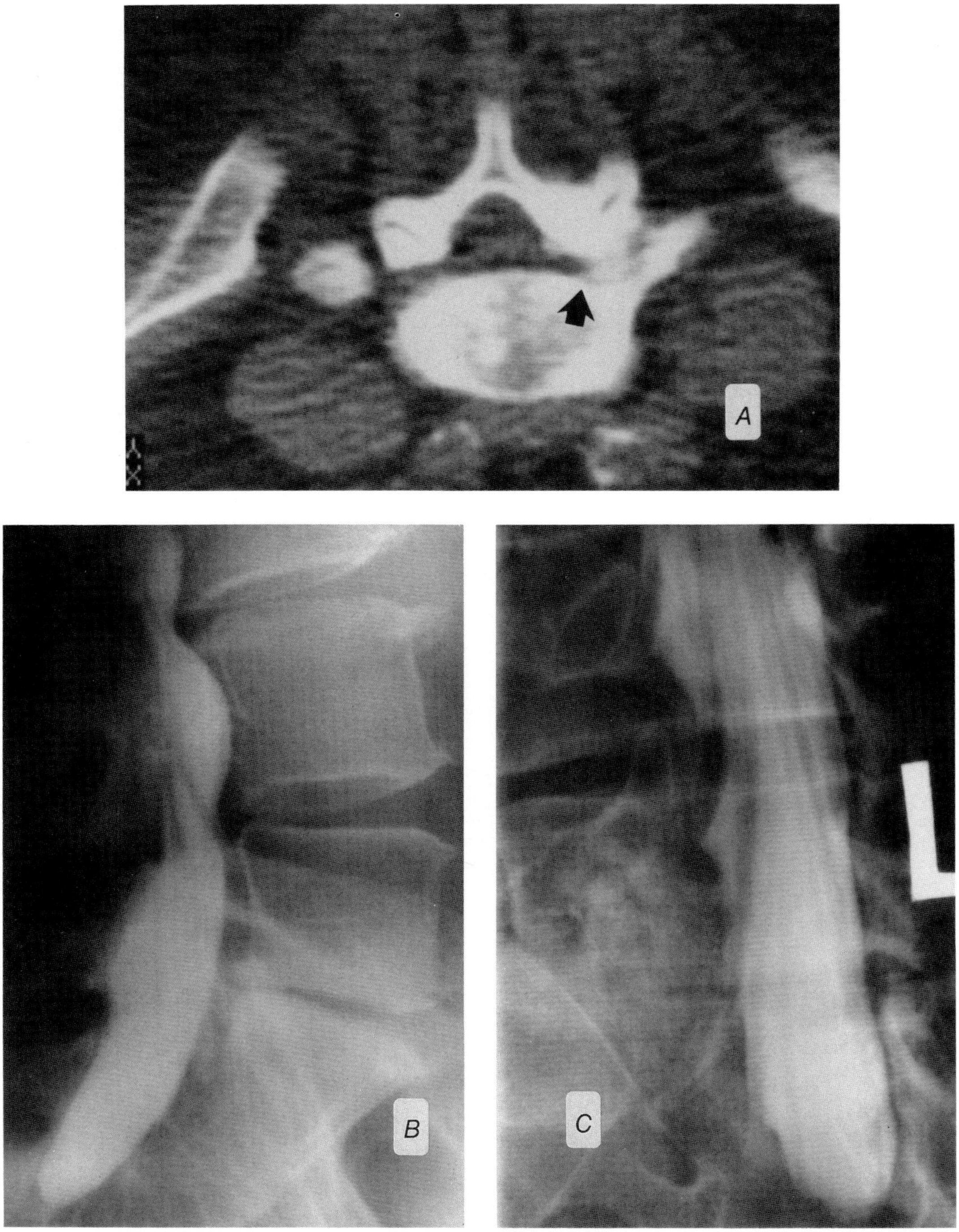

FIGURE 4.22. CT scans are dramatically useful in delineating spinal stenosis and lateral recess stenosis. **A:** This scan documents severe lateral recess stenosis (arrow). This patient's sciatica was not associated with limited straight leg raising and seemed aggravated by prolonged standing or walking. **B and C:** Myelography was normal.

FIGURE 4.23. Lateral recess stenosis is suggested by this parasagittal MRI cut. Although encroachment on the L5-S1 neural foramen is visualized (arrow), its clinical significance can be assessed only with clinical correlation.

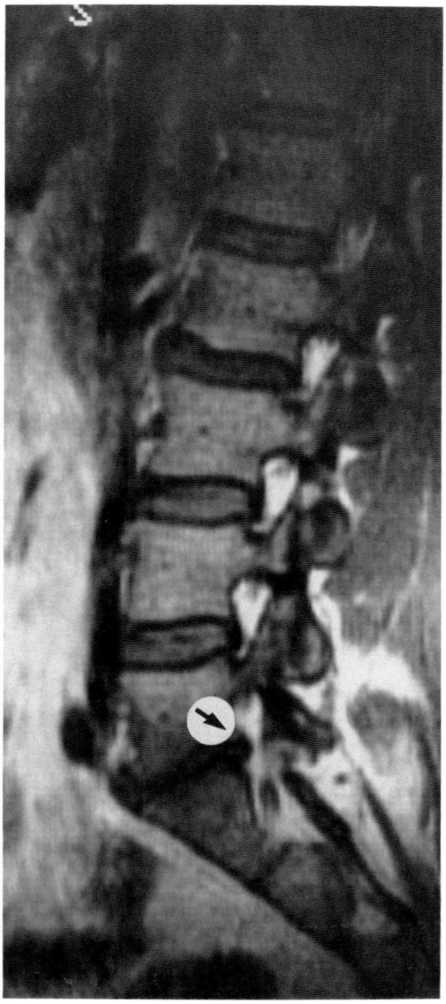

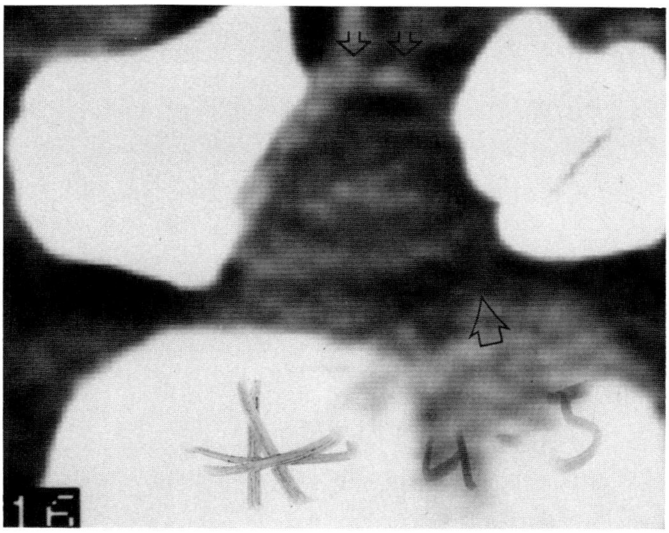

FIGURE 4.24. CT scans become difficult to interpret following discectomy. This scan was interpreted elsewhere as showing a large recurrent disc herniation at L4-L5 (single arrows), the site of previous laminotomy (double arrows). Surgical re-exploration disclosed epidural scarring only, with no disc protrusion or free rupture.

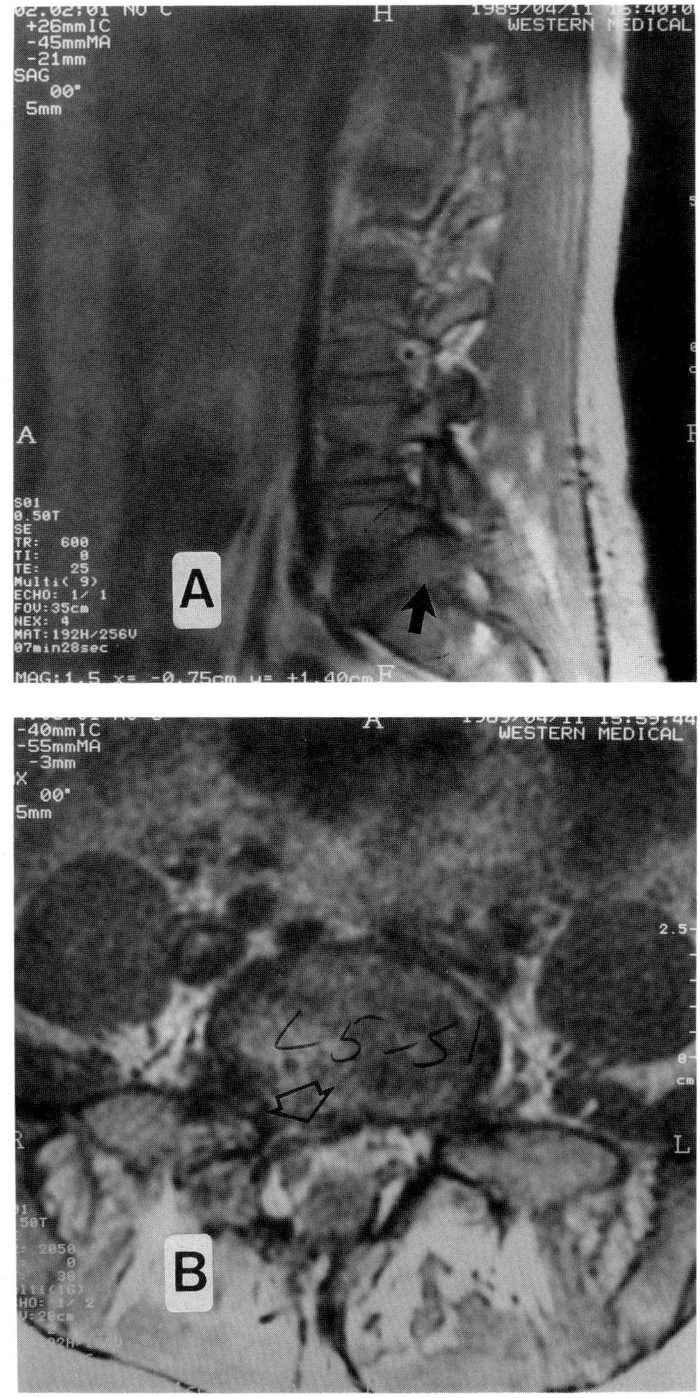

FIGURE 4.25. Postoperative scar can obscure CT or MRI images. This sagittal MRI image (**A**) discloses extensive lateral scar tissue at L5-S1 following unilateral discectomy in a patient with recurrent sciatica. Following Gadolinium enhancement (**B**) the component of epidural scar now enhances, but beneath the scar a sizeable fragment of recurrent herniated nucleus pulposus becomes evident by its lack of enhancement (open arrow).

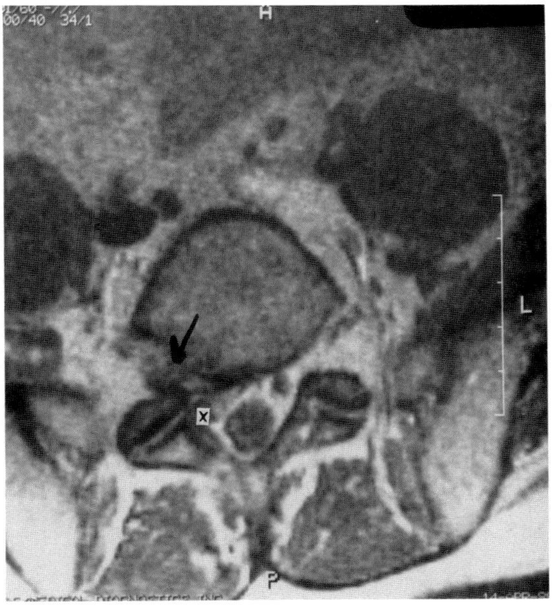

FIGURE 4.26. Transverse MRI images through the L4-L5 space demonstrate a "far lateral" disc rupture. This patient presented with an L4 syndrome of pain and weakness of the right knee with loss of right knee reflex. The "far lateral" disc rupture compressed the L4 nerve root laterally in the neural foramen and only slightly displaced the L5 root within the spinal canal (x).

low thoracic spine to include the conus medullaris and cauda equina, where benign tumors are most likely to be found, most of the benign spinal tumors are isodense with spinal fluid and cannot be visualized on CT scan without intravenous or subarachnoid contrast enhancement. In contradistinction, MRI scans commonly include the upper lumbar and even low thoracic regions and usually dramatically image spinal tumors. For this reason, it can be argued that MRI scanning offers a better modality for diagnosing lumbar disc ruptures, despite its greater cost. With a high-quality MRI scan, the addition of a lumbar CT scan, myelography, or CT/myelography is usually necessary only in atypical or confusing situations, such as in patients with extensive postoperative or degenerative changes. If MRI scanning permits the surgeon to forgo other imaging modalities, its greater expense may well be highly cost-effective, especially since invasive myelography carries a certain inherent morbidity. If primary or secondary (metastatic) spinal tumor is suspected, MRI scan provides clearly superior imaging, detailing the extent of the tumor within the spinal canal and within bone and adjacent soft tissues.

The delineation on CT or MRI scans of mass lesions in the neural canal or far laterally beyond the canal makes it necessary to distinguish between *far-lateral disc rupture* and *nerve root tumor.* Neurofibromas or the more encapsulated neurolimomas may not always be visualized as rounded masses, since they may grow in conformity to their bony confines. Although they grow slowly, they not uncommonly become acutely and persistently symptomatic following trauma, thus closely mimicking the clinical syndrome produced by far-lateral disc ruptures. Many of these tumors enhance following intravenous contrast administration, but disc ruptures do not. CT discography can provide definitive identification of far-lateral disc ruptures in cases of persistent uncertainty. A standard contrast discogram is carried out (see page 88), then a CT scan is obtained while the contrast material is still present in the area of injection. The demonstration of contrast material escape into the far-lateral mass definitively identifies disc rupture and distinguishes it from tumor.

As discussed earlier, both CT and MRI scans can be quite helpful in identifying *spinal sepsis* (see page 65).

Pseudomeningoceles occur rarely following spinal surgery, and in the past have required invasive myelography for diagnosis. CT scans and especially MRI scans can distinguish these spinal fluid collections quite graphically and can demonstrate their size and extent. MRI scans may even be able to document herniation of nerve roots through the ostium of the pseudomeningocele sac.

Adhesive arachnoiditis remains a diagnostic challenge in part because of its pathoanatomic variability and variable clinical presentation. Myelography remains the "gold standard" for imaging the extent, severity, and clinical type (see page 81) of the arachnoiditis. Unenhanced CT scans are incapable of detecting arachnoiditis, but CT/myelography can add to the detail obtained on standard myelography. MRI scans can at times demonstrate clumping of nerve roots or even obliteration of the subarachnoid space, but the specificity and reliability of such imaging have not yet been confirmed (Figs. 4.27 and 4.28). There seems little question that less severe forms of adhesive arachnoiditis probably will not be detectable on even high-quality MRI

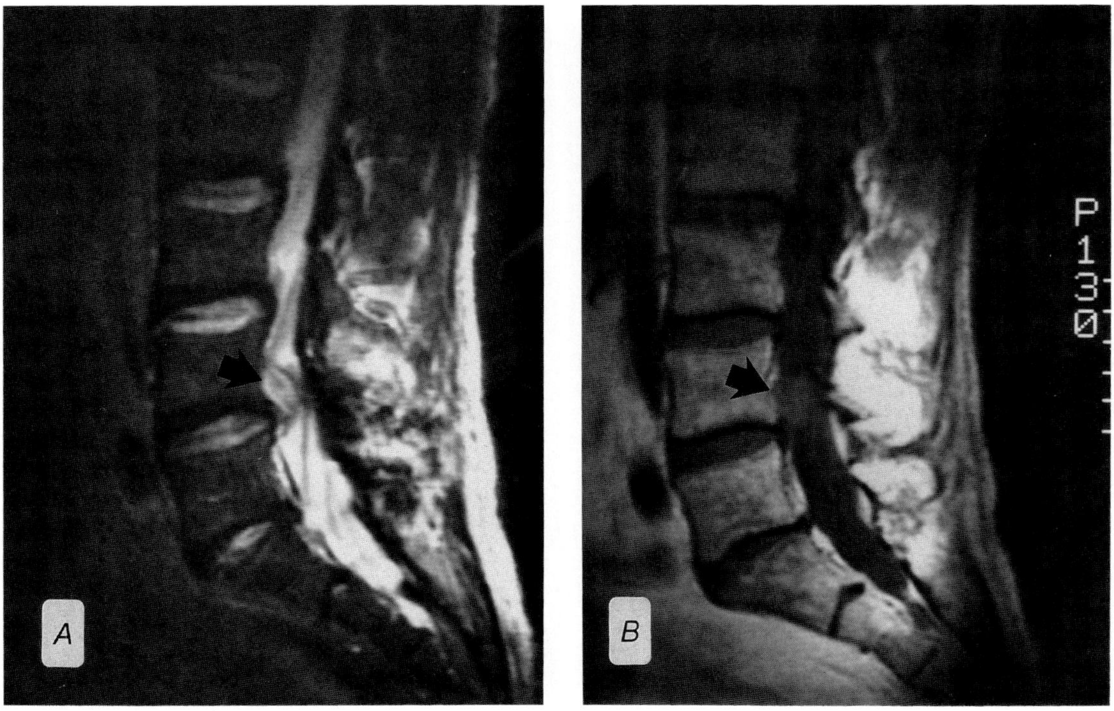

FIGURE 4.27. MRI scans may be capable of demonstrating adhesive arachnoiditis and may better define its extent than myelography, though this remains the most definitive study. Type III or transverse arachnoiditis is demonstrated at the previously operated L4-L5 interspace on these T1 (**A**) and T2 (**B**) images.

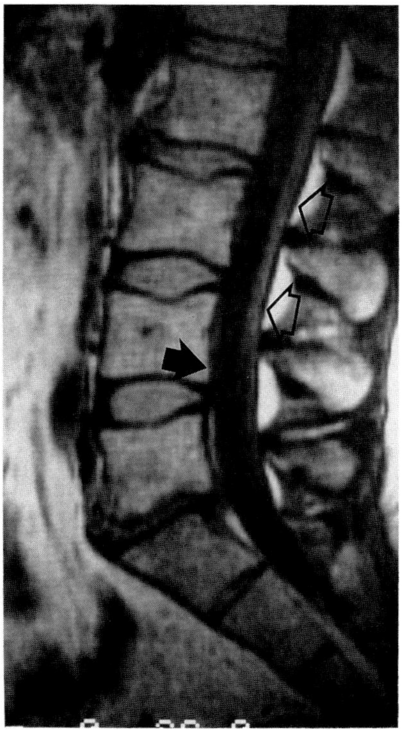

FIGURE 4.28. Type II or annular arachnoiditis is demonstrated less convincingly on this T1-weighted image. Although there seems to be a variation from normal it is less clear whether this represents arachnoiditis or compressive extradural scar.

scans, though it can be argued whether changes of lesser severity are of clinical significance.

CT scans can be of great help in identifying *problems that follow spinal fusion.* MRI scans may delineate soft-tissue components of postfusion problems even better than CT scans, but usually do not give as good bony detail. *Fusion stability* can be confirmed if thin-section CT scans document bone growth with cortical and cancellous continuity across the fused motion segment. However, the identification of gaps between fragments of fusion bone can introduce considerable uncertainty. The gaps may simply be fenestrations within an otherwise rigid interconnection between adjacent vertebral bodies. Conversely, gaps identified on adjacent sections may in fact represent different sections through a nonlinear gap in the fusion bone that wanders completely across the area of attempted fusion and that represents a complete failure of stable bone growth. An overgrowth of fusion bone can be readily visualized, including *kissing pseudarthrosis* between overgrown fusion bone and adjacent spinal segments or hypertrophic bone that causes *spinal* or *lateral recess stenosis.* Fusion pseudarthrosis is not uncommonly associated with localized *soft-tissue hypertrophy,* which can cause nerve root or thecal compression if the hypertrophy occurs within the spinal canal. This type of soft-tissue overgrowth is nicely demonstrated on CT scans and is usually demonstrated in superb detail on MRI scans.

Despite the remarkable *anatomical imaging* that has resulted from CT and MRI scans, *clinical correlation* is not always apparent and may be misleading. As is well demonstrated in degenerative arthropathy, the severity of degenerative changes correlates only poorly with symptomatic significance, so that CT imaging of severe degeneration may be found in asymptomatic patients, and symptomatic patients may show imaging evidence of relatively circumscribed or limited degenerative changes. Anatomic features such as extradural scar, lateral recess stenosis, small pseudomeningoceles, and adhesive arachnoiditis all can occur without causing clinically significant symptoms, and severe symptoms can at times occur as a result of limited abnormalities of these types. Thus, detailed imaging carries with it an increased responsibility on the part of the practitioner to use great caution in interpretation. An extremely common error in interpretation occurs when the radiologist describes a bulging disc on CT or MRI scan, but the practitioner makes no attempt to correlate whether this bulging is a healthy sign of excellent back flexibility or whether this represents a symptomatically pathologic process. The radiologist's description of the disc as "bulging" does not provide the practitioner with any indication of whether that finding is significant any more than would the report of the presence of abdominal gas on an abdominal x-ray. If imaged abnormalities appear likely to be of pathologic significance and they correlate closely with clear cut clinical symptoms, they are likely to be significantly reliable and extremely valuable clinically. In the event of less than ideal clinical correlation or pathoanatomic features, the clinician must be cautious in assuming pathophysiologic significance for anatomic images and additional diagnostic studies (as discussed later) may well be warranted. If MRI scanning permits the surgeon to forgo other imaging modalities, its greater expense may well be highly cost-effective, especially since invasive myelography carries a certain inherent morbidity.

Invasive Radiologic Studies

Myelography

Myelography remains the mainstay of diagnosis of *lumbar disc disease,* even though it has recently been challenged for supremacy by CT scans and MRI scans. The myelographic picture of a true *lumbar disc rupture* is distinctive and fairly reliable diagnostically. A smoothly rounded indentation into the contrast column is visualized in posteroanterior and lateral projection, but is seen at its maximum height on an oblique projection (Fig. 4.29). If the disc rupture is protruding, but still confined by the posterior longitudinal ligament, the myelographic abnormality will conform nicely to the level of the intervertebral disc. If the posterior longitudinal ligament has been perforated, allowing a fragment of disc material to migrate as a *free fragment* in the epidural space, the maximum indentation may be seen to overlie the vertebral body, usually still near an intervertebral disc space. A smaller number of disc ruptures occur in the midline and are consequently best visualized on cross-table lateral views. The myelographic picture of lateral and midline disc ruptures can be mimicked by bony spurring or degenerative changes, so that interpretation of

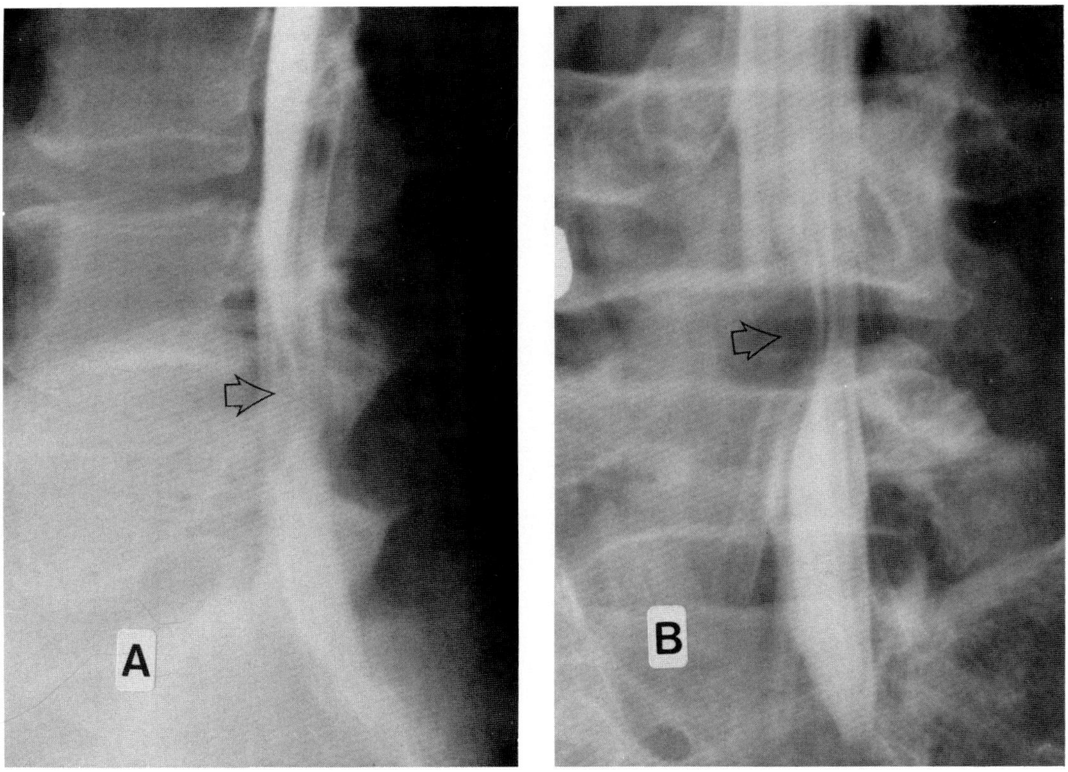

FIGURE 4.29. The classic myelographic picture of a lumbar disc rupture is a relatively smooth defect centered over the intervertebral disc space and indenting the contrast column maximally anterolaterally. This may be visible in a posteroanterior view (**A, arrow**) or a cross-table lateral view, but is seen at its maximum height in an oblique view **(B, arrow).**

myelographic defects must be rendered cautiously in the presence of such bony abnormalities. In any event, the radiographic picture must be correlated in every case with clinical symptomatology, and defects contralateral to a patient's clinical symptoms may well be unrelated to the patient's difficulties. Radiologists especially should be cautious in their enthusiasm for reporting the presence of such extradural defects as "disc ruptures." Only surgical removal of actually ruptured disc material can definitely confirm the diagnosis of disc rupture, and imprudent reporting of myelographic defects as disc ruptures can cause considerable problems for the clinician and valuable fodder for attorneys.

As discussed under adhesive arachnoiditis in Chapter 3, *lumbar adhesive arachnoiditis* occurs in some patients spontaneously and may closely mimic the myelographic picture of disc rupture early in the course of the disease. A myelogram that demonstrates a large defect slightly eccentric to the disc space, or bilateral or multiple-level defects (Type I arachnoiditis), should be interpreted with special caution, since this picture is not typical of lumbar disc rupture and instead is more suggestive of arachnoiditis or multiple-level degenerative changes. More advanced adhesive arachnoiditis causes an extensive irregularity on myelography. When associated with disc rupture, this most commonly takes the form of an irregular filling defect circumferentially around the thecal sac (Type II) or a complete obliteration of the thecal sac in a transverse fashion (Type III). This pattern of arachnoiditis seems to occur more commonly with, and is therefore diagnostically suggestive of, the primary or spontaneous form of arachnoiditis. With Type II arachnoiditis, a central open lumen is often retained, with nerve roots being plastered laterally against the dural walls. Less commonly, the arachnoiditis shows up as a multisegmental irregular filling defect, which may contain within its irregularity loculations of iophendylate (Pantopaque) from previous myelographic studies. Whether arachnoiditis may be a complication of myelography remains unproven, as discussed under adhesive arachnoiditis in Chapter 3. If, however, the incidence of adhesive arachnoiditis in patients with disc rupture proves to be drastically lower following water soluble metrizamide (Amipaque) myelography than following oily iophendylate (Pantopaque) myelography, this will strongly implicate Pantopaque as at least a potentially causative factor in the formation of arachnoiditis, presumably on the basis of an interaction between the contrast material and the local disease process or disc rupture.

In addition to being helpful in patients with primary disc ruptures or other unoperated conditions, myelography is frequently useful in *previously operated patients* with the failed back syndrome. Previously undiagnosed conditions should be carefully sought. *Benign intradural tumors* in the lumbar or thoracolumbar area are uncommon, but when they do occur they may present with a clinical picture quite similar to that typically seen with lumbar disc rupture. Myelography should be nearly 100% accurate in diagnosing these tumors—but only if the contrast material is carried sufficiently high to visualize the low thoracic region, where most of these tumors are found. If the patient's initial myelogram, prior to his "failed" surgery, did not visualize the low thoracic region, special care should be taken to visualize this area if repeat myelography is planned. The roles, strengths, and limitations of CT and MRI scans in diagnosing benign spinal tumors were discussed in the preceding section.

Not all patients who have undergone lumbar disc or other lumbar surgery were subjected to myelography prior to operation. In these patients, myelography may reveal not only a previously undiagnosed spinal tumor, but also evidence of a *disc rupture* at a spinal level different from that suspected clinically prior to the patient's surgery—and consequently not exposed surgically. Even if the correct level of the disc rupture was diagnosed clinically and myelographically prior to initial surgery, the disc rupture may have gone untreated if the *surgery was done at an improper level* because of incorrect anatomic localization at the time of surgical exposure. If the operating surgeon was careful enough to have placed a radiopaque marker at the site of the surgery, the possibility of a misdiagnosed disc rupture or a misplaced operation will be readily apparent should myelography of the failed back syndrome patient disclose a myelographic defect at a spinal level different from that of the surgical marker (Fig. 4.30). Without a surgically placed radiopaque marker, plain radiographs most commonly are unable to confirm the level of previous surgery; myelography may not be able to do so, but CT and MRI scans usually can.

Once disc excision has been performed, some degree of *local alteration* on myelography is quite common *at the operative site*. As demonstrated by myelography, such postoperative changes may be limited to a dorsolateral irregular indentation on the contrast column, a picture that almost certainly reflects scarring secondary to operative intervention, or a dorsolateral smooth outward bulging into the area of bony and ligamentous decompression. More problematic is the myelographic picture of anterolateral irregularity at the previous operative site. If the defect is rough and irregular in contour or extends above or below the interspace level, the possibility of significant intradural arachnoiditis is great. If, however, the defect is relatively smooth and confined to the interspace level, it may not be possible to distinguish radiographically among *recurrent disc rupture*, significant *extradural scar* or *nerve root fibrosis*, and *intradural arachnoiditis*. Extradural or subdural *wound infection* typically gives a more extensive defect that tends to girdle the thecal sac and extend in a rostrocaudal direction for two or more segmental levels. This possibility should always be suspected clinically prior to myelography so that the myelographer can carefully aspirate for pus from epidural and subdural spaces before advancing the needle through the arachnoid membrane and risking subarachnoid inoculation of organisms, with resulting meningitis.

Spinal stenosis may likewise be the reason for a patient's persistent failed disc syndrome (see page 26). This may have been present preoperatively, either in isolation or associated with a superimposed focal disc rupture, and its clinical significance may have been underestimated. In this spontaneous form of spinal stenosis, the myelographic picture is one of multiple-level smooth concentric-filling defects, each adjacent to a vertebral interspace. For these defects to be symptomatic, they must generally narrow the spinal sac by at least 50% of its width. As discussed earlier, CT scans nicely delineate the severity of bony stenosis, and MRI scans document soft-tissue components of stenotic areas perhaps to

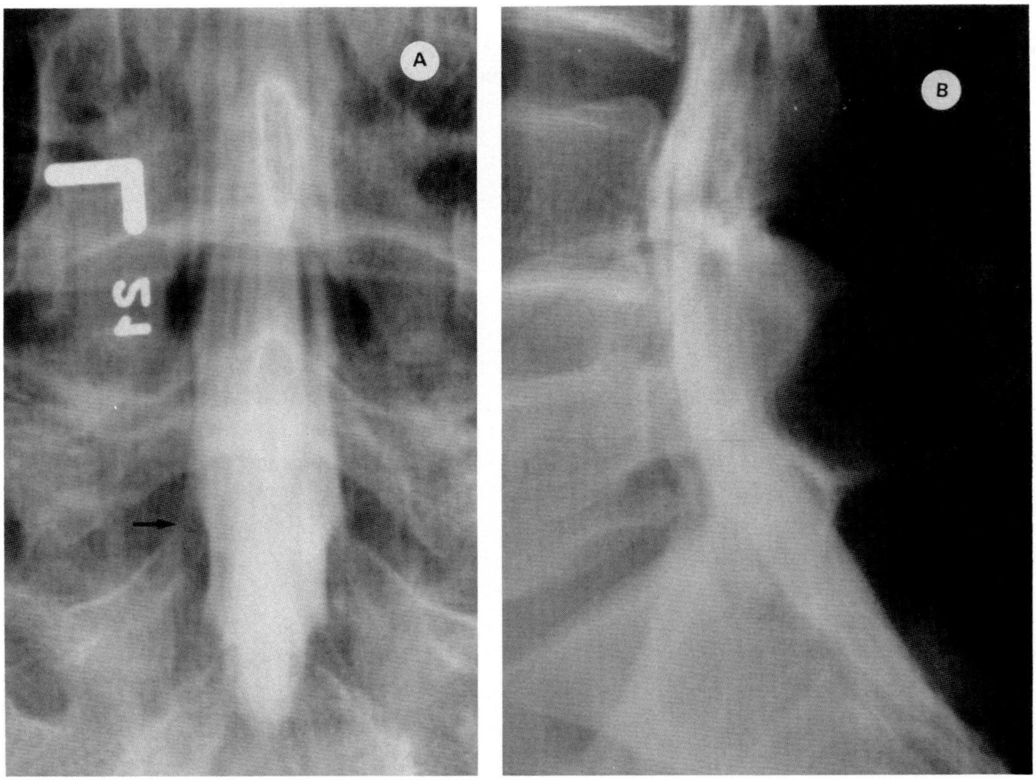

FIGURE 4.30. The level of previous laminectomy and discectomy may be difficult to detect on postoperative plain radiographs and even on postoperative myelography, especially if the surgeon fails to leave a radiopaque metal marker or if a microsurgical bone removal was performed. This woman underwent disc excision at L4-L5. Despite a suspicious blunting of the left L5-S1 nerve root on PA projection **(A, arrow),** a narrowed L5-S1 interspace, and an S1 nerve root syndrome clinically, the lateral projection **(B)** was felt to be normal and the improper level of her operative first intervention was initially overlooked until operative re-exploration disclosed a surgical laminotomy defect at L4-L5 and a virgin disc rupture at L5-S1.

the point of exaggeration, but myelograms definitively image the severity and rostrocaudal extent of compression of the subarachnoid space. An acquired form of spinal stenosis may be seen *following spinal fusion.* In these instances, a more focal and dorsally situated constriction is encountered, often at the level of previous disc excision. Commonly these patients will have undergone bilateral disc excision rather than unilateral excision. Myelography, of course, cannot differentiate whether this constriction is caused by overgrowth of the fusion bone or by secondary overgrowth of scar tissue, and CT scanning may be required. In patients with fusion pseudarthrosis, extensive scar tissue frequently forms beneath the pseudarthrotic line, and the resulting dorsal encroachment seen on myelography can be viewed as a clue to the presence of an otherwise radiographically obscure pseudarthrosis.

Myelography is less reliable and less valuable in the diagnosis of *lateral recess stenosis* than CT scans. Like spinal stenosis, this syndrome causes compression of nerve roots without entrapment or fixation to surrounding structures. Unlike spinal stenosis, lateral recess stenosis usually causes compression of a single root, rather than the entire thecal sac, and thus clinically produces a monoradicular pain syndrome. Because, by definition, lateral recess stenosis causes compression of the nerve root laterally within the spinal canal, myelography is unlikely to show abnormalities, especially in a patient with a narrow thecal sac (Fig. 4.31). Since metrizamide (Amipaque) is less viscous than iophendylate (Pantopaque), it normally gives better

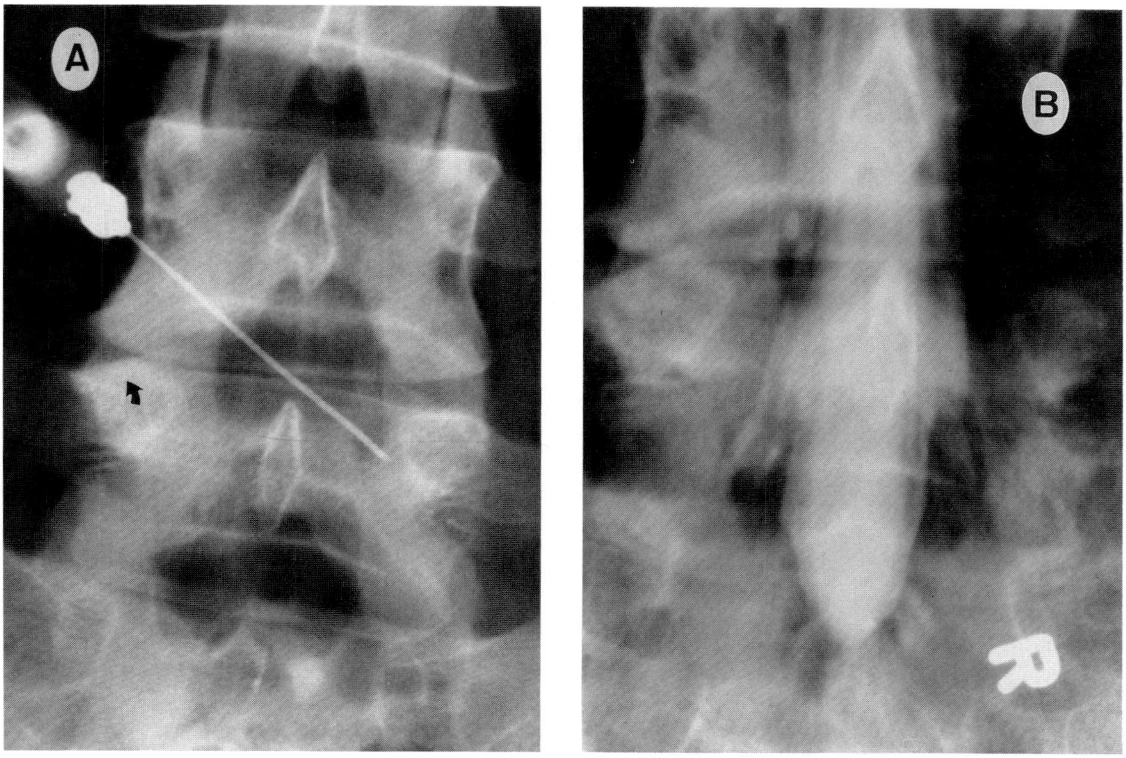

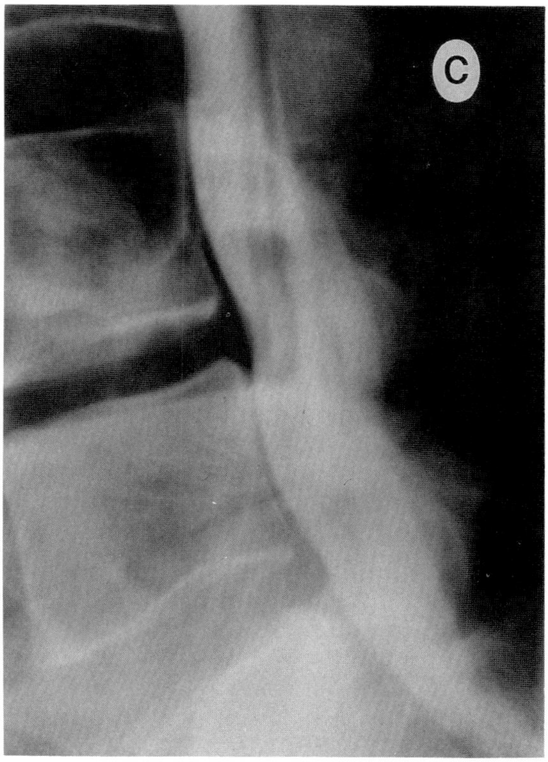

FIGURE 4.31. **A (arrows):** Lateral recess stenosis occurs in association with focal degenerative changes as seen on plain radiographs. **B and C:** Myelography usually shows no abnormality because the compression is far lateral within the spinal canal.

filling of nerve sheaths and thus delineates normal nerve root anatomy farther laterally within the spinal canal. Even so, lateral recess stenosis usually causes little more than amputation of a single nerve root sac, a myelographic finding that carries limited reliability as a diagnostic sign of any symptomatic pathology and that is certainly not specifically diagnostic of lateral recess stenosis. As discussed earlier, CT scanning is probably the diagnostic method of choice in this clinical condition.

Posttraumatic lumbar *arachnoid cysts* may develop following disc excision, especially if the dura is torn intraoperatively. These cystic outpouchings are usually dorsal or dorsolateral and may be difficult to confirm. If they fill with contrast material, diagnosis becomes obvious, especially on lateral or oblique films. Quite commonly, however, the ostium of the cyst is nearly occluded by herniating nerve roots or arachnoid, so that the lumen of the cyst does not fill with contrast medium and is not directly visualized on the myelogram. In these instances, a dorsal or dorsolateral "extradural" smooth myelographic filling defect will be visualized (Fig. 4.32). If an arachnoid cyst is suspected at the time of myelography, but fails to fill with contrast medium, a special technique may be useful. Leaving the lumbar thecal sac filled with iophendylate (Pantopaque) for 24 hours, during which the patient is allowed to ambulate, may allow contrast material to enter the cyst. The diagnosis can then be confirmed radiographically prior to delayed removal of iophendylate.

An extreme form of this problem is the *postoperative pseudomeningocele* (see page 18). This follows a persistent *cerebrospinal fluid (CSF) leak* that often never reaches the skin surface to be diagnosed as an external CSF fistula. Instead, the CSF pools in the extralaminar soft tissues between the lumbodorsal muscles. This fluid-filled cavity eventually becomes smooth-walled and is usually readily seen on

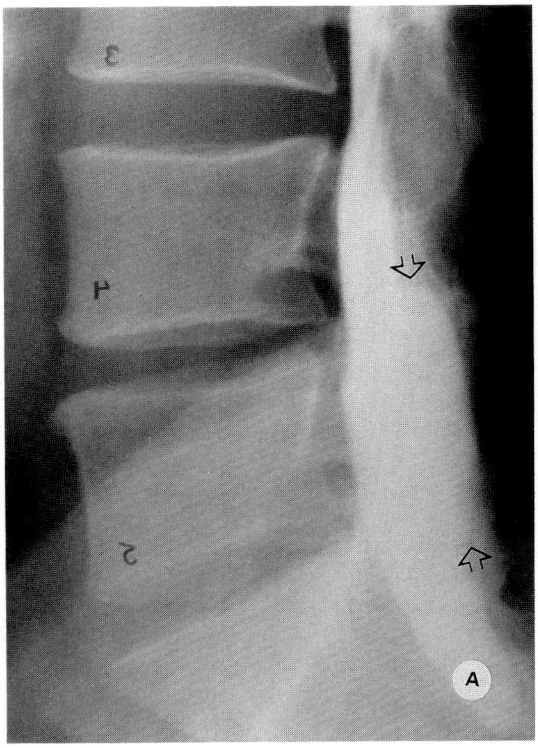

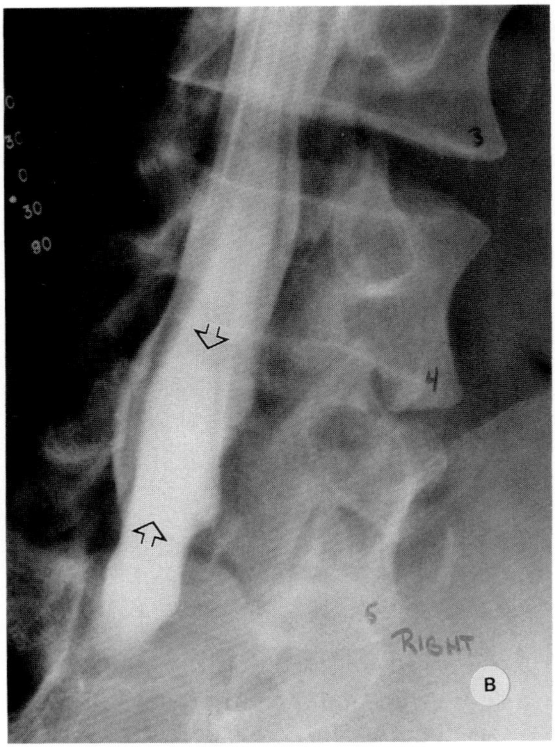

FIGURE 4.32. Postoperative arachnoidal cysts are an uncommon cause of sciatica in the failed back syndrome. This myelogram in PA (**A**) and oblique (**B**) projections documents unusually good filling of such a cyst in a man with persistent low backache and intermittent sciatica, beginning several months following otherwise successful disc excision (arrows). Often, the cyst ostium or opening is occluded by herniating nerve roots that prevent entry of contrast material and myelography demonstrates a filling defect only.

myelography with the patient fully upright, so that turning the patient into the supine position is rarely necessary. CT scanning and, even more impressively, MRI scanning provide definitive diagnosis noninvasively by demonstrating the low-density, fluid-filled cyst dorsal to the lumbar laminae.

Complications of Myelography

The most common complication of myelography is the *post–lumbar puncture (LP) headache.* This form of headache is precipitated by a lowered intracranial pressure and results from continued leaking of spinal fluid through the needle puncture site in the arachnoid or dura. Characteristically, this headache is most severe when the patient is upright, sometimes developing after a delay of several hours to several days. Recumbency improves the headache but frequently does not totally relieve it. Nausea and vomiting may accompany a severe post-LP headache. Low-grade fever is occasionally encountered, as well as mild neck stiffness and aching discomfort in the low back—making it necessary to be wary of the possibility of a low-grade bacterial meningitis. Symptoms may last from a few days to many weeks, the latter being exceptional, while the symptoms of bacterial meningitis usually continue to evolve in crescendo fashion. Treatment for post-LP headache begins with bed rest and vigorous hydration. If nausea and vomiting become severe, or if headaches are particularly severe and unremitting, intravenous infusions of large fluid volumes may be quite helpful. This form of headache often responds best to analgesics, usually salicylates, combined with caffeine to vasoconstrict tense and irritated cerebral blood vessels. In the patient who is nauseated, intravenous continuous infusion of caffeine sodium benzoate (500 mg per liter of 5% dextrose in water or 5% dextrose in quarter normal saline) may be quite helpful.

On rare occasions, post-LP headache may remain quite severe for many days. In these situations, a lumbar epidural *"blood patch"* should be considered. This technique involves placing a lumbar spinal needle into the epidural space at or near the level of the previous myelographic puncture and injecting fresh whole blood that is allowed to coagulate and plug the hole in the dura (Fig. 4.33). A technical difficulty is encountered in ensuring that the needle is in fact in the epidural space and not in the subarachnoid space, since these patients are leaking spinal fluid into the epidural space and have headaches because of low subarachnoid fluid pressure. Once the needle is in place, 10 cc of fresh whole blood are withdrawn from the patient and are injected slowly into the epidural space. Once this fresh blood coagulates, it forms a barrier or patch to help seal the opening in the thecal sac. Some aching low back discomfort is quite common following this procedure. Inadvertent injection into the subarachnoid space can cause severe symptoms of low back pain, meningismus, neuralgia, and even neurologic deficits.[52] I have twice been called to see patients in whom this has occurred.

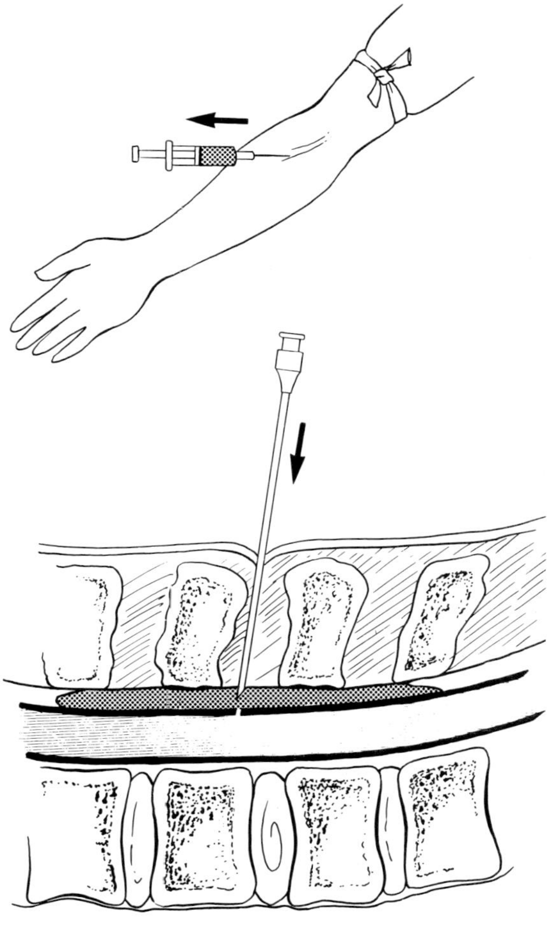

FIGURE 4.33. An epidural blood patch may be used in cases of severe post LP headaches. The internal leak through arachnoid and dura may be sealed by injecting fresh autologous blood from the patient's own veins into the epidural space. The resulting clot effectively plugs the CSF leak.

A potential side effect with *metrizamide (Amipaque) myelography* is a *meningeal reaction* with headache, backache, nausea, and vomiting. This may be severe at times, but can be minimized by keeping the patient semierect following myelography and by vigorously hydrating the patient before and after performance of myelography. Convulsive seizures are uncommonly encountered following lumbar metrizamide myelography, but have been reported with cervical myelography. Despite this obvious evidence of toxicity, lumbar adhesive arachnoiditis seems to be quite rare following metrizamide myelography.

Other potential complications of myelography include *infection, chemical meningitis,* and *nerve root injury.* Fortunately, bacterial meningitis and subdural or epidural abscess are very rarely encountered following myelography and should be avoidable if careful sterile technique is observed throughout. Chemical meningitis is a painful and potentially damaging complication that usually follows inadvertent introduction of irritating chemical agents through the lumbar puncture needle into the subarachnoid space. One unpublished account details a series of such cases that followed the use of myelography needles that had been sterilized in aqueous benzalkonium chloride (Zepherin) solution. When these needles were subsequently used without adequate washing and drying, significant amounts of this antiseptic were introduced directly intrathecally. Other unpublished cases refer to larger volume injections of antiseptic solution. These accidents occurred when the myelographer filled a syringe from a container on the sterile tray in a darkened fluoroscopy room and inadvertently drew up antiseptic instead of iophendylate (Pantopaque). Because of this disastrous complication, good technique suggests that containers of antiseptic solution should not be left on the myelography tray once skin preparation has been completed.

The risk of *nerve root injury* is quite small if local anesthesia is used for myelography, but will be much greater in those rare instances in which general anesthesia is mandated. Nerve roots may be injured at the time of needle insertion, especially if the subarachnoid space is constricted at the site of needle insertion by spinal stenosis, disc rupture, or neoplasm, or if nerve roots are immobilized by extradural scar or intradural arachnoiditis. If iophendylate is used, an even greater risk of nerve root injury is encountered at the time of attempted withdrawal. Iophendylate is much heavier than nerve roots. As long as a pool of iophendylate is present around the needle tip, nerve roots will be relatively safe because they will be displaced away from the needle tip. Once the bulk of the iophendylate has been removed, it becomes easier to suck nerve roots into the open end of the needle. Unduly vigorous suctioning, usually accompanied by protests and complaints of pain from the patient, may then cause nerve root injury. Technical methods of limiting this risk are discussed below.

Technique of Myelography

The procedural technique of myelography has been adequately covered in many radiologic texts and will be reviewed only briefly. There is still controversy as to whether local anesthesia should be injected at the proposed needle site. The argument against using local anesthetics is that the anesthetic injection is as painful as the introduction of the spinal needle and the chance of allergic reaction to the local anesthetic is significant. On the other hand, it has been my practice for two decades to use local anesthesia, for both humanitarian and technical reasons. I have not encountered any documented cases of severe allergic reaction to the anesthetic. If the interspace is properly anesthetized, patients should not find myelography to be a painful procedure. Equally important, however, is the fact that careful local anesthetization allows better patient relaxation and cooperation, while paralysis of interspinous muscles allows the interspace to open wider, thereby facilitating needle insertion. Two anatomic sites are particularly important in planning local anesthesia for myelography or lumbar puncture. A skin wheal should be raised to deaden cutaneous sensation, and approximately 0.5 ml local anesthetic should be placed lateral to the base of the interspinous ligament on each side to paralyze the recurrent dorsal lumbar nerve branches that supply the spinous processes and interspinous muscles. This provides a local field block anesthesia and relaxes the interspinous muscles, allowing the spinous processes to separate widely. If the interspinous space were filled with anesthetic, this would cause lateral distention of muscles and ligaments, which in turn would cause narrowing of the interspinous space.

The vertebral level chosen for spinal puncture is also quite important. The needle should never be introduced at the level of confirmed or suspected disc rupture for fear of damage to an immobilized nerve root or production of a myelographic artifact at the level of maximum interest. Because most disc ruptures occur at L4-L5 and L5-Sl, some myelographers prefer to place the needle at L3-L4. Craniad in the canal, at L2-L3 and above, less available CSF space is present with greater crowding of nerve roots, causing more likelihood of pain on needle insertion and more pain and greater difficulty on attempted fluid withdrawal if non water-soluble contrast is used. Unfortunately, the same clinical inexactitude that makes myelography useful also makes it inadvisable to perform punctures at L3-L4 unless the suspected difficulty very clearly is at L5-Sl. A suspected disc at L4-L5 may in fact be at L3-L4, just where the myelographic needle is placed. If L3-L4 punctures are used, these should always be confirmed fluoroscopically before the needle punctures the dura to prevent inadvertent L4-L5 needle placement.

Spinal fluid samples should always be withdrawn at myelography. Clinical correlations with myelographic defects are extremely important, because not all defects—even some large defects—are clinically significant. Finding an elevated spinal fluid protein or an unexpected pleocytosis can be of great help in assessing clinical correlations, including the presence of intrathecal neoplasms.

With *metrizamide (Amipaque) myelography,* it is no longer necessary to withdraw fluid at the end of the myelogram. Metrizamide is contraindicated in patients with a strong history of a major allergic reaction to iodine, but iophendylate may be safely used as long as it is promptly and totally withdrawn. Occasionally, *allergic parotitis* may be seen following iophendylate myelography, but this is quite rare. Vigorous hydration is important before and after metrizamide myelography to minimize central nervous system and renal toxicity, but convulsions and brain stem injury have been reported after exposure of brain stem or higher brain levels to high concentrations. To minimize brain stem or cortical exposure patients are usually maintained in a semierect posture for six to twelve hours following metrizamide myelography, even though this seems to increase the frequency of post-LP headaches.

Iophendylate should be withdrawn, both because of the potential risk (largely unconfirmed) of late arachnoiditis and because of the potential of inadvertent spillage intracranially with resultant headaches or even CSF pathway obstruction. When iophendylate is withdrawn, care must be exercised not to apply strong suction directly to tender nerve roots. A special multiperforated needle, the Cuatico needle, has been designed to facilitate this process.[53] Unfortunately, this needle also makes the withdrawal of excessively large volumes of spinal fluid nearly unavoidable, so that post-LP headaches seem more common after its use. A technical alternative is to use a 1 ml or 2 ml air cushion in the syringe when withdrawing iophendylate. Interposing tubing between the syringe and the needle to facilitate iophendylate withdrawal under fluoroscopic guidance is extremely valuable. Under fluoroscopic guidance, the patient can be tilted frequently to maintain a pool of iophendylate around the needle tip. The heavier iophendylate droplets actually spread nerve roots apart, away from the needle tip, and greatly lessen the likelihood of aspirating a nerve root against the needle tip, such as often occurs when aspiration is attempted from an intrathecal area filled with spinal fluid only. The risk of post-LP headaches can be minimized in iophendylate myelography by using as small a needle as feasible (generally a 20-gauge needle), by hydrating the patient vigorously postoperatively, and by maintaining the patient at bed rest for 24 hours following the procedure.

Discography

Diagnostic discography remains a controversial tool. However, the release of chymopapain for enzyme discolysis, which also involves injection directly into the disc, led to a heightened interest in diagnostic discography, a technique that I continue to find quite helpful (Fig. 4.34). Discography has classically been done with positive contrast material (*contrast discography*). However, disc injections with local anesthetics (*anesthesia discography*) may also be diagnostically useful if anesthetizing the disc eliminates the patient's back pain. Patients who are severely allergic to iodine-containing contrast materials should not undergo contrast discography, but for these patients the use of diagnostic saline injections may provide information about the volume of the disc, may reproduce local disc pain (or confirm the absence of pain), and therefore may yield sufficient information to influence future therapy. I have never advocated substituting discography for myelography as a principal invasive diagnostic study for patients with low back disease and

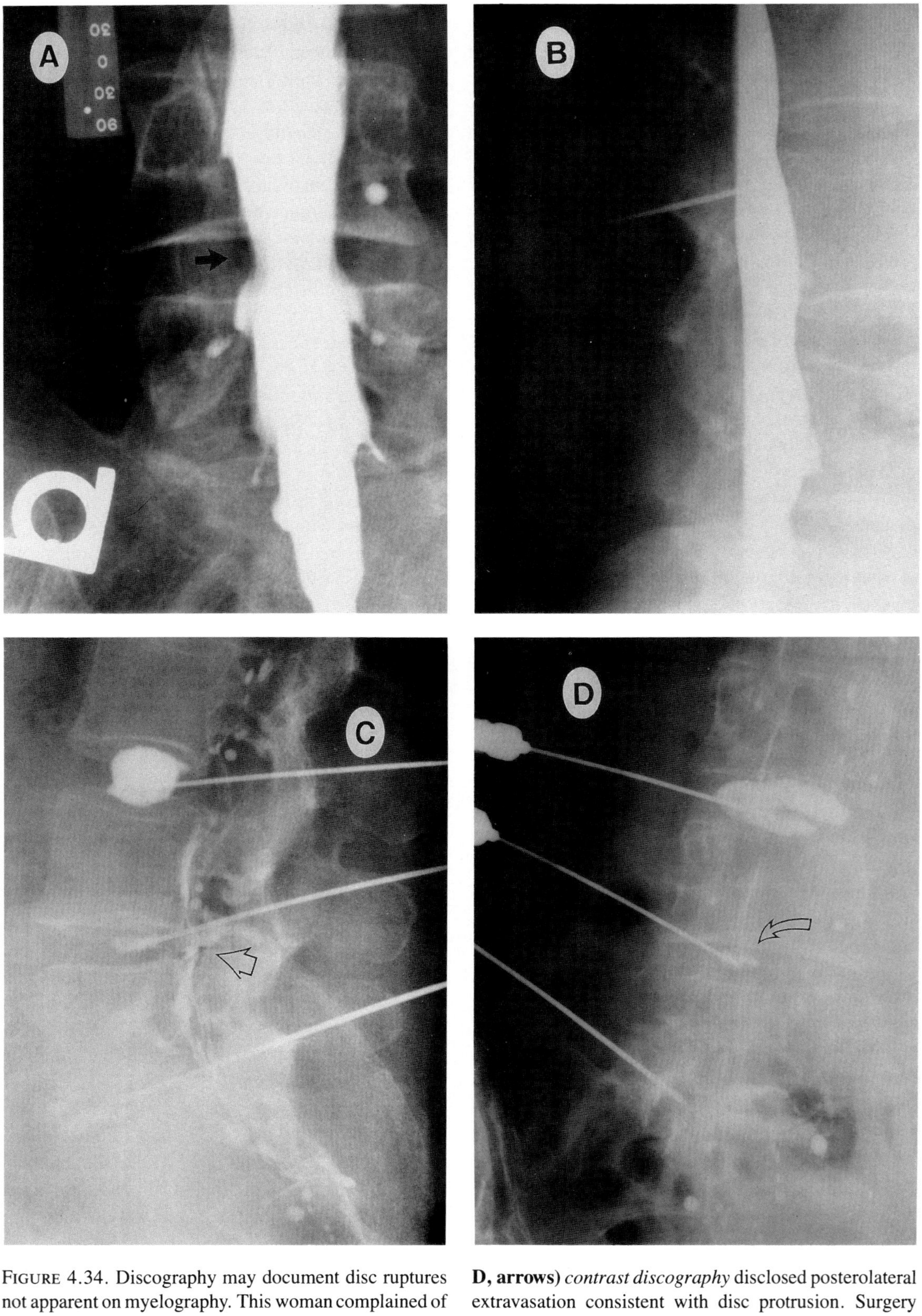

FIGURE 4.34. Discography may document disc ruptures not apparent on myelography. This woman complained of back and leg pain after a fall, but her clinical picture was not convincing for disc rupture. **A and B (arrow):** Myelogram showed a minimal defect at L4-L5, but **(C and D, arrows)** *contrast discography* disclosed posterolateral extravasation consistent with disc protrusion. Surgery confirmed the presence of a disc rupture through the posterior longitudinal ligament laterally within the spinal canal.

sciatica. As I have learned more about the complexity of the diseases affecting the lower back—diseases such as facet syndromes, primary arachnoiditis, and lateral recess stenosis—I have become increasingly wary of this substitution.

In my practice I have used *discography in previously unoperated patients* whose other imaging studies are normal or equivocal, including those possibly harboring far-lateral disc ruptures and whose clinical pictures are diagnostically marginal. Less commonly, I have employed *discography in failed back syndrome patients* who suffer primarily from low back pain. In these patients, injections into adjacent, unoperated discs may document a second or previously misdiagnosed disc abnormality. Injection of a disc that has previously been excised gives an abnormal picture on discography, but the type of abnormality encountered may give useful information, often of a negative nature. Injection of contrast material into a previously operated interspace that shows an abnormally large central cavity of postoperative configuration, no escape of contrast material, and no significant pain effectively eliminates this disc as the source of the patient's continued back pain. However, if the intradiscal injection of contrast material causes severe back pain, similar to the patient's usual pain, the previously operated interspace may still be the source of the patient's pain. Diatrizoate meglumide and sodium contrast material (Renografin) is irritating to body tissues, thus pain following intradiscal contrast injection loses some of its significance if radiographs confirm extravasation out of the interspace through lateral fissures or dorsally through the site of prior disc excision into the extradiscal space. The interspace itself is relatively insensate, so diatrizoate that is injected into a normal, uninflamed interspace and remains contained within that interspace rarely causes more than mild discomfort.

In previously operated patients, *anesthesia discography* may also give useful information if anesthetizing a postoperative interspace largely relieves the patient of long-standing back pain. Anesthesia discography in the lumbar region is more difficult to interpret than anesthesia discography in the cervical region because of the greater amount of discomfort attendant upon needle insertion in the lumbar area. Even if a single inflamed disc is the principal source of the patient's pain, it may be difficult to detect the elimination of this pain if significant local discomfort has been generated during needle insertion. On the other hand, when interspace anesthetization dramatically relieves the patient of his previous pain and produces a temporary, marked improvement in back motion, it is reasonable to assume that the injected disc (whether previously resected or not) is a major source of the patient's disability.

Complications of Discography

Perhaps the most significant *complication associated with discography* is interspace *infection*—a complication I have encountered in two out of nearly a thousand interspaces injected. One of these infections was confirmed at discectomy that followed a few weeks after discography. The other infection led to vertebral osteomyelitis in a normal disc space adjacent to the dicographically abnormal interspace that was operated upon. This led to some diagnostic confusion, as detailed in the following case history (Fig. 4.35):

Case 4

A 44-year-old man experienced abrupt onset of severe sciatica and back pain following a motor vehicle accident. Examination showed apparent dorsiflexor ankle weakness and sensory loss globally over the entire right lower extremity. Protracted nonoperative therapy proved unsuccessful. Myelography showed no definite abnormality. Three-level contrast discography was normal at L3-L4 and L5-S1, but suggested frank disc rupture at L4-L5. At operation six weeks later, a prominent lateral rupture was discovered and was removed. Postoperatively, the patient complained of severe back pain but gradually resumed ambulation. Over the next two months, back pain became slowly and progressively more severe, although leg pain remained much improved. Laboratory studies showed a persistent moderately elevated sedimentation rate and a white blood count that rose progressively from a prediscogram level of 13,000 to a high of 21,000. Postoperative radiographs initially showed no abnormality and good persistence of the interbody bone fusion at L4-L5. Six weeks and twelve weeks postoperatively, the L4-L5 interspace was needled percutaneously and barbotaged with IV saline. Cultures were negative aerobically and anaerobically. On the second occasion, intradiscal methylprednisolone acetate (Depo-Medrol) was placed but produced no improvement. Two weeks following the second injection, a 14-day course of chloramphenicol (Chloromycetin) was given empirically by the patient's family physician with dramatic improvement in the patient's pain and return of his white cell count to prediscogram levels. Repeat radio-

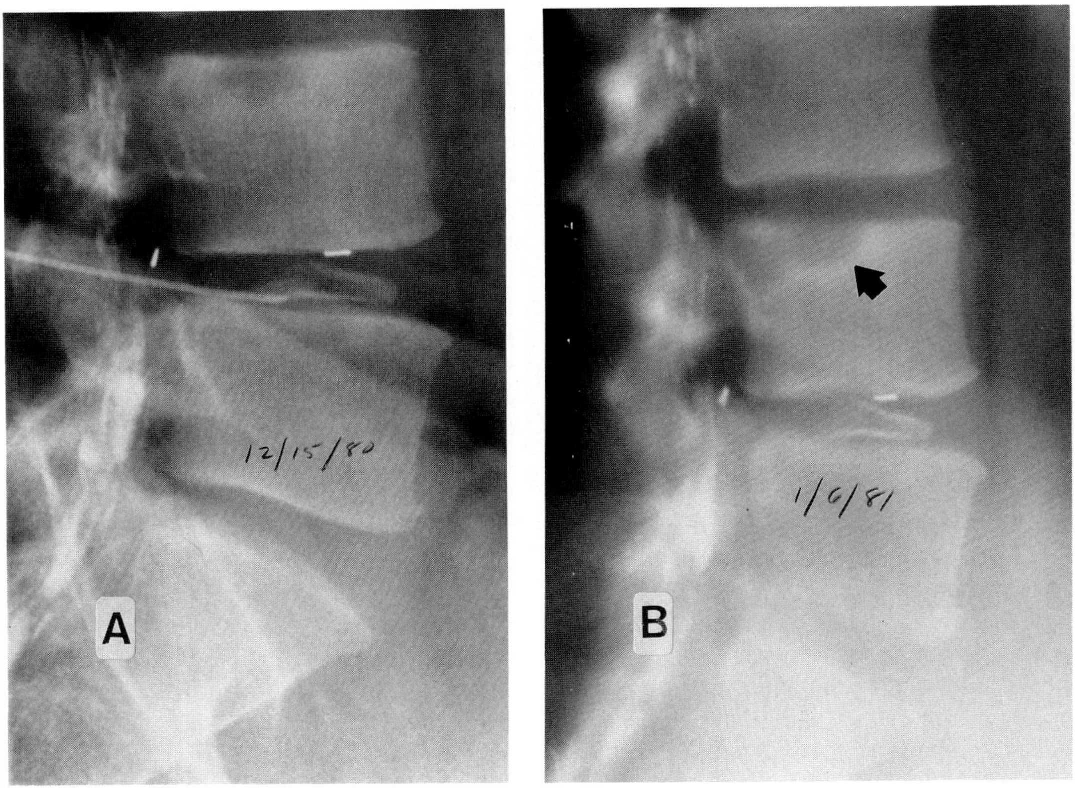

FIGURE 4.35. Disc space infection and osteomyelitis are potential complications of discography. This patient, presented as Case 4, underwent three-level discography that confirmed disc rupture at L4-L5. **A:** Delayed postoperative back pain was initially attributed to the operative site, but diagnostic injection and barbotage for culture at the level of the interbody bone plug failed to confirm disc space infection. **B (arrow):** Later radiographs disclosed osteomyelitic destruction at L3-L4 site of discography instead.

graphs at the conclusion of this course of antibiotics demonstrated osteomyelitic destruction of the body of L4 adjacent to the L3-L4 interspace.

An additional three weeks of chloramphenicol was given because of the documented osteomyelitis. Six months later, radiographs showed bony healing and white cell count remained normal.

A more common complication following discography is *post-LP headache,* if discography is done by a direct posterior approach, since this approach entails multiple punctures through the dura and arachnoid. This complication should not follow discography done by a posterolateral approach.

Discussions of the complications of discography frequently contemplate the possibility of *mechanical damage* to the intervertebral disc or to lumbar nerve roots. Unless sepsis has been documented, there has been to my knowledge no documentation of disc injury from discography alone. Nerve roots certainly could be injured during discography, since the posterior approach entails transfixing the thecal sac and the posterolateral approach necessitates placing needles in close proximity to the extradural nerve roots. This complication, however, is largely avoidable if discography is done carefully and under local anesthesia.

Interpretation of Discograms

Discography should always be done under *local anesthesia,* not general anesthesia. The added risk to nerve roots under general anesthesia has been alluded to already. Equally important is the diagnostic significance of the patient's *pain response to discography,* a response that would be totally unavailable under general anesthesia (Fig. 4.36). As mentioned earlier, the presence or absence of pain on disc injection may be diagnostic even without injection of contrast medium.

Three diagnostic factors should be assessed in

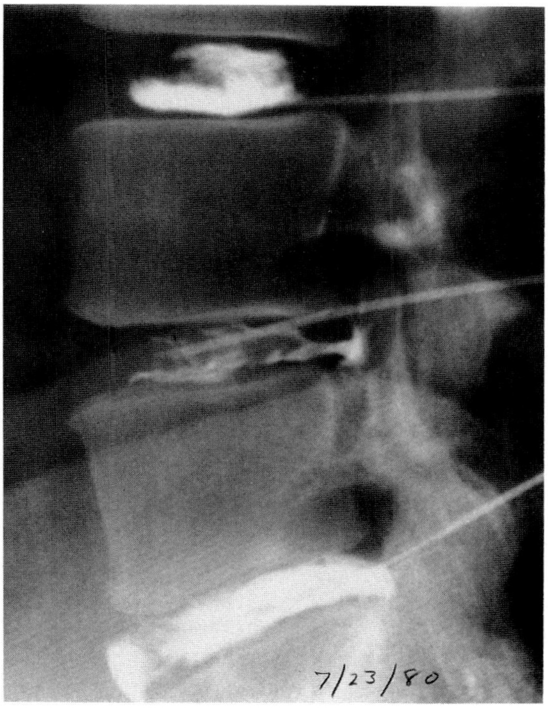

FIGURE 4.36. Discographic abnormality of two types was documented in this man who complained of persistent back pain. Injection at L3-L4 was painless and radiographic picture shows a normal disc. Injection at L5-S1 was also painless even though the radiographic picture shows degeneration and extensive filling. This was felt not to be a symptomatic degeneration. The injection of L4-L5 demonstrates posterior protrusion and elicited severe complaints of back and leg pain. Surgical exploration confirmed disc rupture at this level.

interpreting contrast discography: (1) the *volume* of material injected, (2) the *radiographic picture,* and (3) the *pain response*. The normal lumbar disc will usually accept less than 2 ml of aqueous contrast material, generally 76% diatrizoate meglumide and sodium (Renografin 76), and will have the radiographic appearance of a central ball, pancake, or double pancake. Injection of a normal disc should elicit a dull aching discomfort in the lower back but no pain. A disc that is degenerated will often accept 2 ml or 3 ml of contrast material without extravasation, and radiographs will show extensive central filling. Many degenerated discs are asymptomatic, and injection of these should elicit little or no pain. Injections into those degenerated discs that are, in fact, inflamed and a source of pain frequently elicit severe pain in the lower back, buttock, or groin. This pain is usually relieved within 60 seconds by intradiscal injection of 1 ml or 2 ml of 1% or 2% lidocaine (Xylocaine). Lumbar discs that are protruding markedly are usually associated with obvious sciatica on injection, while discs that are frankly ruptured allow free extravasation of contrast material, which is usually seen radiographically as posterolateral extravasation and which is almost universally associated with severe pain. Patients in whom a disc ruptures laterally within the spinal canal or in whom the thecal sac is quite narrow or foreshortened commonly have normal myelograms despite classically abnormal discograms. *CT scans* done at the end of contrast discograms add anatomic precision and can distinguish clearly among contrast extravasated into ruptured fragments still contained beneath spinal ligaments, free extravasation into adnexal tissues, and protrusion of nuclear material into far-lateral disc ruptures.

A *false positive discogram* can occur even in a previously unoperated interspace if diatrizoate escapes through a small fissure in the annulus into the epidural or paraspinal soft tissues. The escaping contrast material will allow injection of a greater than normal volume and will cause local irritation and pain that may mimic the patient's customary pain. Radiographs and CT scans should be helpful in distinguishing this type of abnormality, since they should disclose extravasation without protrusion of the contrast-filled nuclear portion of the disc backward into the spinal canal.

Diagnostic contrast injections into *previously operated discs* always give abnormal results, but several different types of abnormalities may be encountered (Fig. 4.37). If the surgical fenestration in the posterior annulus and posterior longitudinal ligament remains open, contrast material will extravasate into the spinal canal and will be evident radiographically and by the patient's complaints of severe pain caused by the irritating contrast material coming in contact with pain-sensitive structures. On the other hand, after successful disc excision the surgical fenestration often seals completely. Injection into a disc that has healed normally will reveal a large volume central cavity with no significant posterior bulging and with little or no discomfort on injection. Discs that remain the source of pain due to chronic irritation or inflammatory discitis will cause the patient severe, predominantly back pain on injection even if the surgical fenestration is nicely closed.

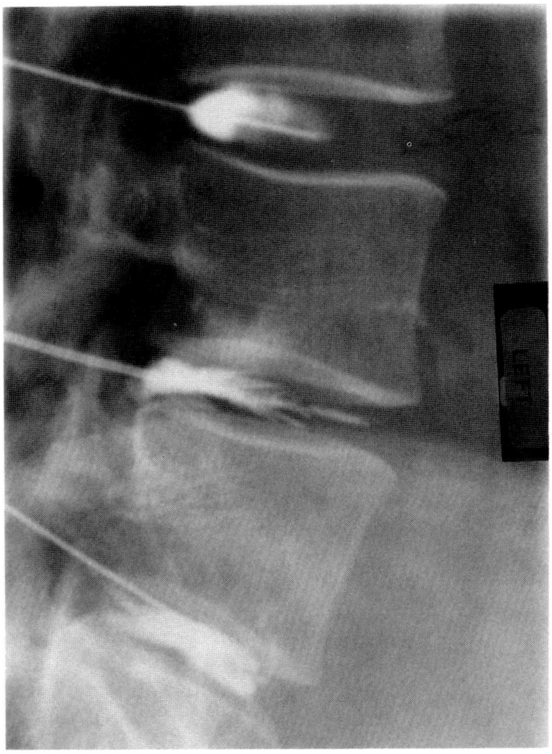

FIGURE 4.37. Discogram is always abnormal following disc removal. This discogram documents extensive filling but no posterior extravasation at the previously operated L4-L5 interspace. This injection was painless and the patient's pain was subsequently confirmed to arise from a facet syndrome instead. Discography at L5-S1 and at L3-L4 was painless and radiographically normal.

Techniques of Discography

The two principal *techniques for lumbar discography* are a *posterior, midline, transdural approach* and a *posterolateral, oblique, extradural approach* (Fig. 4.38). Disc injections are performed with the patient lying on a fluoroscopy table. Normally it is my practice to inject all three lower lumbar, or at least both L4-L5 and L5-S1, discs, because these account for the majority of disc ruptures and because it is extremely useful to have normal disc injections to compare with the abnormal disc injection, both radiographically and in the patient's subjective assessment of the pain that results.

The *posterior, interspinous, transdural approach* is no longer commonly used, but may be valuable if the lumbosacral disc cannot be reached via the posterolateral approach. Skin wheals are raised with a local anesthetic in the midline just caudal to the tips of the spinous processes of L3 and L4 and approximately 2 cm lateral to the tip of the spinous process of L5, depending on which levels are to be injected. The patient is positioned prone with a bolster under the anterior pelvis. After skin wheals have been raised, a local field block is produced by blocking the recurrent nerves to the interspinous muscles and ligaments near the base of the spinous processes on each side and by placing a small additional amount of anesthetic in the interspinous ligaments (see page 88). The more caudal, laterally placed needle is directed medially toward the L5-S1 interspace, and its tract is infiltrated locally. One-and-a-half-inch long 18-gauge needles are inserted just caudal to the spinous processes of L3 and L4 and are aimed in a slightly rostral direction. A third such needle is placed in the lateral tract aimed in a slightly caudomedial direction. Under fluoroscopic control, 22-gauge spinal needles of 3 1/2- or 5-inch length are inserted through the guide needles to the posterior annulus of the disc. Careful fluoroscopic guidance is important if multiple dural punctures are to be avoided. Each needle is then advanced into the nuclear center of the disc and cross-table lateral and overhead posteroanterior (PA) radiographs are taken for radiographic confirmation of placement.

When a *lateral extradural approach* is used, the patient is positioned on his side with neck, hips, and knees flexed to open the posterior margin of the interspaces. A single skin wheal of local anesthetic is placed 6 cm to 10 cm lateral to the spinous process of L4 and two skin wheals, approximately 2 cm apart, are placed 6 cm to 10 cm lateral to the L5 spinous process, just above the iliac crest. After local anesthetic infiltration, 6- to 8-inch 20-gauge needles are passed under fluoroscopic guidance lateral to the facets at L3-L4, L4-L5, and L5-S1 and just caudal to the transverse processes of these vertebrae. These needles pass in close proximity to the exiting nerve roots, and care must be taken to avoid damaging these nerves. When the needles impinge at the dorsolateral "corner" of the intervertebral disc, the operator should confirm this localization with biplane fluoroscopy or radiography before penetrating through the annulus into the nuclear center (Fig. 4.39). A failure to do so increases the likelihood of multiple needle punctures into the disc, allowing extravasation of contrast material or medications.

Biplane radiographs to confirm intradiscal place-

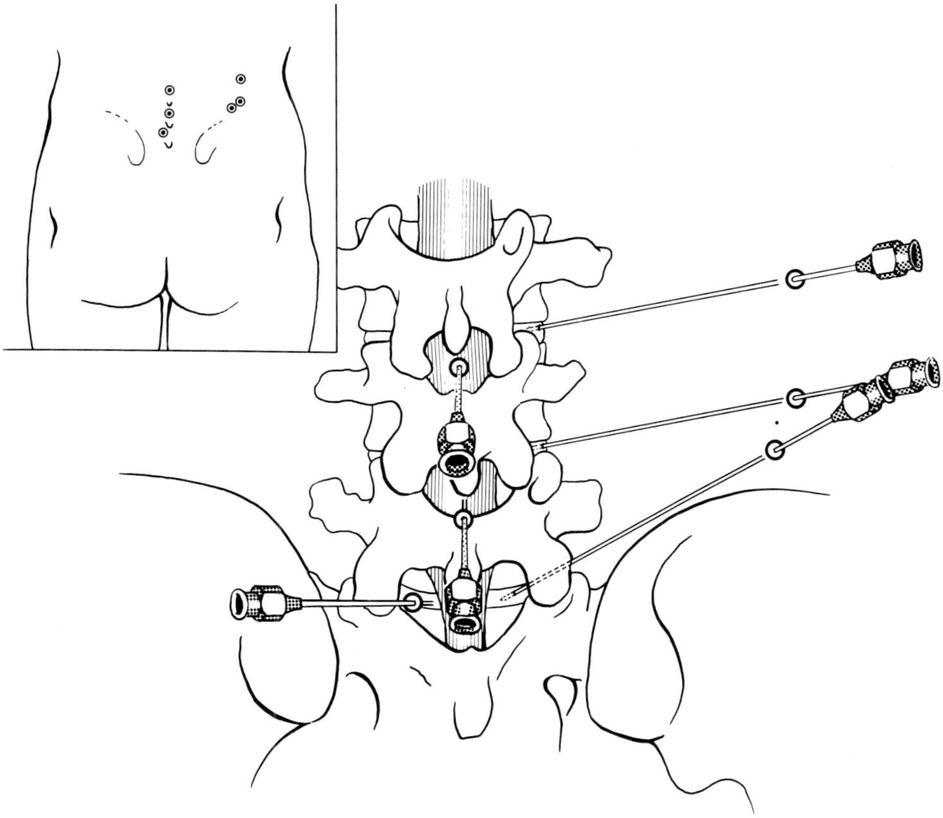

FIGURE 4.38. Lumbar discography may be performed by a posterior transdural approach or a posterolateral extradural approach. The needles in the midline of this drawing have been inserted transdurally, with the lowest needle angled to match the angle of the lumbosacral disc. The needles on the right were introduced by a posterolateral approach, sparing the dura but passing near the nerve roots paraspinally. The inset shows the location of skin wheals for each set of needles.

ment should always be taken before *disc injection.* Once the needles are placed within the discs, the fluoroscope or radiographic tube is positioned for lateral views. One disc space at a time is injected in rapid sequence with a volume not to exceed 2 ml or 3 ml of contrast material, usually 76% diatrizoate meglumide and sodium (Renografin 76) because of its greater density and better radiographic visibility. For clarity of detail, in addition to accurate localization, it is often useful to take one small coned-down view and a larger full lumbar view following each injection, especially when fluoroscopy is being used to obtain the radiographs. Between injections the patient is quickly questioned about how much pain he felt and the location of that pain. If the pain is unbearably severe, a PA radiograph should immediately be taken so that local anesthetic can be injected intradiscally at the painful site before proceeding to the remaining injections. If a single disc space is strongly suspect clinically, it is usually wise to leave injection of this disc space for last.

I frequently couple *anesthesia discography* with *contrast discography* by injecting 1 ml each of 1% lidocaine (Xylocaine) and 0.5% bupivacaine (Marcaine) intradiscally into the abnormal disc at the conclusion of contrast discography. If this dramatically relieves the patient of preexisting pain for several hours, useful information is gained. Patients who are strongly allergic to iodinated contrast media or who object to contrast discography because of previous painful experiences may be candidates for *anesthesia discography without prior contrast injection.* In a truly abnormal or inflamed disc, even injection of local anesthetics will often produce an initial burst of pain, but the rapid subsidence of preexisting back pain is diagnostically a most useful aspect of anesthesia discography. Following anesthesia discography, the patient is questioned about

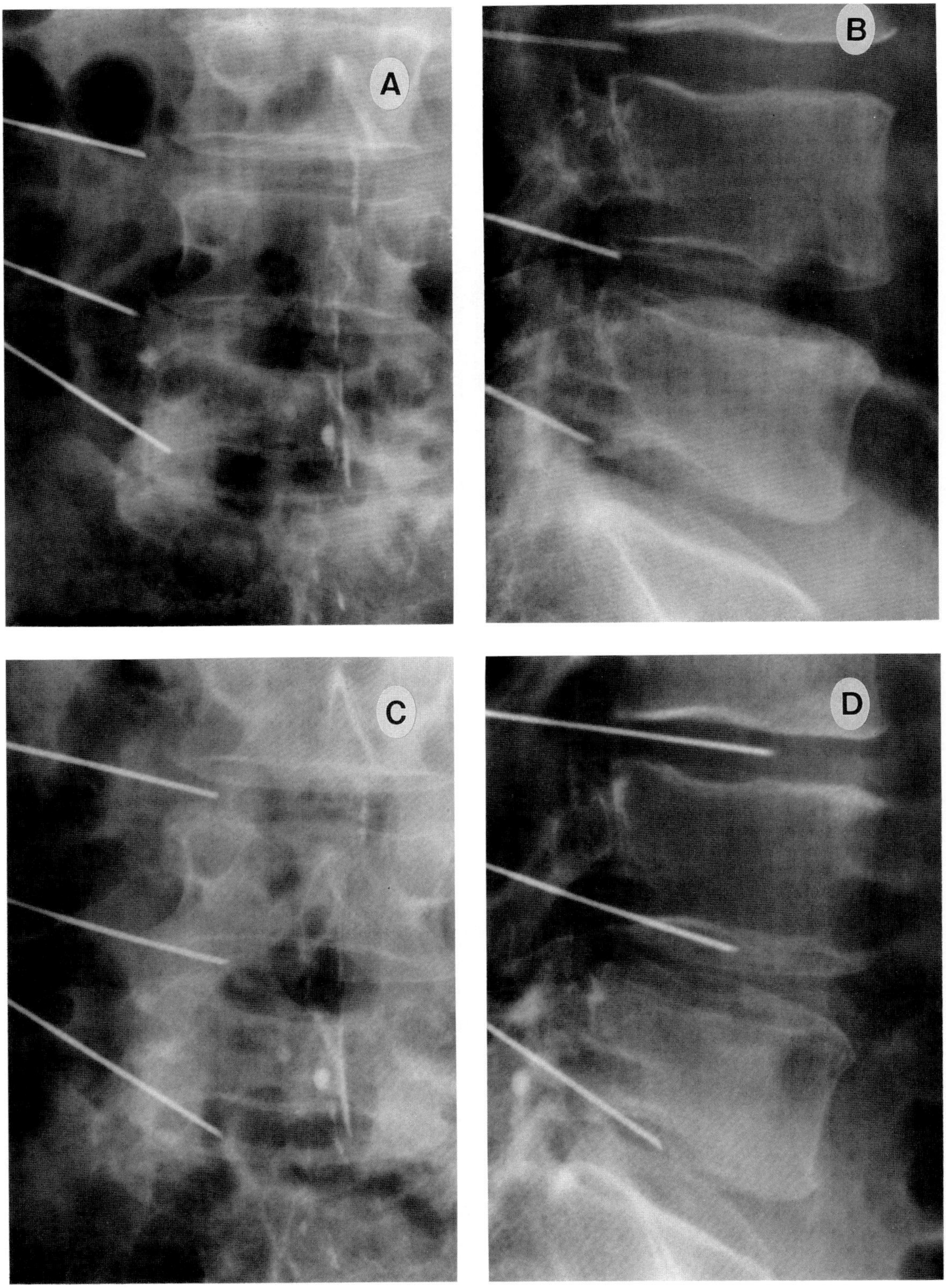

FIGURE 4.39. Multiple penetrations into the disc during discography can lead to extravasation of contrast material and confusing results. Biplane radiographs should be taken with needles at the corners of the disc (**A and B**) to confirm proper localization before penetration into the disc space (**C and D**).

pain relief obtained both within the next few minutes and over the subsequent several hours. After needle withdrawal, range of back motion is retested. A significant improvement in pain and in range of motion following anesthesia discography strongly implicates the injected disc as a major source of the patient's pain. Before removing the needles a decision should be made whether the patient should receive therapeutic intradiscal steroid injection (see Chapter 6).

Epidural Venography

Lumbar epidural venography is a logical radiographic extension of myelography, but has been made totally obsolete by CT and MRI scanning. Myelography delineates radiographically the space within the bony spinal canal that is occupied by the thecal sac but leaves unvisualized the epidural space. In the normal anatomical state, a considerable proportion of the *lumbar epidural space* is occupied by a plexus of veins, often referred to as *Batson's plexus*. Lumbar epidural venography attempts to fill these veins in the hope of delineating epidural mass lesions by visualizing filling defects in the epidural veins (Fig. 4.40).

Lumbar epidural venography was first accomplished by *transosseous injection* of lumbar epidural veins with contrast medium. Unfortunately, this test not only proved to be extremely uncomfortable for the patient but also gave unpredictable filling of the epidural plexus. A more recent evolution is epidural lumbar venography done by way of *retrograde catheter* insertion. The femoral vein is punctured unilaterally or bilaterally and a *Seldinger technique* is used to pass a catheter over a guide wire in retrograde fashion into the venous tree. Under fluoroscopic control, the catheter is manipulated into ascending lumbar veins and contrast medium is injected either unilaterally on the side of major

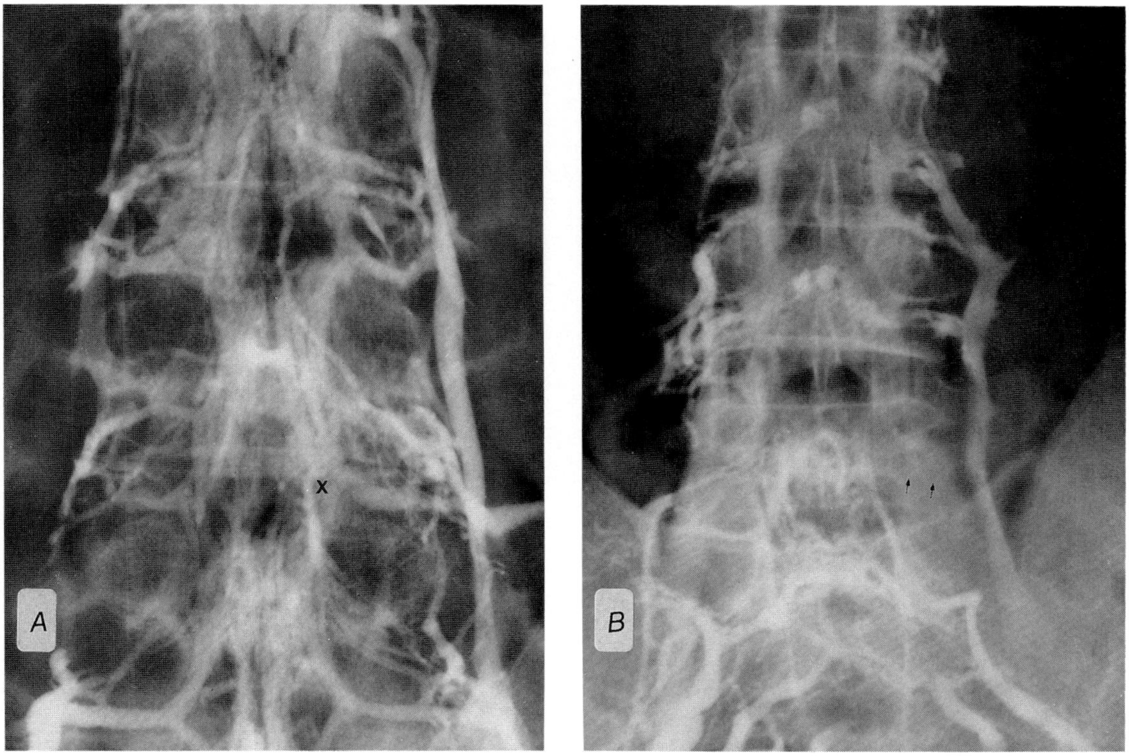

FIGURE 4.40. Lumbar epidural venography fills the veins in the epidural space and surrounds the lumbar vertebrae. **A:** Compression and nonfilling of the epidural veins (x) would occur in the presence of a disc rupture but is not seen in this normal study. To be reliably interpretable, contrast material must fill the veins both rostral and caudal to the area of interest. **B:** A flow-related artifact is seen in this "false positive" radiograph that was initially interpreted as representing disc rupture, although this was not confirmed by operative exploration. Arrows point to an area of nonfilling in a radicular vein caudal to the site of the presumed disc rupture.

symptoms or bilaterally. Radiographic "subtraction" techniques are often helpful in visualizing the contrast-filled venous plexus.

The goal of epidural venography is to delineate mass lesions in the lumbar epidural space. Before a study can accurately be *interpreted as abnormal,* the following two technical conditions must be met: (1) adequate venous filling must be demonstrated, and (2) there must be a focal area of nonfilling of veins in the epidural space. Epidural venography is of little value in attempting to document the presence of recurrent disc rupture at a previously operated site. During the course of disc excision, epidural veins are commonly coagulated and most often remain nonfilling on subsequent epidural venography.

Epidurography

Another radiodiagnostic study has been offered as an alternative to lumbar epidural venography. *Epidurography* also attempts to fill the epidural space that lies beyond the capability of myelography to visualize (Fig. 4.41). This study, which has also been made obsolete by CT and MRI scanning, involves direct injection of water-soluble contrast material into the epidural space. This is accomplished by passing a catheter through the sacral hiatus and manipulating its tip under fluoroscopic control into one or both lateral epidural spaces or "gutters." Water-soluble contrast material injected at this site infiltrates between epidural fat globules and veins and usually neatly outlines lumbar nerve roots. If adequate filling is obtained, mass lesions can be delineated by focal filling defects and by visualization of distortion and shifting of nerve roots. Following surgery, postoperative scarring may interfere with catheter placement or with adequate filling, making interpretation difficult. The test is perhaps somewhat easier to perform than epidural venography, but it is approximately equally unpleasant for the patient.

Radioactive Isotope Scans

Radioactive isotope scans are occasionally useful in the diagnosis of patients with the failed back syndrome. Scans done with radioactively tagged diphosphonate are capable of demonstrating abnor-

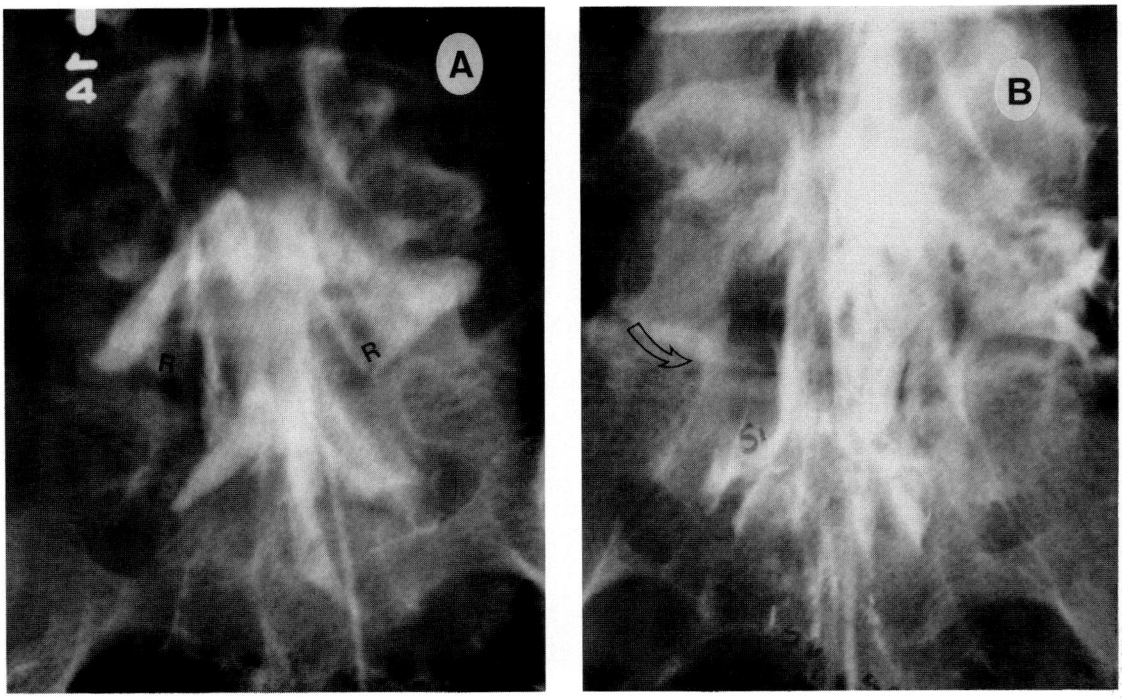

FIGURE 4.41. Epidurography is designed to disclose mass lesions in the spinal canal that do not impinge upon the thecal sac. **A:** The normal epidurogram shows good delineation of both S1 nerve roots (R). **B:** This epidurogram shows displacement of the S1 nerve root medially and nonfilling of the lateral epidural space at L5-S1 (arrow) in a patient whose myelogram showed no obvious abnormality. Confirmatory discography at L5-S1 was classically abnormal for lateral disc rupture and surgical exploration was likewise confirmatory.

mal uptake in areas of *active arthritis.* Since inflammatory and degenerative arthritis are high on the list of differential diagnostic possibilities for patients suffering chronic back pain, isotope scans may at times be useful supplements to plain radiography by delineating the degree of biological activity or active inflammation in a given disc, facet, or sacroiliac joint.

On occasion, plain radiographs may show minimal or equivocal changes, and documentation of clearly abnormal isotope uptake may help to confirm the diagnosis of *pseudarthrosis of a spinal fusion.* Symptomatic pseudarthroses are often associated with an element of local inflammatory reaction. If this process is sufficiently severe, it may be detected by a local increased uptake on radioisotope scanning. Unfortunately, the diagnosis of pseudarthrosis and the establishment of the true symptomatic nature of a pseudarthrosis are both sufficiently imprecise that no clear documentation is available about the percentage of patients whose symptomatic pseudarthrosis can be documented on isotope scanning. Nonetheless, a positive scan can be a helpful confirmatory test, although a negative scan certainly does not exclude the possibility of a pseudarthrosis that causes symptoms either through local inflammation or through secondary subjacent scarring in the epidural space.

Metastatic carcinoma of the lumbar spine remains a worrisome though uncommon cause of back pain that may be misdiagnosed or overlooked in the failed back syndrome patient. Bone scans with radioactive technetium or other isotopes may detect abnormal uptake even before radiographic changes have become diagnostic.

Scanning with *radioactively tagged autogenous white blood cells* may be useful in detecting occult infection.[54] Postoperative infections are usually readily diagnosed clinically, but they occasionally present as diagnostic problems. Bone scans may or may not be positive in the presence of osteomyelitis, and white cell scans may prove to be a useful supplement.

Diagnostic Injections

Diagnostic injection of anesthetics plays an important and underused role in the diagnosis and management of patients with previously unoperated back disease, but plays an even more important role in the treatment of failed back syndrome sufferers. These patients usually have already undergone excision of one or more lumbar discs, with or without spinal fusion. Since their pain persists, or has recurred despite previous surgery, the likelihood is great that the etiology of their pain is something other than classic disc protrusion.

Diagnostic anesthetic injections are useful in *three groups of patients* who suffer from failed back syndrome: (1) those in whom diagnostic radiography discloses no abnormality, (2) those in whom diagnostic radiography is only equivocally abnormal, or the relationship between the abnormality and the patient's symptoms is unclear, and (3) those who present with clinical pictures suggesting diagnoses in which diagnostic anesthetic injections may be helpful but do not require diagnostic radiography for confirmation. In all three of these patient groups, diagnostic anesthetic injections can be extremely useful in diagnosing painful conditions not diagnosed on radiography, in confirming the clinical relevance of radiographic abnormalities, and in confirming a clinical diagnosis without radiography, especially diagnosis of conditions that involve local tender areas.

Six major types of diagnostic anesthetic injections will be considered. (*Anesthesia discography* was discussed earlier in this chapter and will not be discussed again here.) Diagnostic injections into *local tender areas* are chiefly useful in patients with low back pain and postfusion problems. Diagnostic injections into *facet nerves* and *joints* or *sacroiliac joints* are likewise useful for patients with back pain, even though both disorders cause radiation of pain to the buttock and posterior thigh. *Lumbar sympathetic ganglion blocks* are most useful for patients with leg pain of a type suggesting sympathetically mediated pain. *Epidural* or *paravertebral injections, nerve root injections,* and *intrathecal* or *spinal anesthetic injections* are more useful in patients with leg pain, but are occasionally employed for patients with predominantly back pain.

Local Tender Areas

Diagnostic anesthetic injections into local tender areas are useful in patients with back pain who are suspected clinically of having periosteal or muscular *trigger point pain* (see page 21), *fasciitis* (see page 21), *ischiogluteal bursitis* (see page 22), painful *neuromata* (see page 25), or *coccydynia* (see page 56). Periosteal trigger points and areas of fasciitis occur most commonly along the posterior iliac crest or sacroiliac ligaments, but may occur in interspinous ligaments, laterally over the iliac crests, or at points of muscle attachment to fusion bone. Painful neuromata that cause a failed back syndrome are almost exclusively encountered at the site of donor bone removal for spinal fusion. The midline incision used for laminectomy generally does not interrupt nerve fibers, so the chance of neuroma formation in the midline of the back is quite small. Painful and locally tender areas associated with *pseudarthrosis* may occur either over a pseudarthrotic line through the body of the fusion or at the upper end of the fusion at points of impingement on adjacent normal bone—so-called *kissing pseudarthrosis*. Ischiogluteal bursitis and coccydynia produce characteristic clinical symptoms, and both have in common pain and tenderness that are especially prominent when the patient sits. In ischiogluteal bursitis, the area of maximum tenderness usually directly overlies the ischial tuberosity and may be best palpated with the hip flexed or the patient seated. The point of maximum tenderness in coccydynia is usually at the point of attachment of the coccyx to the sacrum and may be most easily apparent on bidigital palpation with one finger in the rectum and one finger on the cutaneous surface of the coccyx.

Diagnostic injection of these tender areas calls for a similar *technique* in each instance (Fig. 4.42). After locating the area of maximum tenderness, the skin is prepared with antiseptic solution and an intracutaneous wheal of 1% lidocaine (Xylocaine) is raised. Additional lidocaine is injected incrementally as the needle is advanced through the skin wheal into the center of the tender area. For most injections, a 22- or 25-gauge needle is preferred, but in areas of previous surgery, scarring may make manipulation of a 25-gauge needle difficult. The needle length required will vary with the patient's adiposity and may range from a standard 1.5-inch injection needle to a 3.5-inch lumbar puncture needle. I find that a pediatric 2.5-inch LP needle is often useful. Once the center of the area of maximum tenderness has been needled, injections may proceed using lidocaine only, lidocaine mixed with the longer-acting anesthetic bupivacaine (Mar-

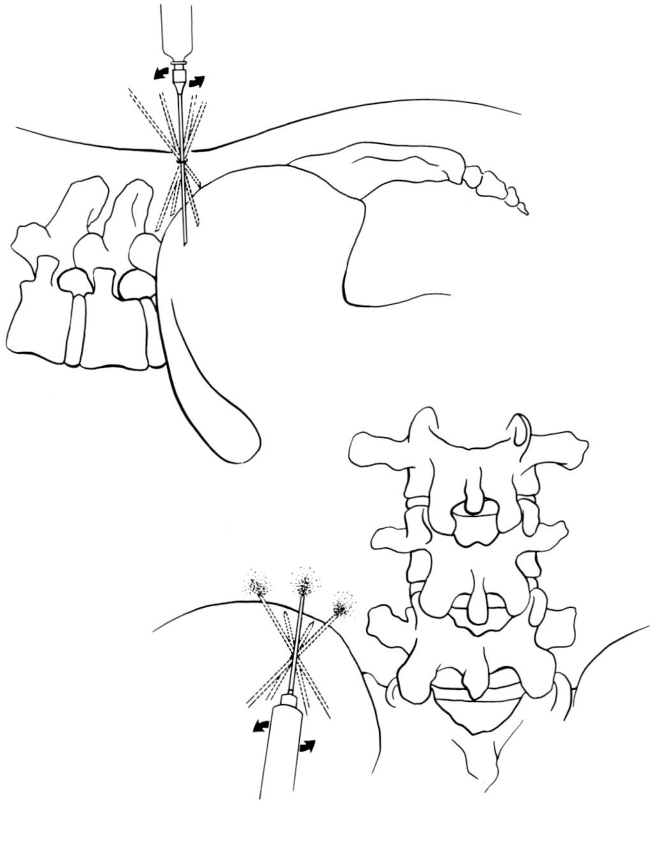

FIGURE 4.42. Periosteal trigger points should be injected in the direct center of the area of tenderness and in the surrounding, immediately adjacent tissues. Most trigger points occur at sites of ligamentous attachment to bones, especially along the posterior iliac crest. The center of tenderness is usually in or adjacent to the periosteum and injections should be placed as close to the bone as feasible. The operator should keep in mind the three-dimensional nature of the area, injecting both above and below the area of maximum tenderness, as well as around this area.

caine) (0.5% or 0.75%), or with lidocaine followed by injection at the same site with bupivacaine. After initial injection of the center of the tender area injections are made circumferentially at four to eight points around the margin of the area. In patients with periosteal trigger points or tender pseudarthroses, the area of maximum tenderness will be adjacent to bone, and injections should be placed quite close to the bone, infiltrating the periosteum surrounding the center of maximum tenderness. Full anesthetization may require that some injections be given at deeper levels than others. At the conclusion of the diagnostic injection, most or preferably all local tenderness should have been eliminated. Prior to needle withdrawal, one should consider the possibility of simultaneous therapeutic injection of depository corticosteroids or prolotherapy solution (see the discussion on corticosteroid and anesthetic injections of local tender areas and prolotherapy in Chapter 6). With the area anesthetized, the patient is asked to bend, move, sit, or perform other functions that would normally be painful. The immediate impact on pain is assessed in terms of approximate percentage reduction of the patient's overall pain problem (i.e., the reduction of his local pain and tenderness and the improvement in his range of motion). Relieving such a local area may bring the patient welcome relief but may still leave him disabled by more diffuse pain, pain at other sites, or persistent pain on motion. Assessment by the patient of longer-term functional improvement after he leaves the office is equally important and is often aided by having the patient make written notes of the amount of relief and the time of pain return. On rare occasions, diagnostic injections give long-lasting relief of a painful tender area, but much more commonly pain recurs after one to two hours if only lidocaine was used or after six to ten hours if bupivacaine was used.

Facet Nerves and Joints

Diagnostic anesthetic injections into facet nerves or *joints* may be quite useful in the diagnosis of the facet syndrome (see pages 19 and 64).[50] It has become apparent clinically and from CT scans that many patients previously diagnosed as having lumbar disc disease instead suffer from a painful facet syndrome. This syndrome may be suggested by a characteristic clinical history and by specific features of the physical examination. Plain radiographs and CT scans may demonstrate obvious abnormalities of the facet joints but do not provide the necessary clinical correlation between radiographic abnormality and clinical symptomatology. Myelographic and discographic abnormalities are not produced by this syndrome except in rare instances when extreme hypertrophy or deformity of the facet is so severe that it impinges on the thecal sac. In most patients with facet syndrome, diagnostic injection is the only way to obtain clinical confirmation of the diagnosis—short of definitive surgery.

Facet joint injections are often beneficial for patients, but they also provide graphic instruction in *human physiology* for the clinician. When a needle penetrates a facet joint or its capsule, the patient experiences pain ipsilaterally in the lower back and strongly in the buttock and posterior thigh. Needling the annulus of the intervertebral disc produces pain in a similar pattern, but contact with a lumbar nerve root elicits pain felt most strongly distally in the leg or foot. Thus the clinician who uses a needle to perform invasive diagnostic or therapeutic procedures on patients with failed back disorders has the opportunity to fully appreciate the distinctions between "mechanical" and "sciatic" back and leg pain drawn in Chapter 3.

Diagnostic anesthetic injections in the facet syndrome may be performed *unilaterally* in patients with unilateral low back, buttock, and posterior thigh pain, especially if plain radiographs show unilateral facet abnormalities. More commonly, patients complain of translumbar or bilateral back pain, and these patients require *bilateral* injection. If radiographic abnormalities or previous back surgery at a single level suggests the possibility that a single pair of facets is involved, the injection may be limited to the two nerves on both sides that supply this *one pair of facet joints* (Fig. 4.43).

On the other hand, if there is no strong reason to suspect symptomatic abnormality at a single facet level, diagnostic injections are performed at *multiple levels* with anesthetization of two or three of the lower lumbar pairs of facet joints (L5-S1, L4-L5, and often L3-L4) (Fig. 4.44). If adequate anesthetization of all six facet joints (three on each side) fails to produce significant relief of pain, the likelihood of symptomatic facet syndrome is considerably reduced. Exceptions to this rule are extremely rare but may occasionally be encountered, as illustrated by the following case:

Case 5

A 27-year-old fashion model developed increasingly severe back and left leg pain following lifting. Bed rest therapy was pursued for two months after a myelogram showed no abnormality. During this period, pain remained severe and a mild but definite footdrop developed. Diagnostic discography showed a classic lateral disc rupture at L3-L4, but was normal at L4-L5 and L5-S1. Disc excision relieved her of radiating leg pain and footdrop, but mid to upper lumbar back pain slowly increased. Pain was characterized by a constant deep aching pain and a sharper secondary pain on bending. Bending produced an audible click in the mid lumbar region but radiographs, including flexion/extension films, showed no abnormality other than postsurgical changes at L3-L4. Anesthesia discography at L3-L4 temporarily reduced the deep aching component of pain, but intradiscal steroid injections gave no lasting relief. A modified interbody bone fusion gave only partial improvement in the deep pain but no improvement in pain on motion. Diagnostic anesthetization of the L3-L4 facet gave a modest improvement in overall pain. Posterolateral fusion with the aid of Harrington rods was then performed at L3-L4. Following this, she regained some mobility of her back, but deep aching pain and pain on motion still prevented her from pursuing an active exercise program despite a conscientious effort on her part.

Repeat myelography, repeat discography at L4-L5 and L5-S1, and diagnostic anesthetization of the facet joints at L4-L5 and L5-S1 showed no abnormality and gave no pain relief. Anesthetization of the L2-L3 facet, however, gave dramatic relief of the severe deep aching pain and distinctly improved her range of motion. A series of phenol interruptions of the facet nerves coupled with intrafacet steroid injections has given her long periods of relief of the deep pain component and has permitted her to begin a restorative back exercise program for the first time in four years.

Facet nerve injections may also be diagnostically useful *following spinal fusion* (Fig. 4.45). Even if the spinal fusion involved destruction of the facet joints, fusion of these joints, and interruption of the facet nerves, facet nerves do regenerate and eventually reinnervate the fusion bone. Some patients may later develop painful pseudarthrosis or painful avulsion of muscular or ligamentous attachments to

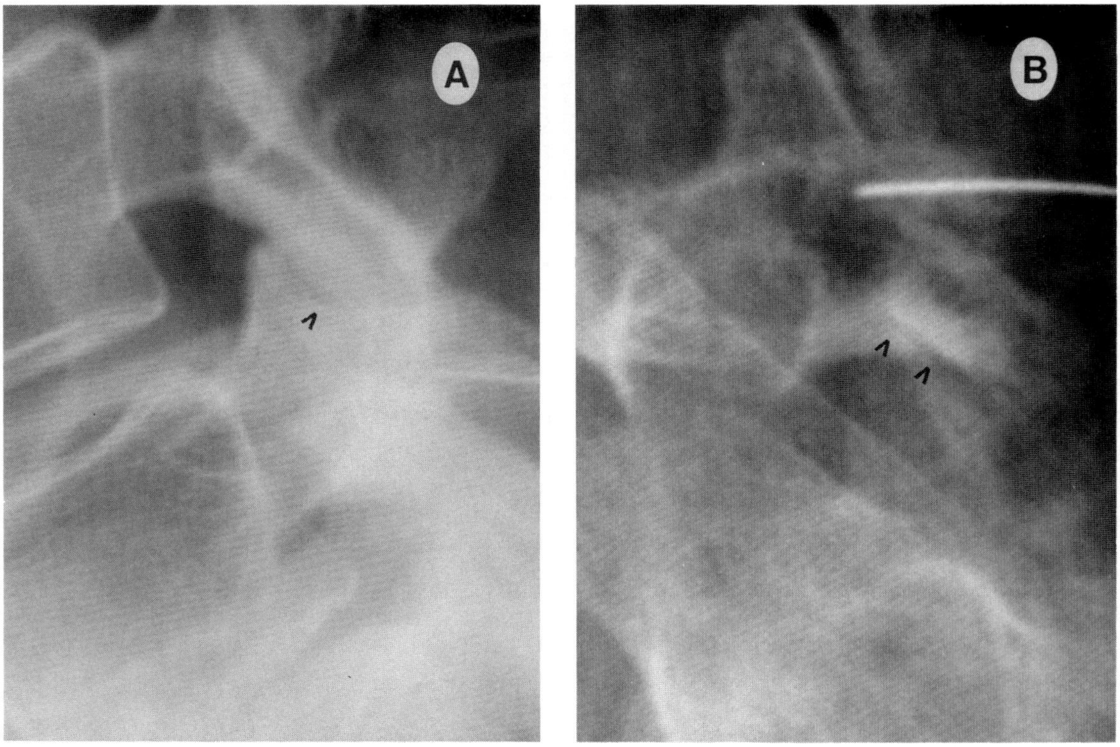

FIGURE 4.43. Injection of the nerves to a single sclerotic and deformed facet (v's) can be done with one skin wheal and two separate placements of the same lumbar puncture needle. Needle tips are positioned above and below the target facet. Radiographs are taken with the patient in the **(A)** lateral and **(B)** oblique positions with the needle tip first below, then above the L4-L5 facet.

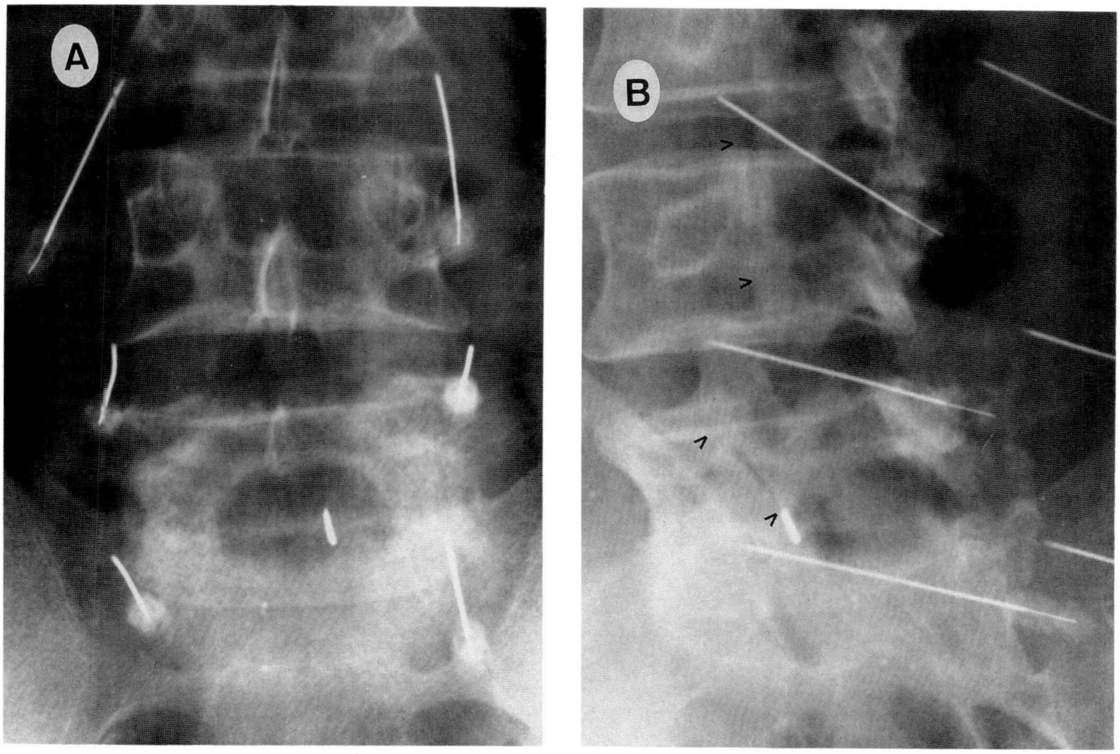

FIGURE 4.44. Injection of two or more pairs of lumbar facets involves multiple needle placement to interrupt both superior and inferior nerves to each facet. Needle tips should be positioned just above the upper facet, just below the lower facet, and midway between adjacent facets. These radiographs demonstrate anesthetization and phenol facet rhizotomy at L4-L5 and L5-S1 bilaterally. Radiographs are taken in **(A)** posteroanterior and **(B)** oblique patient positions. V's mark rostral and caudal ends of L4-L5 and L5-S1 facets.

the fusion bone from trauma or exertion. Pain from these sites will be transmitted along the facet nerves, and interruption of these nerves can be helpful in documenting such fusion-related causes of low back pain in the failed back syndrome. When facet nerves regenerate, their anatomic location may be altered somewhat, but usually the more proximal segment of the nerve retains approximately its normal position relative to the neuroforamen.

Diagnostic and therapeutic injections into facet nerves and into facet joints employ a similar *technique*. Both are usually done with the patient prone on a fluoroscopy table. Since each facet is innervated by a pair of nerves, one entering the rostral end of the facet and the other entering the caudal end, anesthetization of a single facet requires interruption of two nerves. Injections of local anesthetics directly into facet joints are sometimes performed, but this may fail to anesthetize the facet capsule, and anesthetic may extravasate medially through the joint into the epidural space, producing confusing anesthesia of nerve roots. The rostral and caudal facet nerves arise from a single common branch from the nerve root as it exits through the neuroforamen. Interrupting this common branch midway between two adjacent facets will thus anesthetize the rostral half of the caudal facet and the caudal half of the rostral facet. After antiseptic skin preparation, skin wheals are raised 6 cm to 8 cm lateral to the lumbar midline at the rostral and caudal ends of the facets, or pairs of facets, that are to be injected. One skin wheal and one 22-gauge lumbar puncture needle may be placed at each site under fluoroscopic control, or a single skin wheal may be raised and a single needle may be inserted first rostral then caudal to the target facet through the same skin wheal. Under fluoroscopic guidance, needle tips are inserted just caudal to the lowest facet joint to be injected, midway between two adjacent target facets and just rostral to the most rostral facet that is to be injected. The needles are placed 2 mm to 3 mm

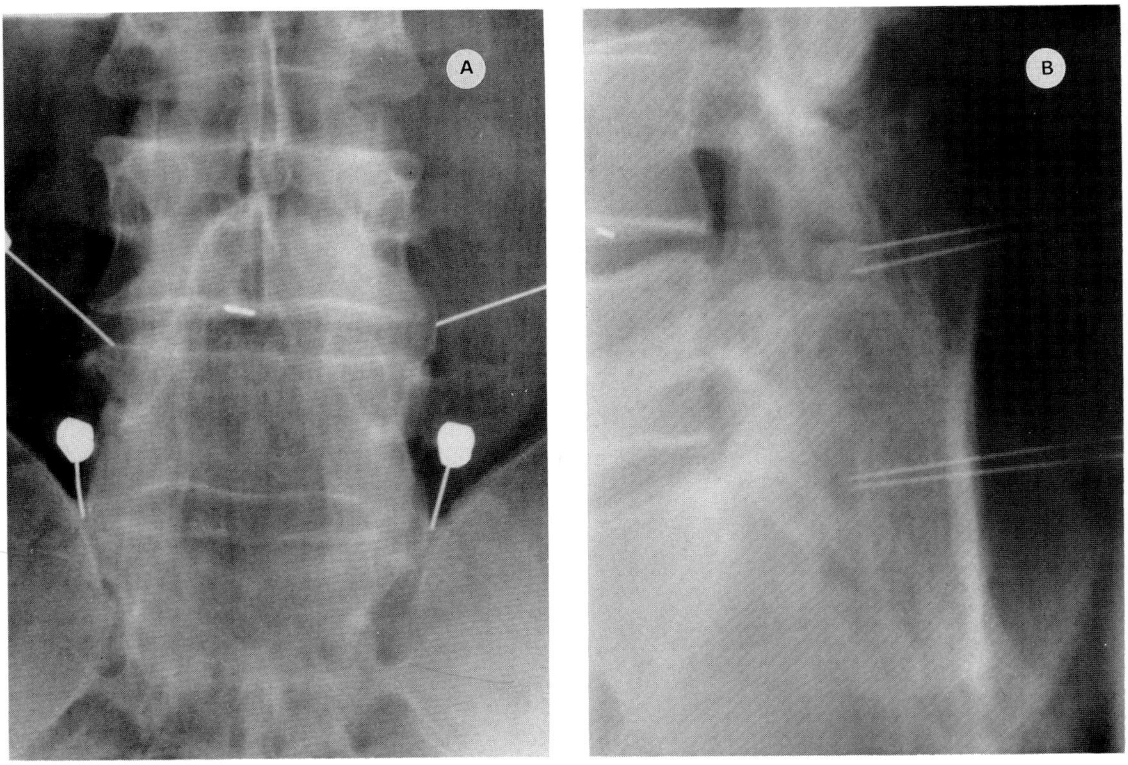

FIGURE 4.45. Facet nerve blocks can be diagnostically useful following spinal fusion in patients suspected of painful pseudarthrosis or avulsion of scar and muscular attachments from the fusion bone, as seen here on PA **(A)** and lateral **(B)** radiographs. Low back pain and percussion tenderness persisted in this young man after he fell several years following spinal fusion. Successful diagnostic anesthetization of recurrent facet nerves supplying the fusion led eventually to prolonged improvement through the use of local steroid injection in addition to a back brace.

lateral to the pedicles and are penetrated to a depth of 4 mm or 5 mm superficial to the dorsal rim of the neural foramen, as seen on lateral radiographs. Needle position is confirmed fluoroscopically and recorded for the permanent record with posteroanterior, lateral, and right and left oblique projections. The oblique projections most clearly delineate the facet joints and confirm with certainty needle placement relative to the rostral and caudal extent of these joints. Once needle placement is confirmed and documented, 2 ml of lidocaine (Xylocaine) or lidocaine and bupivacaine (Marcaine) are injected at each needle site prior to needle withdrawal or therapeutic injection.

Permanent radiographic records are extremely important if a series of facet nerve procedures is to be performed on a given patient. This is especially true if diagnostic facet anesthetization yields dramatic pain relief and subsequent therapeutic injection therapy or radio-frequency (RF) lesioning is planned. Adequate anesthetization of facet joints cannot be tested from the cutaneous surface and can be assessed only in terms of pain relief. It is extremely frustrating to be unable to reproduce an initial dramatic response to injection and not have confirmatory radiographs available to lessen the possibility that failure of the second procedure is due to placement of the injection needle at a different site.

Once the facets have been injected and needles have been withdrawn, *the patient should be tested immediately* for range of back motion and should be questioned about spontaneous pain and pain on movement. Immediate, dramatic relief is occasionally seen and is important diagnostically. However, the *longer-term result* over several hours should also be assessed, since the excitement and discomfort of the injection may confuse the patient's immediate assessment of his response. For this reason, it is valuable to employ bupivacaine (Marcaine) along with lidocaine (Xylocaine) to give a more lasting anesthetization. Patients should be instructed to assess their level of pain and tolerance of back bending over the period of several hours during which anesthesia is likely to persist. The combination of good pain relief followed by rapid recurrence of symptoms is confirmatory of a therapeutically useful response to diagnostic injection. The patient should be specifically questioned and cautioned about the possibility of induced numbness and weakness in the leg or legs. If this occurs, the patient may fall and be injured. Furthermore, the presence of analgesia or anesthesia in the leg seriously confuses the results of facet nerve injection, since one is unable to tell whether pain relief results from facet anesthetization or from anesthetization of nerve roots.

Sacroiliac Joint Injection

Unilateral or bilateral lumbago, often with radiation of pain from lower lumbar or posterior pelvic areas into posterior thighs or upper lumbar areas, may derive from *arthralgia,* or joint pain, originating in the *sacroiliac (SI) joints.* This possibility is especially likely if forceful pelvic twisting motions or percussion with fist or rubber hammer over one or both SI joints triggers pain. Radiographs and isotope scans may or may not be abnormal, but diagnostic anesthetic block may be useful in drawing clinical correlations.

Diagnostic anesthetic injection of the SI joint can be done with or without radiographic or fluoroscopic confirmation, but x-ray guidance can help to localize the joint, and intraarticular contrast injection provides absolute confirmation that the joint has been injected. The joint is approached with a 20- or 22-gauge spinal needle in a medial to lateral direction from anesthetic skin wheals 2 cm to 3 cm lateral to the midline of the upper sacrum, thus allowing the needles to pass beneath the overhanging posterior margin of the iliac bone. One to 5 ml of lidocaine (Xylocaine), bupivacaine (Marcaine), or a mixture of both is injected for each joint, then the patient is assessed for relief of spontaneous pain, pain on pelvic twisting, and pain on percussion.

Sympathetic Ganglion Blocks

Sympathetically medicated dysfunction in the failed back patient is usually manifest as a characteristic type of leg pain, often termed *causalgia* or *reflex sympathetic dystrophy.* The pain is nearly always associated with painful hypersensitivity and is frequently associated with dystrophic swelling, joint stiffness, discoloration, altered sweating, or loss of skin integrity (i.e., the dystrophic component of reflex sympathetic dystrophy). The pain is usually described as a constant burning pain, sharply aggravated by activity or skin contact. Not uncommonly, however, the pain syndrome is atypical or not characteristic, and a correct diagnosis may not be possible without diagnostic anesthetic blocks. Furthermore, in this condition early diagnosis is extremely important, since early therapy has a greatly improved chance of success—and successful early therapy may require only one or more diagnostic anesthetic blocks.

The *technique of lumbar sympathetic ganglion anesthetic injection* requires fluoroscopic guidance. One or more 3.5-inch or longer 22-gauge needles are passed through skin wheals 6 cm to 10 cm lateral to the midline, and their tips are placed close to the sides of the target lumbar vertebrae, penetrating (on lateral views) nearly to the ventral aspect of the body. L2, L3, and probably L4 sympathetic ganglia project to the lower extremity, each ganglion lying at or just caudal to the intervertebral disc. Mixing contrast material with the local anesthetic permits confirmation that the anesthetic remains in the retroperitoneal space and reaches all of the desired sympathetic ganglia. The effectiveness of sympatholysis, or interruption of sympathetic outflow, is usually confirmed by monitoring increases in skin temperature or blood flow in the injected limb. Relief of pain and hypersensitivity once good sympatholysis has been achieved confirms that the pain was sympathetically mediated.

Nerve Roots

Diagnostic anesthetic injection of *nerve roots epidurally or paravertebrally* is chiefly useful in failed back syndrome patients who suffer from *sciatic pain* radiating into the lower leg. (Midline epidural anesthetic injection not aimed at specific nerve roots is discussed in the next section.) Patients with unilateral low back pain or with buttock and posterior thigh pain in addition to back pain are less likely to be relieved by nerve root blocks. Patients with bilateral lumbar pain or bilateral low back, buttock, and posterior thigh pain rarely benefit from or experience temporary pain relief from nerve root diagnostic injections, because this type of pain usually does not arise primarily from nerve roots and rarely arises from a structure innervated either by a single nerve root or by two or three adjacent nerve roots.

Intraspinal, epidural nerve root blocks may not be possible in a patient who has undergone standard posterior fusion unless a midline fenestration has been left, but should usually be possible following a posterolateral or transverse process spinal fusion if no fusion bone has been placed over the posterior midline. Even following spinal fusion, *paraspinal nerve root blocks* can usually be performed.[55] The S1 and S2 nerve roots can usually be reached through the sacral foramina, since these are rarely covered with fusion bone (Fig. 4.46).

In patients with previous single-level back surgery or with patterns of sensory or motor loss suggesting single nerve root involvement, nerve root anesthetization at a single level is usually done before proceeding to anesthetization of two or more adjacent nerve roots. If a nerve root is entrapped and irritated by intraspinal epidural scar tissue, anesthetizing that root further laterally in the paraspinal area may fail to interrupt centripetal transmission of pain impulses and may fail to provide pain relief. On the other hand, dense epidural scarring may preclude satisfactory anesthetization of a nerve root by intraspinal needle placement. Anesthetization of a nerve root cannot be considered to be of diagnostic quality unless high-grade analgesia of the appropriate nerve root cutaneous territory is achieved. If anesthetization of a single nerve root gives clear-cut relief of pain, additional therapy at the same session may be considered: local steroid injection or attempted mechanical disruption of adhesions through forceful fluid injections or forced straight leg raising. If the pain relief achieved is incomplete or insufficient, despite adequate nerve root anesthetization, repeat nerve blocks simultaneously at the same level and at an adjacent level should be considered. Not uncommonly, two adjacent nerve roots are painfully involved in scar tissue, and good pain relief is not achieved until both roots are anesthetized simultaneously. If relief from pain is not achieved, despite good anesthesia, injection of one

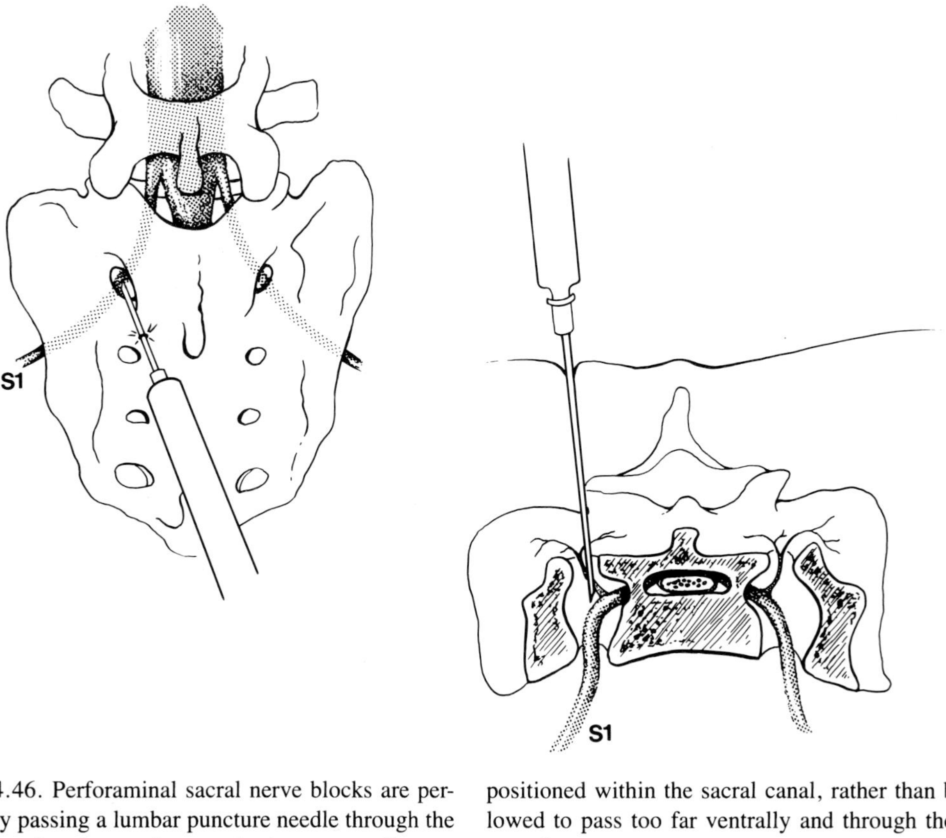

FIGURE 4.46. Perforaminal sacral nerve blocks are performed by passing a lumbar puncture needle through the appropriate dorsal neuroforamen in the sacrum. For optimum nerve root anesthesia, the needle tip should be positioned within the sacral canal, rather than being allowed to pass too far ventrally and through the ventral neuroforamen.

or more adjacent nerve roots should be considered, since the single nerve root initially anesthetized in this instance is most likely not the source of the patient's pain.

Unfortunately, diagnostic nerve root anesthetization is *not absolutely accurate* since, as mentioned above, pain in a single nerve root may originate proximal to the point of nerve injection and may yet be amenable to ablative therapy. For these patients, spinal, intrathecal blocks may be useful.

Standard technique dictates that diagnostic nerve root blocks should be done with *radiographic control* (Fig. 4.47). The patient is usually positioned prone on the fluoroscopic table. The lumbar skin is prepared with antiseptic, then one or two skin wheals are raised with lidocaine (Xylocaine). To perform *intraspinal epidural blocks,* the skin wheal is placed either in the lumbar midline over the appropriate interspinous space or slightly to the contralateral side. Under fluoroscopic control, a 20- or 22-gauge spinal needle is introduced with the aid of incremental local lidocaine injections and is positioned through the interlaminar space in an oblique direction aimed as far laterally and caudally as possible. The needle tip should lie adjacent to the nerve root as it curves laterally to exit through the neuroforamen at the next lower level. Contact with the nerve root will elicit radiating sciatic pain, which should mimic the distribution of the patient's customary pain. Lateral fluoroscopy should confirm placement of the needle near the neuroforamen. Care must be taken not to injure the nerve root at this point in the procedure, and needle advancement should be avoided once the nerve root has been anesthetized for fear of injuring the root. Once the needle is in place, it is wise to obtain permanent radiographs for the patient's record and for future reference. Incremental injections of 0.25 ml or 0.5 ml volumes of lidocaine with or without bupivacaine (Marcaine) are then made while sensory testing is carried out on the appropriate limb. It is best not to exceed a volume of 1 ml of anesthetic, since this is likely to spread to adjacent nerve roots and result in a confusing picture. If appropriate anesthe-

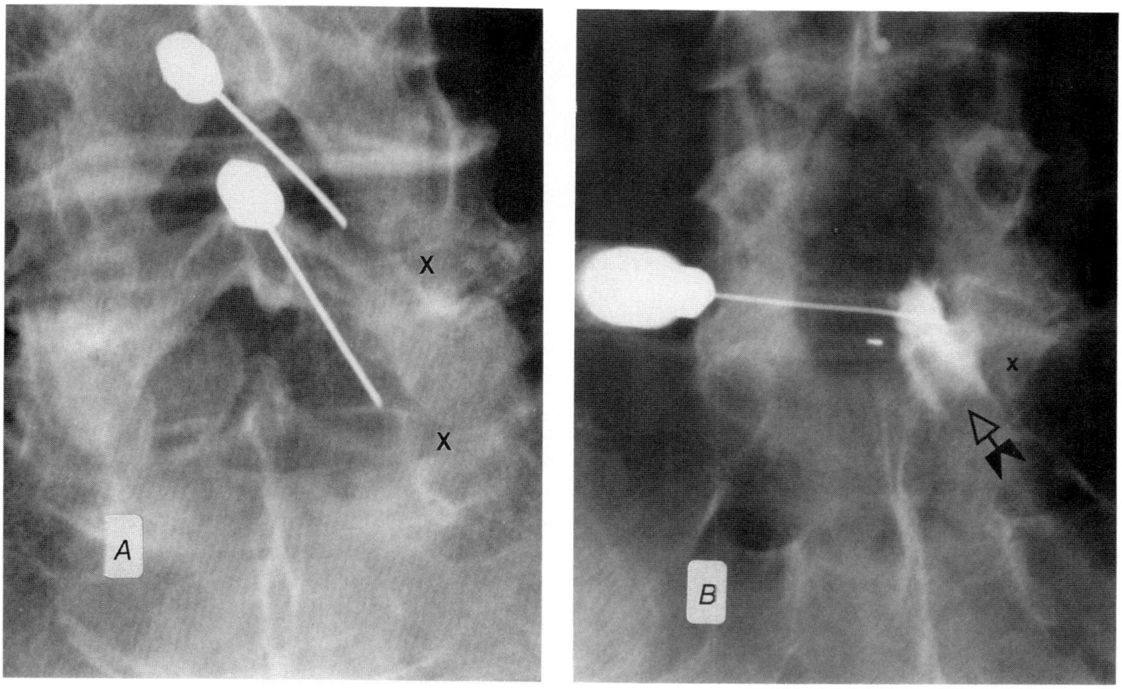

FIGURE 4.47. **A:** Lumbar epidural nerve root block is performed by placing needles under fluoroscopic guidance laterally in the spinal canal through the interlaminar spaces or through a surgical defect in a posterior or posterolateral fusion. The needle tip should be positioned adjacent to the nerve root as it swings around the pedicle (x) on its way to exit laterally through the neuroforamen. **B:** Proper positioning can usually be documented by eliciting paresthesiae with needle placement and appropriate sensory loss with injection of an anesthetic. Injection of a water soluble contrast agent can be used to confirm injection of anesthetic around the nerve root (arrow).

sia does not rapidly develop, especially in a previously operated interspace, it may be informative to inject 0.5 ml of 60% diatrizoate meglumide and sodium (Renografin 60) or other water-soluble contrast agent for fluoroscopic confirmation of the distribution of the anesthetic agent. When scar tissue is present, occasionally contrast injection will disclose that the anesthetic solution escapes to the contralateral side or migrates rostrally or caudally to an adjacent nerve root.

When a *paraspinal nerve root block* is planned, the skin wheal should be raised 4 cm to 6 cm lateral to the midline on the appropriate side and at a level even with the tip of the spinous process adjacent to the desired interspace. Under fluoroscopic control and with incremental injection of local lidocaine (Xylocaine), a 20- or 22-gauge needle is introduced just lateral to the facet mass and is guided by fluoroscopy with the patient prone and in the oblique position to a point just lateral but adjacent to the neuroforamen, keeping in mind that this nerve root would be more likely to have been injured by a disc rupture at the next most rostral disc space (see page 9). As the needle approaches the neuroforamen, caution should be observed to avoid damaging the nerve root, but close approximation to the nerve root, yielding tingling or electric sensation in the appropriate distribution in the leg, usually heralds a successful block. Once the needle position has been documented by permanent radiographs, 2 ml of lidocaine or lidocaine with bupivacaine (Marcaine) are injected and sensory testing is carried out on the appropriate limb. Paraspinal injections are unlikely to spread to adjacent nerve roots but may be distal to the source of nerve root irritation and therefore may produce anesthesia without pain relief, even when the appropriate nerve root has been injected.

Intrathecal or Epidural Spinal Injections

Intrathecal or epidural spinal injections may be used to produce unilateral or bilateral temporary sensory loss in the lower extremities. Epidural anesthetization of individual nerve roots was discussed in the preceding section. More extensive epidural spinal blocks are occasionally used diagnostically and are commonly employed as a therapeutic maneuver (see the discussion of epidural injections in Chapter 6).

Epidural spinal blocks are accomplished by placing a lumbar puncture needle or indwelling catheter in the midline epidural space. Lidocaine (Xylocaine) or bupivacaine (Marcaine) injected at this site usually produces bilateral sensory loss, with relatively less severe motor loss. In patients with a failed back syndrome, epidural scarring may interfere with spread of the anesthetic solution, resulting in a patchy or asymmetric area of analgesia. This unpredictability limits the usefulness of epidural spinal blocks as diagnostic procedures, since intrathecal spinal blocks yield more predictable and controllable results. When epidural spinal anesthetic injections are employed, care must be taken to ensure that the injection is indeed into the epidural space and not into the subarachnoid space. Epidural injections usually employ larger amounts of anesthetic than is needed for subarachnoid injection to ensure transdural penetration. The solutions used are usually isobaric to spinal fluid, so inadvertent subarachnoid injection may produce a dangerously extensive, dense spinal anesthesia. Patients with lumbar *adhesive arachnoiditis* may have no CSF at the needle puncture site, making it difficult to guard against subarachnoid puncture. Large volume injections into areas of arachnoiditis may cause local nerve root compression and injury that can be severe and permanent.

Unilateral or "one leg" spinal *subarachnoid blocks* are useful for patients with sciatica in whom individual nerve root blocks have yielded negative or equivocal results. These blocks are especially useful diagnostically for patients with unilateral low back or leg pain in whom intrathecal chemical rhizotomy or thoracic cordotomy is contemplated. Both of these therapeutic procedures cause more widespread interruption of afferent sensory pathways than does one- or two-level surgical rhizotomy. Thus, nerve root blocks are more appropriate and better predictors of the utility of the more specific surgical intervention of surgical rhizotomy, whereas spinal intrathecal diagnostic blocks may more truly represent the type of sensory interruption that might be achieved with chemical rhizotomy or cordotomy. A special modification, graded differential diagnostic spinal block, will be discussed separately later. All diagnostic anesthetic blocks, of course, have in common the limitation that their effect is only temporary, and even an excellent temporary pain relief may not correctly predict a lasting beneficial result of surgery because of late recurrence, altered patterns of pain, or development of central deafferentation pain.

Bilateral intrathecal spinal blocks are less frequently employed in failed back syndrome sufferers. Perhaps the greatest usefulness of this diagnostic procedure is a negative one: Patients who fail to obtain pain relief even after bilateral spinal anesthesia throughout the lumbar and sacral region are unlikely to benefit from any afferent sensory ablative (destructive) procedure. In these patients, the source of pain and distress most likely lies within the spinal cord or brain, perhaps a central deafferentation pain, though a considerable component of emotional suffering above and beyond the sensory input component of pain may be involved. Patients with bilateral low back, buttock, and posterior thigh pain or patients with bilateral sciatica are the occasional candidates who might benefit from bilateral intrathecal diagnostic spinal blocks. One is generally quite reluctant to consider bilateral thoracic cordotomy or bilateral chemical sensory rhizotomy because of the significant frequency of complications and the limited chance of successful pain relief with these more extreme procedures. In those instances in which such radical therapy is planned, it may be useful to precede therapy with a bilateral diagnostic intrathecal spinal block. In addition, patients occasionally may be suspected of suffering from painful pseudarthrosis, bilateral painful epidural scarring, or adhesive arachnoiditis for which the surgeon is reluctant to consider reparative or restorative surgery because of the uncertainty of diagnosis and the uncertainty of achieving satisfactory pain relief. For these patients also, bilateral intrathecal spinal block may encourage or discourage the decision to proceed with surgery. Patients are usually not considered for this type of diagnostic injection if their pain is suspected to arise from focal meningeal inflammation, early arachnoiditis without spinal block, or bilateral nerve root inflammation. Under these conditions, surgical intervention usually has little to offer. If relief is to be obtained, it is more likely to be obtained from systemic or intraspinal pharmacologic therapy. In these situations, the risks and diagnostic uncertainties of intrathecal spinal block are rarely warranted, and are certainly not warranted until an adequate trial of pharmacologic therapy has been undertaken. Only if pharmacologic therapy fails would I consider this form of diagnostic injection, and often would perform this test primarily for its predictive value in ascertaining failure of further local therapy.

Unilateral intrathecal anesthetic blocks are done with the patient in the lateral position. I generally prefer a hyperbaric anesthetic solution, which settles downward in the lighter-density spinal fluid, so I position the patient with the painful side down. Use of a hypobaric solution, lighter in density than spinal fluid, would require positioning the patient with the painful side uppermost. *Bilateral intrathecal spinal blocks* are performed either with the patient in a prone Trendelenburg position (head lower than pelvis) or as two separate unilateral one-legged spinal blocks performed at the same sitting. With the former technique, hypobaric anesthetic solutions must be used. With the latter technique, either hypobaric or hyperbaric solutions are used, and the patient must be turned carefully and quickly following establishment of the first side analgesia to prevent unwanted distribution of the anesthetic agent into higher lumbar or upper spinal areas.

Once an *anesthetic block* is in place and its effectiveness has been confirmed by careful sensory testing, the patient is asked to assess the degree of pain relief that he has experienced. The distribution of sensory loss is important, since this should cover the patient's painful area if relief is to be expected. If a dense spinal block has been induced, including motor paralysis, it may not be possible to test the patient for improvement in range of motion, although some assessment can be obtained by having the physician perform straight leg and bent leg raising maneuvers on the anesthetized patient.

Forced straight and bent leg raising maneuvers are sometimes done as a *therapeutic measure,* but should be done with care so as not to leave the patient with greater pain when the anesthetic wears off. An alternative is to perform a spinal block with a dilute solution, achieving analgesia with little motor weakness. This is not always easy to accomplish and has the drawback of giving results that are at times equivocal. This is particularly true if complete pain relief is not obtained, leaving the physician with uncertainty as to whether the failure to obtain relief was due to the patient's disease or due to an inadequate study. At the conclusion of a spinal diagnostic procedure, the patient is confined to bed until full motor and sensory functions have returned to the lower extremities. He is encouraged to remain at bed rest for an additional period of six to twelve hours to lessen the risk of post-LP headache. Intrathecal spinal diagnostic blocks may be performed on an outpatient basis if the patient is accessible enough to home that prolonged traveling in the vertical position is not required.

Graded differential diagnostic spinal anesthetic blocks are a special variation of this technique that can be useful in attempting to assess the origin of a patient's pain and his likelihood of responding to therapeutic measures. This test is performed with the same basic technique as just described, usually employing a unilateral block. An attempt is made to induce graded depths of anesthesia over a specific set of lumbar nerve roots, with sensory testing and assessment of pain relief at each step of the procedure. An ideal graded differential diagnostic block should produce the following levels of neuroblockade:

1. Placebo
2. Autonomic block with little or no hypalgesia
3. Hypalgesia without analgesia or motor involvement
4. Dense analgesia or anesthesia with limited motor weakness
5. Complete spinal blockade

Depending on the degree of pain relief obtained, it may not be necessary to proceed through all stages of the test, but it is always wise to proceed at least one stage beyond the point at which the patient claims total relief. Some patients will then remark, "that feels even better than the last time." The usefulness of this test is that it is said to separate *organic* from *inorganic* pain. Whether any test is capable of this distinction and whether such a distinction ever actually occurs are uncertain. What is certain is that this test helps to differentiate patients whose pain is easily interrupted from those whose pain is more difficult to interrupt. Patients in the former group may have relatively little painful sensory input with significant secondary distress or may merely be potent "placebo reactors." Patients in the latter group may have severe or extensive nociceptive input from damaged tissues—input that is difficult to interrupt. On the other hand, they may have central deafferentation pain arising from within the spinal cord or brain, or they may in fact be reacting principally at a cortical level because of significant psychiatric disease or frank malingering.

Neuroblockade with the most dilute anesthetic, blocking autonomic input without blocking small fiber pain input, could conceivably alter *causalgic pain* in the lower extremities, although such pain is difficult to document with certainty.

The *level of anesthesia achieved* in a graded differential diagnostic spinal block is determined by the concentration of anesthetic agent injected. The area of sensory involvement is determined by the volume injected. The depth of neuroblockade should be confirmed by using the patient's subjective assessment of induced warmth, by careful and repetitive sensory testing to assess both area and depth of sensory impairment to light touch and pinprick, and by requesting voluntary movement. The actual concentrations of anesthetic necessary to achieve optimum results vary with factors such as the degree of perineural scarring present in that particular patient. I have generally used tetracaine (Pontocaine) as the anesthetic agent, mixing this with 10% dextrose solution for a hyperbaric procedure. The following concentrations generally give satisfactory results: (1) for autonomic blockade, 1 mg tetracaine per 2.5 ml dextrose (0.4 mg per ml solution); (2) for hypalgesia, enough tetracaine added to the remainder of the first solution to make a 1.5 mg per ml solution; (3) for analgesia or anesthesia with minimum motor weakness, enough additional tetracaine to make a solution of 2.5 mg per ml concentration; (4) for complete sensory and motor blockade, enough additional tetracaine to make a concentration of 4 mg or 5 mg per ml. If bilateral blocks or multisegmental blocks are anticipated, larger volumes of dextrose and tetracaine should be employed for the initial solution. To perform a one-legged spinal block covering two or three nerve root segments, injection of 0.5 ml increments is usually satisfactory. It is worth reiterating that if significant subarachnoid scarring is present, results may be quite variable, with unpredictable distribution and penetration of the anesthetic agent.

5

Noninvasive Therapy

In dealing with medical problems, two basic questions must always be addressed: *"What is it?"* and *"What should be done about it?"* Although this statement seems insipid, it is especially worthy of repetition in a discussion of the failed back syndrome. All too often, the myriad symptoms and specific etiologies that constitute this dreadful diagnosis are greeted by the practitioner with a sense of despair. The patient is all too often offered a diagnosis of sorts, but no offer of therapy is forthcoming: "Yes, you've got a real problem"—period. Other patients are shoveled aside to whatever practitioners are willing to tackle their cases, and if none are available locally, many patients are referred to distant cities. As discussed in Chapter 1, this is unfortunate and unfair to both the patient and the recipient physician, who cannot easily undertake an integrated and continuing therapeutic program at a distance. Equally frequent is the unhappy situation in which a more or less precise diagnosis of the cause of a patient's failed back syndrome is met with a stereotypical and at times inappropriate response: "You've got back trouble. We'll operate next week!" This approach overlooks one key word in my two short opening questions. The question is "What *should* be done about it?" rather than "What *can* be done about it?" A variety of therapies are available for the failed back syndrome sufferer, and the management of these patients requires a carefully tailored therapeutic program based on the patient's needs, which may heavily tax the physician's or surgeon's knowledge, experience, intuition, and patience.

The *indications for the therapeutic approaches* that I present can be given only in general terms because they are evolved from a quarter century of experience with a wide variety of patients, each with a particular nuance of pain, disability, and physical disorder. As alluded to earlier, my basic therapeutic approach is to seek that form of therapy that will be effective for a given patient at minimum cost, including risk, time, pain, and dollars. The diagnostic scheme that I present is based on the assumption that many disorders can be effectively diagnosed using a generalized and almost exclusively symptomatic approach. What makes this approach effective is that many of the noninvasive therapies are useful for a variety of specific disorders. An estimate of when these therapies may be effective can be gained with reasonable accuracy without the need for elaborate specific confirmation beyond a symptomatic diagnosis. Even if a specific diagnosis has been made for a failed back syndrome sufferer, noninvasive therapies frequently remain the preferred first line of treatment. For some patients, these therapies may be the only reasonable therapies to apply. For some patients, the reasonableness of noninvasive therapy unfortunately does not guarantee that it will be effective, but implies rather that more dangerous and more invasive therapies may carry no greater chance of success despite a clearly increased risk of harm or symptomatic worsening for the patient. As stated earlier, I do not consider the undue prolongation of ineffective noninvasive therapy to be good conservative therapy when more effective invasive therapies are available. Only careful consideration involving the active participation of physician and patient can determine when invasive therapies should be added to noninvasive therapies. The appearance of new symptoms or findings and the abject failure of noninvasive therapies in patients in whom invasive therapies offer hope of improvement clearly suggest the need for invasive therapy. On the other hand, many patients obtain at least partial symptomatic and functional improvement with noninvasive therapy; for them, the decisions about when to add invasive therapies and which therapy to recommend tax both the science and the art of medicine to its fullest.

Noninvasive therapies fall into *five major groupings:* enforced inactivity, enforced activity, noninvasive analgesic methods, pharmacologic methods, and psychologic approaches. Each of these categories is discussed in this chapter.

Enforced Inactivity Therapy

Bed Rest

Bed rest well deserves its widespread recognition as one of the mainstays of *therapy for many acute conditions* that affect the lower back. When tissues are acutely inflamed, continued stress of those tissues through weight bearing or activity may lead to progressive symptomatic worsening with increased pain and prolonged disability. Bed rest is particularly helpful in acute flare-ups of pain that are predominantly confined to the lower back and usually benefits patients with leg pain caused by actual disc rupture. Almost any activity in which the patient is sitting or standing, even an activity involving almost exclusively the upper extremities, requires at least tightening of the back muscles, if not their active contraction, to produce motion or to maintain a vertical posture. Pain may ensue whether the source of inflammation is the discs, facet joints, spastic muscles, inflamed nerve roots, or a host of other specific etiologies. As a relatively nonspecific and relatively safe therapy, bed rest is often one of the early procedures of choice in patients with episodic, disablingly severe pain. When bed rest is coupled with many of the other noninvasive therapies, a high proportion of episodes of acute back or leg pain can be successfully treated with this as the basic therapeutic modality.

Of course, bed rest is not without *risks and limitations*. At any age, bed rest predisposes patients to *venous stasis* in the lower extremities, and the incidence of venous thrombosis or thromboembolism increases progressively as the duration of bed rest increases. For the *elderly patient,* bed rest poses additional risks because the geriatric patient is more prone to develop atelectasis, osteoporosis, and urinary retention with enforced, prolonged bed rest. For the patient with *arthritis,* the enforced inactivity may lead to progressive stiffening and may leave the patient with even greater pain when resumption of activity is attempted. For all patients, enforced inactivity leads to *progressive muscle weakness or even atrophy.* After a period of prolonged bed rest, patients frequently find that their increased muscular weakness predisposes them to back pains. Their weakened muscles are no longer capable of providing adequate support and stabilization for their musculoskeletal structures, and weakened muscles may become painfully intolerant of activities that require exertion greater than that muscle is capable of producing. *Postural hypotension* may also be seen following prolonged bed rest, but this is rarely a lasting problem.

Two major *limitations of bed rest* are the tendency of some physicians to *prolong its application* beyond its period of usefulness and the *imprecision* of this method of therapy. Bed rest therapy is imprecise because there are no firm guidelines on when an adequate trial has been undertaken or even when bed rest therapy should be recommended at all. The patient with *chronic, unremitting back pain* from the failed back syndrome is not a good candidate for bed rest therapy.[56] The chronicity of his pain makes it unlikely that he will rapidly achieve significant pain relief from recumbency, and prolonged recumbency may lead to increased pain through increased muscle weakness or arthritic stiffness. Daily rest periods of an hour or so may be useful for these patients if this rest gives them relief. If they remain equally uncomfortable with or without bed rest, the period of rest then becomes useful principally for any value it provides in allowing psychologic fortification. Bed rest should not be allowed to become a "crutch" for these chronic sufferers when a crutch is undesirable.

For many chronic failed back syndrome sufferers, enforced activity provides the best road to recovery, but this road may be strewn with stumbling blocks of discomfort and the unpleasant necessity of self-will and self-discipline. At this point in the medical course, both the patient and the phy-

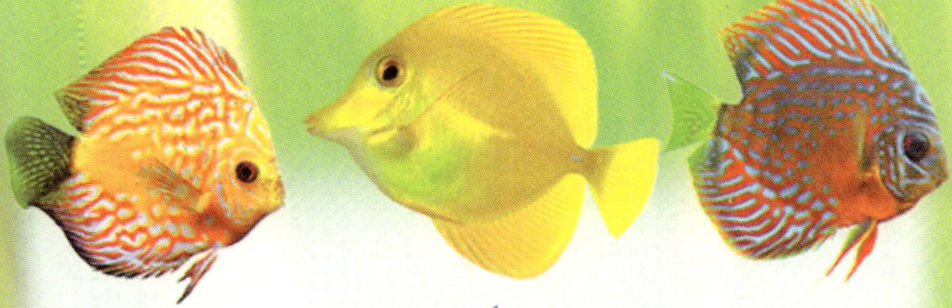

A Special Note...

sician may have become accustomed to thinking in terms of bed rest, but bed rest should be *proscribed,* not prescribed, when an activity program is indicated.

Patients with chronic failed back syndromes are also prone to *acute, episodic pains.* It is these painful episodes that are more appropriately and usually more effectively treated with bed rest. Acutely spastic and painful muscles, acutely and painfully stretched joint capsules, and acutely painful separations of adhesions at a fusion bone or around nerve roots are all conditions that frequently respond dramatically to enforced inactivity. The healing process begun by the body flowers best with careful nurturing. Tissues that are inflamed or separated require rest, time, and proximity for recovery. In these acute situations, enforced inactivity is closely analogous to strapping a twisted ankle or casting a broken arm. However, with both back problems and sprained ankles, a time is reached when a transition must be made from enforced inactivity to enforced activity. If enforced inactivity is continued too long, the pain of injury may merge into the pain of stiffness. Some conditions, notably trigger points, fasciitis, and ischiogluteal bursitis (see the discussion of low back pain in Chapter 3), are notoriously refractory to bed rest.

Recent studies now strongly suggest that episodes of *acute lumbar pain* are best managed if *bed rest is limited* to the first two or three days, after which a cautious and graded activity program should supersede.[56] Longer periods of rest may be necessitated by severe symptoms following major trauma, but these can usually be obviated by supplying the patient with a back support as he resumes ambulation. *Sciatica* due to recurrent or new lumbar disc ruptures does seem to respond well to bed rest, which should be continued for several days after acute pain subsides in order to encourage healing of the disc rupture. On the other hand, if relief does not begin to appear within seven or eight days, other diagnostic or therapeutic intervention is usually warranted. If pain relief has not been obtained within two weeks, few patients will obtain good relief by further prolongation of bed rest as the only therapy. Thus, patients who have obtained some relief of sciatica by the end of the second week, but who still have sufficient pain at rest or with brief excursions out of bed, should be offered additional therapeutic or diagnostic intervention. A similar conclusion should be reached about the patient who rapidly obtains good pain relief with bed rest but who consistently relapses shortly after resuming weight-bearing activity.

The *psychologic risk* of enforced inactivity in bed must be weighed in every case. This is particularly true in chronic failed back syndrome sufferers. As discussed under psychogenic factors in Chapter 3, psychologic factors play an important role in the etiology and management of these patients. Factors such as motivation, self-image, depression, and secondary gain must all be carefully assessed in arriving at a diagnosis and in planning therapy. Enforced bed rest guarantees that the patient will be dependent, usually at the expense of his image of self-worth and usefulness. Forcing a patient to accept a dependent and "worthless" role may be quite destructive in situations in which the therapist is struggling to improve a patient's sense of motivation and worth. If this is the price that the patient must pay for successful bed rest therapy, the price may well be worth the product. If, however, prolonged bed rest yields little benefit and instead leads to significant psychologic deterioration, the patient has been harmed rather than helped.

Bed rest therapy can take two forms: *intermittent* or *complete. Intermittent therapy* involves having the patient retire to bed one or more hours once or several times daily. This can be done on a regular schedule, but is usually done purely on the basis of aggravated symptoms. This form of therapy provides both physical and psychologic relief from the stress of aching discomfort and is particularly valuable when coupled with a vigorous restorative program of back activity. Even without a restorative program, intermittent bed rest may provide pain relief more safely than anodynes for the patient who is chronically limited by a failed back syndrome but who is not sufficiently crippled by the disease to be incapable of some degree of useful activity. Intermittent bed rest is of much less usefulness for the patient with acute low back or sciatic pain of crippling severity. For these patients, bed rest therapy is often indicated as the first or only major therapy. For a patient with a disc protrusion or a severe muscle spasm, bed rest should be indeed *total* and *complete.* I usually try to impress upon patients that there is a significant difference between 23 hours a day in bed and 24 hours a day. Each time these patients resume weight bearing, even briefly, tissues in the delicate stage of early healing may be disrupted, and muscles that are beginning to relax may be thrown back into painful and protracted spasm. For my patients, I often draw an analogy between bed rest therapy for a disc rupture and the growing of young plants:

> If you are waiting for tiny seedlings to grow in your garden and once a day—only once a day—you come by and stomp on that seedling, you would hardly be surprised to find that its growth is slow and your garden fails to produce. The same is true of healing tissues around a disc rupture. Each time you sit up in bed, dangle on the side of the bed, or stand up, you apply several hundred pounds of levered weight against your disc, so there should be little surprise if you fail to improve when you continue to punish your disc in this fashion.

Bed rest should be done in a *proper bed.* A mattress that sags or is uncomfortable will not permit proper back alignment or muscle relaxation. A firm mattress or boards under a mattress are essential. Bed rest can often be made more comfortable if the hips are maintained in slight flexion, sufficient to flatten the normal lumbar lordosis. This can be done in a hospital bed by raising the head 5 degrees, raising the knees 15 degrees, and placing the feet at a height equal to or slightly greater than the knees. At home, this can be accomplished by propping the calves on pillows. Care should be taken that the pillows are placed under the calves, not under the knees, since popliteal compression can interfere with venous drainage and increase the risk of thrombophlebitis. A small pad or rolled towel under the mid lumbar region may also be a great comfort. This simple device is also quite useful for women with back problems who attempt to engage in sexual intercourse—although that form of bed rest therapy is not the specific subject of this section. An alternative method of accomplishing recumbency with modest hip flexion is hammock sleep. This technique is not widely used, but it has its enthusiastic advocates.[57]

Just as the patient has a major responsibility in maintaining adequate bed rest, the *physician* also has a special *responsibility* when placing a patient at bed rest. Because complete bed rest therapy is usually undertaken for patients with acute sciatica sufficiently severe to consider hospitalization, it must be kept in mind that these patients may continue to worsen despite bed rest therapy. In fact, these patients are at greater than average risk of developing further neurologic damage. This damage is likely to dictate more aggressive diagnostic or therapeutic intervention, such as early myelography or early surgery, if the progress is rapid and the neurologic deficit becomes severe. The physician in charge has a greater responsibility to his hospitalized patient to monitor neurologic function by daily physical examination, in addition to monitoring the effect on pain relief. The physician also has the responsibility of gauging on a day-to-day basis how long to continue complete bed rest, when to allow the patient limited ambulation, when to initiate aggressive diagnostic studies, and when to abandon bed rest therapy before it becomes wastefully and perhaps destructively prolonged. The physician must be sensitive to the decision as to how stringently to require adherence to a program of complete bed rest. In practice, complete bed rest therapy becomes most difficult when the time comes for bowel evacuation. Requiring a patient to perch on a bedpan (and no bedpan I know of was engineered to fit the human rear end comfortably) may cause more aggravation, muscle tightness, and back strain than allowing the patient out of bed once daily for a brief visit to a bedside commode.

A major consideration in deciding on bed rest therapy is whether this should be undertaken *at home or in the hospital.* Home bed rest therapy is less expensive to society if not to the patient, whose hospital costs may be paid by third-party carriers, though this treatment option is increasingly being denied financial coverage by third-party payors. Bed rest therapy is inherently costly for wage earners because of the loss of work time and income, so the cost of home versus hospital bed rest therapy becomes even more consequential. *Home therapy,* of course, offers an environment that is often more pleasant and a diet to which the patient is accustomed. On the other hand, home bed rest therapy is usually difficult to carry out with any degree of completeness. Many patients have no one to stay with them both day and night to provide bedpans or bathroom assistance, make meals, and run errands. If the patient has small children, the problem is further complicated by their presence in the sickroom and their demands for attention—both the children's vocal requests and the parent's perception of the children's needs. On the other hand, *bed rest in the hospital* can usually be carried out with adequate assistance for the patient and without the demands of children. Also, medication is more readily available to supplement bed rest therapy in the hospital. An important, intangible benefit of hospital therapy is the greater likelihood of patient compliance with strict bed rest in the strange and forbidding atmosphere of a hospital, under the supervision of watchful nurses. Also, knowing the cost and commitment of effort that goes into hospital bed rest provides the patient with persuasive additional inducement to maintain a strict program of bed rest therapy.

Traction

Two types of traction are frequently employed as part of enforced inactivity therapy in the management of painful back disorders: *pelvic traction* and *leg traction or Buck's traction.* Tilt board or hanging traction is employed in home or outpatient programs, and some pain clinics and professional athletic trainers are enthusiastic about the use of this method in young, otherwise healthy patients.

A *twofold rationale* is often given for the usefulness of traction in painful back disorders. First, traction tends to separate vertebral bodies and open neuroforamina. This facilitates the return of protruding discs to a more normal position for subsequent healing and helps to decompress nerve roots. Second, traction applies countertension against back muscles that are tense or even in spasm. Stretching a muscle that is in spasm is one of the oldest known forms of therapy for muscle spasm and often helps relax the painful and sustained muscle contraction. From my experience with pelvic traction, I have conceived of a *third rationale* for its usefulness, one that I feel is probably its most helpful aspect. Since common forms of traction are done with the patient recumbent in bed, and since removal of a pelvic or leg traction device is a cumbersome prospect, I contend that traction aids greatly in the therapy of acute painful low back conditions by keeping the patient in bed. There is little doubt that enforced bed rest is a powerful tool for the management of these acute conditions, and any form of therapy that aids in achieving the goal of complete or near complete bed rest is likely to be beneficial therapeutically.

Pelvic traction is usually accomplished by using a wide lumbar belt or a lumbar band that resembles a garter belt (Fig. 5.1). Ropes or straps pass from the belt on each side of the patient toward the foot of the bed. There the ropes are attached to both ends of a 14- to 20-inch spreader bar that keeps the ropes from cutting inward into the patient's legs. From the center of this spreader bar, a single rope passes through a pulley, and weights are applied at its down-hanging end. For home use, a foot board or even a ladder-back chair at the foot of the bed can be substituted for a formal pulley. Depending on the weight of the patient, 20 to 40 pounds of traction are applied. With lighter patients and heavier weights, it becomes important to raise the foot of the bed to prevent the patient from being pulled out of bed, thus defeating the purpose of traction.

Buck's traction is applied by placing a band of felt, canvas, or cloth along one side of the patient's calf and foot, looping the material below the foot, and applying it to the opposite side of the calf. The material is then strapped or taped into place, and weights are attached by ropes and pulleys to the loop of material below the foot. Prefabricated devices are also available, consisting of foam rubber and canvas "boots" that strap on to the patient's foot and lower leg and have built-in attachments for traction weights. With either system, traction may be applied with one weight per leg or one weight applied through a spreader bar to both legs. Occasionally, unilateral Buck's traction is applied, but generally bilateral traction is preferred. The weight employed commonly ranges from 10 to 15 pounds per leg.

Hanging traction is less commonly employed in the treatment of low back pain and sciatica than traction therapy that is applied with the patient recumbent in bed. Hanging traction can be performed either with the patient inverted (head down) or with the patient's head elevated. In hanging traction, the lumbar area is stretched by having the weight of the patient's own body provide the distracting force.

Hanging traction with the patient's head elevated can be done either with the patient lying on a tilting table or frame or with the patient ambulatory and using crutches. With either technique, the upper body is stabilized and the lower body is allowed to hang dependent to provide the traction weight against the lumbar spine. When patients are placed on tilting frames or beds, a chest harness or underarm straps are attached to the top of the bed or frame and the bed is elevated 45 to 60 degrees, or occasionally as high as a full 90 degrees. Ambulatory hanging traction can be accomplished by having the patient use crutches, thus supporting the upper torso and allowing the pelvis and lower limbs to hang dependent during at least a portion of the time spent

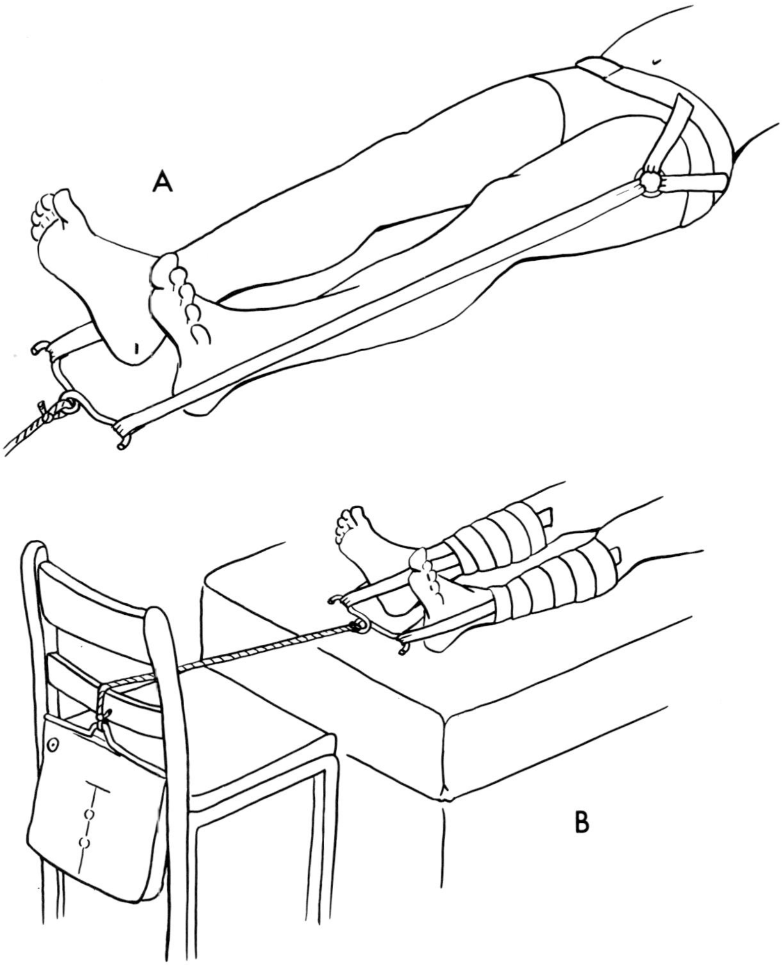

FIGURE 5.1. Lumbar traction is usually accomplished either **(A)** with pelvic traction or **(B)** with Buck's leg traction. Leg traction may be applied to one leg or to both. When used at home, the rungs of a ladder-back chair can serve nicely instead of an expensive pulley. The waterbag weights are attached to the traction by a spreader bar to prevent ropes from cutting into the patient's leg.

in ambulation. This technique does not permit constant traction, since crutch walking does require full weight bearing on the lower extremities during the period of time when the crutches are moved forward. Nonetheless, this technique has the advantage of permitting the patient to be out of bed. It can occasionally provide enough additional pain relief and psychologic support to permit a patient to remain active and even gainfully employed despite persistent low back pain.

A more strenuous variation of this technique is *hanging traction with the patient inverted.* This form of traction seems to be at least relatively contraindicated in older patients. It seems to have enjoyed its earliest popularity in certain pain clinics and athletic clubhouses and is now available in the form of commercially available devices sold in sporting-goods stores. The principle behind this form of traction is the inverse of the more commonly employed pelvic traction. In inverted hanging traction, the lumbar area is stretched by having the weight of the upper torso dependent below the lumbar spine and using the torso to provide the weight for traction. In its gentler form, this is accomplished by having the patient supine on a tilting bed or frame with both feet or legs attached by straps to the foot end of the bed or frame. The bed is then tilted to an angle of 30 to 75 degrees with the patient's head and torso dangling below and stretching the lumbar spine. A more vigorous version of hanging traction involves having the patient hang upside down from an exercise bar that he holds onto with flexed knees. For this form of traction to be useful, patients must be sufficiently limber and agile to be able to position themselves on the exercise apparatus; therefore, I doubt that this form of traction would be practical for the patient severely disabled by back pain.

Differences of opinion exist about optimum *time durations for traction therapy,* but one principle seems well-established: Once applied, traction should be left in place for a minimum of one hour to permit gradual relaxation of back muscles. This is especially important, since initial application of traction may be painful for a few minutes before pain relief ensues. A common schedule is to use traction for one hour q.i.d. (every four hours for four times a day). Long applications of traction sometimes become irritating to the skin or to a patient's psyche. However, I frequently counsel my patients that using pelvic traction is somewhat like baking a cake: The more sugar you put in the cake, the sweeter it is, and the more you use traction, the more benefit you are likely to obtain.

Traction therapy has *limitations.* Not all patients benefit from traction therapy. Some patients find that traction consistently aggravates their pain. Improperly applied traction that distorts the patient as it pulls is particularly likely to be troublesome. Leg traction is relatively contraindicated in patients with severe sciatica, since leg traction is more likely to cause sciatic stretching and may therefore aggravate sciatic pain and even cause nerve injury. Leg traction has the potential disadvantage of causing stasis of venous return in the feet, thus accentuating the possibility of venous thromboembolism. This can be partly thwarted by wrapping both the calf and foot in elastic bandages.

Back Supports

Another variation of the therapeutic theme of enforced inactivity is the use of *back supports, corsets, or braces.* A somewhat bewildering variety of specific types of corsets and braces are commercially available. It is not my intent to endorse any specific brand, but rather to discuss general categories of support devices. The simplest type of back support device is the *lumbar* or *lumbosacral belt*—a four- to six-inch wide band of elastic material that fits around the waist. These devices do little to impede back flexion and extension, but serve as reminders to patients to limit their back activities and provide some comforting pressure or counterirritation. *Corsets* and *girdles* provide more back support than lumbar or lumbosacral belts. Surgical corsets are available in varying lengths and with or without steel stiffening stays. Many women, however, prefer to use corsets or heavy girdles designed as women's undergarments for comfort and sartorial style. Corsets and girdles do restrict back motion modestly in addition to providing comforting and reassuring pressure and compression. The restriction of back motion can be improved further by the addition of a formed plastic insert, such as can be obtained with the "Warm Form" back support. *Rigid back braces* provide yet greater stabilization and can be applied with or without compression of the mid lumbar area, a feature that may be important in patients with tender backs. Short steel braces such as the chair-back brace or the Norton-Brown brace still permit some upper trunk mobility, while full-length back braces such as the Taylor brace, Orthomold hyperextension brace, or specially molded fiberglass or plaster bivalved body jackets provide immobilization as complete as can be accomplished with an ambulatory patient short of internal fixation (Fig. 5.2).

Back supports are extremely useful in patients with *acute episodes* of *back pain,* especially if these episodes are relapsing in nature. They are particularly helpful when patients feel constrained by economic or other considerations from undertaking a period of immobilization in bed. Patients who are capable of functioning in society or at work with the aid of a back support should, if at all possible, couple the use of a back support with an exercise program to prevent deterioration of the back. Back supports are useful if they permit patients to be less dependent on dangerous medication, but should be used with caution in patients who remain incapacitated and who continue to ingest significant amounts of analgesics even while wearing back supports.

Back bracing may be beneficial for patients, even if they prove refractory to weaning from the back support, by providing *diagnostically useful information* or *delayed healing.* Documentation of pain relief through external bracing and support strongly supports the contention that internal bracing through spinal fusion might achieve a similar degree of pain relief. In patients who have already

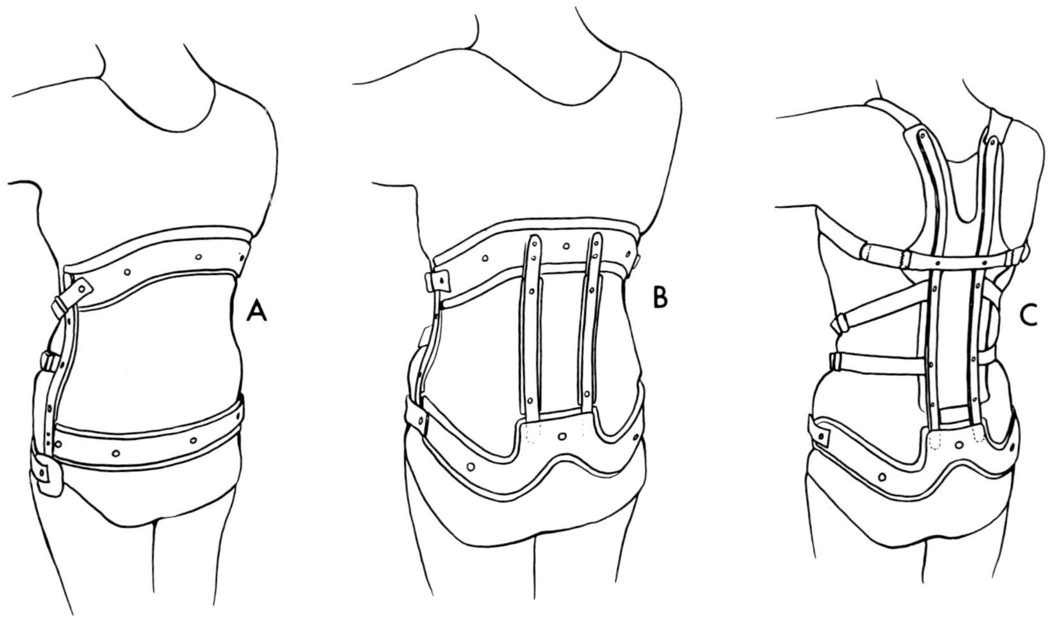

FIGURE 5.2. Steel back braces supply better support for the lower back in ambulatory patients. Among the most popular versions are **(A)** the Norton-Brown brace and **(B)** the Knight spinal or chair back brace. The Taylor brace **(C)** gives even more support than the first two because it includes support for the upper back, as well as the lower back.

undergone spinal fusion, pain relief from the addition of an external support strongly suggests a problem with the fusion, such as kissing pseudarthrosis or unstable pseudarthrosis, or a problem adjacent to the fusion, such as juxtaposed arthritis or facet disease. For some patients, strict full-time use of a back brace for three to six months may finally allow an area of bony instability or pseudarthrosis to heal and stabilize. When this occurs, the patient may be able to discontinue use of the brace without recurrence of back pain. A full-length brace or body jacket is usually necessary to provide sufficient stabilization to allow healing and "cure" of a painful pseudarthrosis or bony instability. Patients who fail to obtain pain relief from a corset or girdle should not be discarded as candidates for spinal fusion surgery until they have been given a trial of one or more months with a full-length brace.

The *type of back brace* selected should be tailored to the patient's specific condition, generally relying on the least rigid and most flexible system that will provide useful symptomatic relief. However, back bracing should not be discarded as ineffective unless an appropriate and sufficiently rigid support has been used. For most patients, a lumbosacral corset or lightweight back brace will suffice. However, some patients who fail to obtain relief with light supports will achieve dramatic pain relief through the use of a full-length brace or body jacket.

Back supports, like enforced inactivity in bed, have their *limitations*. They may aggravate arthritic stiffness or lead to progressive muscle weakness, and thus may be deleterious in the long run, especially with chronic use.

Enforced Activity Therapy

Enforced activity therapy and enforced inactivity therapy have both opposite and identical goals and are mutually antagonistic, yet supplementary, as therapies. Although the short-term goals of inactivity and activity obviously are diametrically opposed, the long-term goals of each therapy are the same: restoration of ailing backs. It is contradictory to prescribe enforced inactivity and enforced activity at the same time, but these therapies work well in selected instances when used alternately and are essential supplements to each other when used serially, if the patient is to recover useful function. As discussed earlier, enforced inactivity carries with it the risk of aggravation of arthritic stiffness and worsening of muscle weakness, both of which can lead to the prolongation of back pain and disability. Patients suffering acute and severe episodes of low back pain usually will not tolerate enforced activity for the first one or two days, yet must graduate from a program of enforced inactivity through a program of enforced activity if they are to return to a fully functional status.

Patients who work frequently comment that they are so tired at the end of a workday that they certainly do not need back exercises. Unless patients are engaged in heavy physical labor, however, this is usually a fallacious assumption, and it often develops that the patients become excessively tired precisely because their muscles are not strong enough. Furthermore, back muscles are not made stronger by sitting at an office desk, walking about, or submitting to the routine stress and tension of the workplace, even though "tiredness" may result.

The *transition between enforced inactivity and enforced activity therapies* continually poses a problem for health care practitioners dealing with patients with the failed back syndrome. Urging a patient into activity that is too vigorous for his aching anatomy too soon may simply intensify the pain and psychologic disability through fear of further pain. On the other hand, the transition to enforced activity is rarely easy for patients, and all patients should be cautioned to expect some discomfort during the early stages of the transition. I counsel my patients: "If you're not tired and a bit achy at the end of each day, you've been goofing off!" For some patients with less severe back problems or who have partially recovered following enforced inactivity, a combination of *alternating therapies* may be useful. For these patients, wearing a back brace or support during wage earning and home working hours can sometimes effectively be coupled with a cautious exercise program during other hours of the day. Knowing when to make the transition is extremely difficult, often severely tests the art of the clinician, and for maximum success requires full cooperation and understanding on the part of the patient. Even after two decades of trying to fathom the mysteries of the timing of this transition, I still depend heavily on a trial-and-error approach. In general, patients who still complain of severe back pain at rest and who require strong analgesics while at rest are probably not ready to undertake a vigorous back-strengthening program, but they may benefit greatly from a more gentle program emphasizing back stretching or limbering. In contrast, many patients continue to have pain when they attempt the activities of daily living precisely because they need a program of enforced activity to loosen and limber tight muscles, joints, and ligaments and to strengthen and increase endurance in the weakened and flabby muscles of the back and extremities. To deny these patients a program of enforced activity is to thwart or prolong their recovery—even though the transition from enforced inactivity to enforced activity may be an uncomfortable or even painful experience requiring considerable self-discipline on the part of the patient.

The following case report illustrates the development of a painful flabby back syndrome and its ultimate successful therapy through enforced activity:

Case 6

A 45-year-old industrial worker had suffered intermittent low backaches since childbearing in 1959. In 1978, she injured her back in a fall at work experiencing predominantly sciatica. Pain gradually worsened despite phenytoin (Dilantin), carbamazepine (Tegretol), and several anti-inflammatory drugs. She finally found it necessary to discontinue work, but bed rest at home and in the hospital brought no significant relief. A myelogram in March 1979 showed a large anterolateral defect at L5-S1 on the left. She underwent disc excision with modified interbody bone fusion. Sciatica was immediately relieved. Postoperatively, she wore a chair-back brace for four months. Recovery was assisted by indomethacin (Indocin) and perphenazine plus amitriptyline (Triavil). She was able to return to full employment at her industrial job in August 1979.

Twelve months later she reinjured her back when she slipped at work. She continued half-time work with the aid of indomethacin, then ibuprofen (Motrin), but back discomfort persisted. In December 1980, discography was normal at L4-L5 but caused severe back pain when L5-S1 was reinjected, even though the injected contrast material did not extravasate outside of the disc space. Intradiscal lidocaine (Xylocaine) and bupivacaine (Marcaine) gave prompt relief of back pain, and intradiscal methylprednisolone acetate (Depo-Medrol) gave sufficient relief so that she was able to return to full-time employment in January 1981.

She was seen again in July 1981 complaining of increased aching and tiredness of her back. She found it necessary to return to a reclining lounger immediately after each working day. Her physical activity, outside of the job, was extremely limited, with no sports, exercises, or other regular schedule of activity.

She noted that sex relations with her husband often left her with a backache for the subsequent 24 hours. She was diagnosed as having a flabby back syndrome secondary to enforced inactivity necessitated by her back condition and secondary to her sedentary life-style. Diazepam (Valium) 5 mg during the morning and afternoon improved the aching back tension at work, but a schedule of regular exercises and limited sports activity gradually strengthened her back and brought freedom from backache and tiredness.

Exercises

A fundamental consideration in those forms of enforced activity aimed at improving muscle strength and endurance is that *voluntary muscle contraction* is a prerequisite. As a result, no amount of activity by a therapist or any person other than the patient will improve muscle strength unless the patient initiates voluntary muscle contraction. Supervision of an exercise program is extremely useful to monitor compliance, to tailor specific exercises to specific stages of recovery, and to minimize painful overexertion or improperly performed and potentially detrimental activity. This supervision need not be constant, and patients must be taught and encouraged to continue their activity programs on their own and for many hours more than those few hours spent directly with the therapist each week. As a result, home exercise programs for muscle strengthening and improvement in endurance are frequently even more effective than hospital-based programs, as long as adequate supervision is provided.

Exercise therapy can have *three different goals,* and exercises should be prescribed in a specific fashion depending on which goal is intended. *Muscle stretching exercises* are helpful in relaxing muscle spasms and in improving back limberness, but do little or nothing to improve strength or endurance. *Back strengthening exercises* are important in obtaining long-term relief from conditions such as periosteal trigger points and the flabby back syndrome, and are essential after prolonged immobilization or external bracing. Exercises designed to *improve endurance* emphasize more frequent repetitions against gradually increasing resistance and are an important part of a restorative or back-hardening exercise program.

One goal of enforced activity therapy is the *limbering* and *stretching* of back and hip muscles, ligaments, and joints, which are particularly beneficial for muscles in painful spasm, as is well-known to anyone who has suffered a charley horse in a calf muscle. Limbering and stretching are also helpful in reversing painful stiffness and in improving range of motion. In the transition from enforced inactivity, this type of exercise is usually prescribed first, before exercises aimed at muscle strengthening. The classic back-limbering exercises are those known as *Williams' exercises*—a group of exercises so widely employed that there is now considerable variation in the specific exercises that are included in the group. The basic group of exercises is done with the patient supine and emphasizes (1) one leg or both leg hip flexion with knee flexed or extended, and (2) pelvic tilts to flatten the lumbar lordosis (Fig. 5.3). Since these exercises are done in a nonweight-bearing position, they can be started while the patient is still on bed rest therapy. They should not be started, however, until the patient is free of sciatica, since persistent sciatic root entrapment can lead to severely increased pain with attempted limbering exercises. Some therapists include sitting lumbar flexion exercises with the Williams' group, but these are generally too difficult for patients to perform early in their exercise programs and it seems more proper to include them with the group of back-strengthening exercises. Another group of exercises can be properly included along with the Williams' exercises as principally limbering exercises: *quadripedal exercises,* done with the patient in a crawling position. In this position, the lumbar spine is not weight bearing, and the hips and knees begin in flexion. The patient crawls about or rocks forward and backward onto his haunches and tilts his pelvis to straighten the lumbar curve; essentially the same exercises are done as in the basic Williams' exercise group. By doing these in the quadripedal position, more physical activity is generated with better toning of arm, neck, and trunk musculature (Fig. 5.4).

Muscle-strengthening programs can take a *variety of forms.* The gentlest forms of back-strengthening exercises do not involve the use of weights or mechanical devices and do not even require back bending. *Tonic back exercises,* with neither flexion nor extension, can help to improve back muscle strength even while patients are restricted from back movement following spinal fusion or injuries that necessitate rigid orthoses. Back muscles can be strengthened isotonically by simple voluntary contraction in a fixed position or by exercising upper extremities asymmetrically with respect to the patient's center of gravity. A seated or standing patient who exercises by raising both arms extended in front of him must tighten trunk muscles to avoid toppling over, and so is engaging in a simple and gentle form of back strengthening. A simple yet gentle exercise that does require back bending and that incidentally helps to improve limberness as well as strength can be performed while the patient is brushing his teeth. This involves forward bending at the waist with knees held rigid to reach as far down as is slightly uncomfortable, relaxing momentarily, then "bouncing" for an extra downward stretch. This is followed by elevating the trunk into a hyperextended position, where a backward "bounce" is also taken. Twenty to 50 such repetitions once or twice daily can have a remarkably salutary effect on back muscles.

Exercises such as standing forward bending and prone hyperextension of the back muscles work to *move body parts against gravity* (Fig. 5.5). After the patient is able to perform these exercises easily and with minimal discomfort, he may graduate to a regimen of cautious *weight lifting* if desirable. Many patients find exercising alone to be boring, and motivation to continue quickly fades. Job-related activity will provide adequate muscle strengthening for many patients but by no means for all, especially those engaged in sedentary occupations. *Sports activities* offer the prospect of a more pleasant approach to enforced activity and are a useful adjunct to rehabilitation of the back if properly applied. However, many sports endeavors do not involve motions that benefit the back, and many others involve the necessity or at least the risk of sudden twisting, bending, or stressing that may severely aggravate a fragile and slowly healing back. In the long run, there is no question that the patient who is able to exercise regularly and wisely whether at work, at play, or at home has by far the best chance of maintaining a healthy back. It should be added parenthetically that despite the enthusiastic advocacy of some nonmedical publications for conjugal nocturnal activities as therapy for back disorders, this form of activity, whether therapeutically enforced or voluntary, is only one of the minor adjunctive therapies for the failed back syndrome sufferer that I advocate.

Manipulation

Spinal manipulation can be considered a form of enforced activity, one that entails limbering or straightening of the lumbar spine. Formalized spinal manipulation as practiced by *chiropractors and osteopathic physicians* may, at times, be of great benefit to sufferers from painful back conditions, but short-term relief does not always last, and some studies suggest that equally good results can be achieved by nonmanipulative physical therapy.[58-61] Unfortunately, spinal manipulation can also aggravate back pain, can cause further rupture of protruding discs, and can cause severe vertebral or neurologic problems if unsuspected malignancies are present in the vertebrae or neoplasms are present within the spinal canal.[62] Because of the generally limited "medical" training included in the chiropractic curriculum, I customarily refer my patients who might benefit from manipulation therapy to osteopathic physicians, whose more extensive medical training is reassuring. Ideally, patients undergoing spinal manipulation therapy for back disorders should be monitored carefully neurologically and should be advised to report immediately to their physicians any increase in sciatic pain or neurologic deficit such as paralysis, sensory loss, incontinence, or urinary retention—all complications that may result on rare occasions from manipulation therapy.

An even more vigorous approach to manipulation therapy is spinal or sciatic *stretching* or *manipulation under local, regional, or general anesthesia.* Most commonly, this entails forced straight leg raising done after an epidural or subarachnoid anesthetic block or while the patient is still under spinal or general anesthesia at the conclusion of back surgery. The rationale for this therapy is that stretching or disruption of perineural adhesions may relieve pain or neurologic deficits, with the corollary assumption that the patient can prevent the re-formation of these same adhesions through active exercise, perhaps aided by anti-inflammatory medications. I am not aware of convincing proof of the effectiveness of these maneuvers, but I consider them to be relatively innocuous and at least potentially useful. I occasionally apply them to patients with chronic sciatica of unknown etiology in whom diagnostic studies have failed to disclose recurrent disc rupture or neoplasm or in patients with a failed back syndrome upon whom I have just performed open surgical neurolysis, frequently with local instillation of depository corticosteroid. My clinical impression, based on rather limited personal experience, reinforces my expectation that such stretching maneuvers probably add little to the long-term benefit that the patient derives.

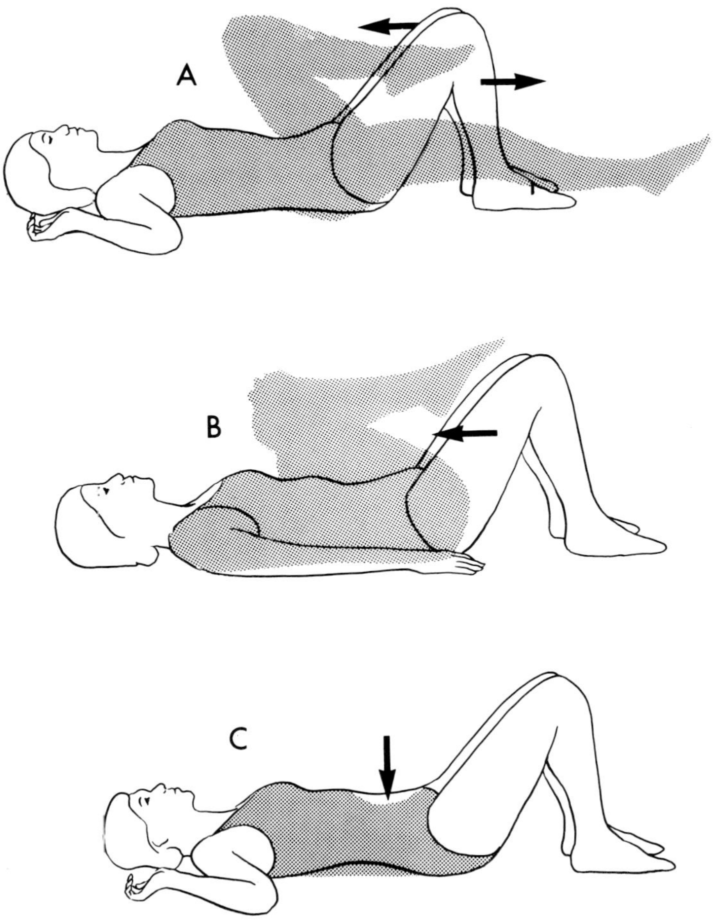

FIGURE 5.3. Williams' back limbering exercises appear in a number of variations. Their goal is to improve flexibility of the low back without weight bearing or muscle strengthening. The basic exercise group includes **(A)** alternating one leg flexion, one leg extension; **(B)** simultaneous flexion of both legs; and **(C)** supine back flattening. Other variations include one leg or two leg flexion beginning from a legs-extended supine position.

Topical and Transcutaneous Therapy

Noninvasive adjuvant therapies provide useful supplements to both enforced inactivity and enforced activity. Among the most commonly employed are various cutaneously or transcutaneously applied analgesic therapies, including topical applications of thermal or radiant energy, surface cooling, mechanical stimulation (massage), or topical medications. Less commonly employed are the transcutaneous or intracutaneous techniques of neurostimulation and acupuncture.

Thermal: Heat and Cold

Topical applications of thermal energy or heat are usually employed for their analgesic and muscle-relaxing properties. Locally applied heat brings a soothing warmth and tends to improve circulation in the skin and at least the more superficial muscle layers beneath. In addition, *topical heat applications* to the back require recumbency, which further adds to muscle and psychic relaxation and pain relief. This combination of inactivity, local soothing, and improved circulation can be extremely effective as an aid in the therapy for local muscle spasm or unpleasant muscle tension. Many practitioners distinguish between warm applications and hot applications; the point is to emphasize the potential danger of excessive heat. Repetitive applications of heat may lead to local impairment of thermal sensitivity. Some patients welcome the pain associated with excessive heat because it provides analgesically effective counterirritation. However, if the local heat is excessive, cutaneous burns can

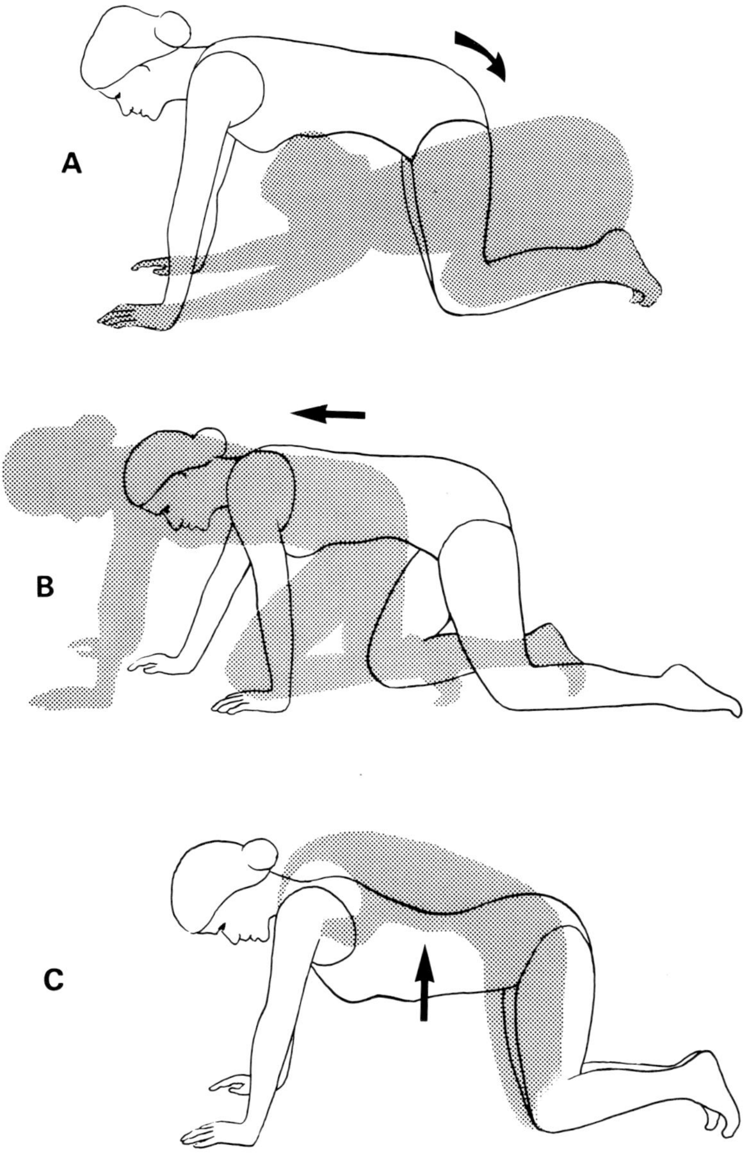

FIGURE 5.4. Quadripedal low back exercises are really variations of the Williams' exercise group done on all fours. Although these exercises employ the same basic back-limbering motions as the Williams' exercises, they also require more upper extremity exertion and overall more muscle activity in the trunk and limbs to support partial weight bearing. Examples include **(A)** all-fours crouching, **(B)** crawling, and **(C)** back arching.

easily result, which only aggravate the patient's problems—despite Oriental enthusiasm for moxibustion (see page 127). Even if damaging heat levels are not reached, repetitive applications of heat usually lead to brownish discoloration of the local skin—a feature that should be noted in the physical examination of patients with the failed back syndrome.

At home, *local heat application* can be done most efficiently through the use of an electric heating pad set on low or medium heat (Fig. 5.6A). It provides a continuous source of heat at a safe temperature. A certain mystique has grown about the use of moist heat rather than dry heat. In treating back pain, remember that the applied moisture does not penetrate through the skin. Moist heat is indeed effective if local skin problems such as infection or open wounds are present, but these are rarely encountered in failed back syndrome sufferers. Moist heat also develops some of its mystique from hospital

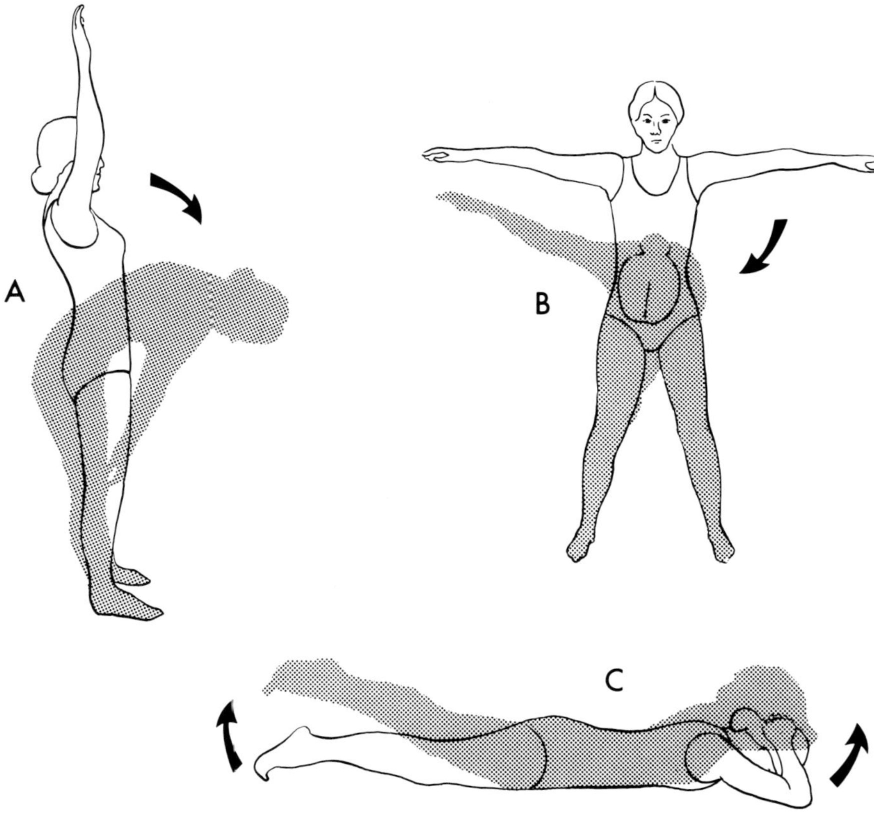

FIGURE 5.5. Back strengthening exercises force the back muscles to lift the weight of the body; hand-held weights can be added later. Among the most popular exercises are **(A)** standing forward bending, **(B)** standing, forward twist, and **(C)** prone, back arching.

use (Fig. 5.6B). For safety reasons, electric heating pads are rarely used in hospital settings, where heat packs are often used instead. Soaking such a heat pack in very warm water permits the pack to store a greater amount of heat, which is then released over a longer period of time. An alternative source of local heat application that is acceptable for hospital use is a small pad through which warm water is circulated from a small bedside heater. Like electric heating pads, these devices provide a continuous source of safe heat, although they may be less durable and more prone to breakdown than electric heating pads and require periodic refilling with water (Fig. 5.6C).

Topical cold applications are useful for their analgesic or counterirritating effect. They are particularly beneficial in an extremely acute situation or for the first 24 hours after an invasive needle procedure. The local numbing cold actually produces hypalgesia, at least in the skin and probably in tissues below the skin. Like applications of heat, applications of cold must be made with caution to prevent thermal injury or *frostbite*. Cold applications can be in the form of cold compresses, crushed ice in a waterproof sack with a dry or wet cloth between the ice and the body, or sprayed-on applications of ethyl chloride. The ethyl chloride spray must be handled carefully because it can easily produce frostbite and local tissue necrosis. Occasionally, cold applications are coupled with local massage through the use of ice cubes or "ice cube lollipops." The latter are made by inserting one or more tongue blades or short sticks into a glass or cup of water, then freezing it with the tongue blades protruding for later use as handles.

Radiant Energy

Topical applications of radiant energy usually employ *ultrasound* or *diathermy,* a high-energy radio-

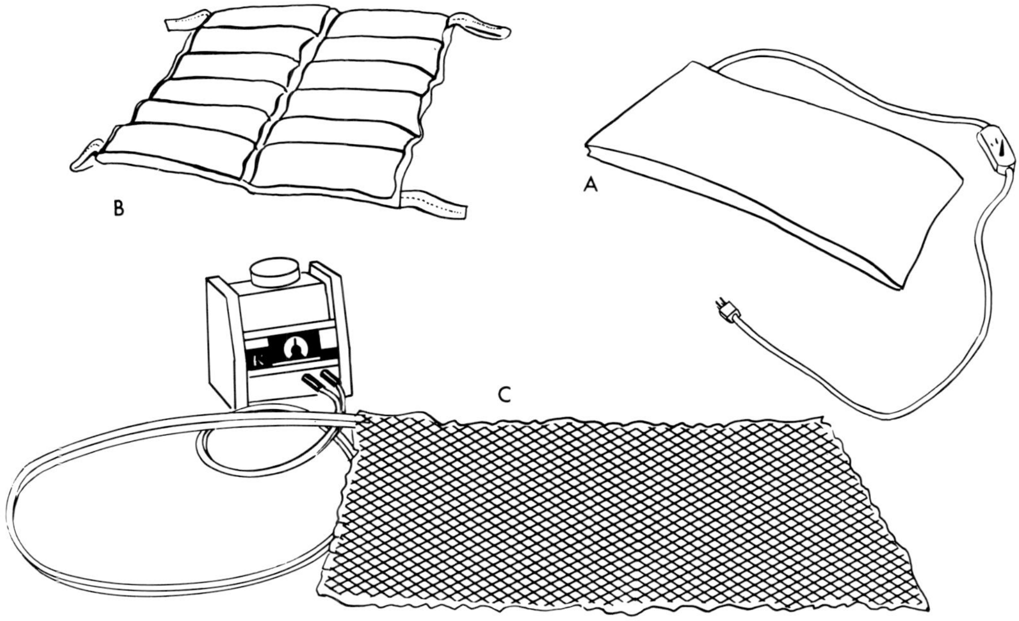

FIGURE 5.6. Local applications of heat to aching backs have been recognized as valuable since antiquity. **A:** Electric heating pads supply continuous warmth and are ideal for home use. **B:** Moisture adds little to heat application for backaches, but the moisture stores more heat in warm packs often used in hospitals. **C:** A newer device for local heat application, which meets hospital safety codes, is a warm-water pad with a remote heater and water circulation.

frequency radiation. These forms of radiant energy penetrate deeper into the body than simple topical thermal applications and cause heating in deep, as well as superficial, tissues. Like topical heat applications, they also produce their beneficial effect by inducing local soothing and muscle relaxation. These devices are not usually available for home use, but are frequently employed in physical therapy departments or at the patient's bedside in a hospital setting.

Massage

"Laying on of hands" has symbolized healing for many centuries. For patients with a failed back syndrome, a laying on of hands to perform back massage or massage of leg muscles in painful spasm also brings welcome relief—although only rarely are miraculous cures reported. Rolling, rubbing, pressing, kneading, and gently pounding tender back areas help to relax tight muscles and improve local circulation. The psychologic support inherent in body contact and personalized therapeutic attention also plays a key role. Spinal manipulation is a specialized outgrowth of massage therapy, which has as an additional goal the relocation of minimally but painfully subluxed bony alignments in the treated area. As discussed earlier (see page 121), this form of therapy carries more risk than simple back massage but may also be effective in providing pain relief. Massage is often facilitated by the application of emollient ointments or liquids such as rubbing alcohol. These help to protect the skin by controlling the degree of skin friction and friction-generated heat.

Topical Medications

Various analgesic *liniments* may also be applied before, during, or at the conclusion of massage or independent of massage. Many of these formulations include salicylates in the hope that a part of their effectiveness will include local penetration to provide a local analgesic effect. Most liniments have in common a local irritating effect that creates a sensation of warmth or heat in the area. This acts as a counterirritant to help block awareness or central transmission of nociceptive or painful receptor inputs. If care is taken not to induce skin blistering or allergic reactions, liniments are another readily available and frequently helpful adjunct to the therapy for painful backs and extremities.

Acupuncture and Transcutaneous Neurostimulation

Related to the use of counterirritating liniments are the more sophisticated techniques of *acupuncture* and *transcutaneous neurostimulation (TNS).* Although acupuncture has been in clinical use for several millennia and arguments still echo as to precisely how these topical analgesic therapies produce a beneficial effect, the general principle seems to have been scientifically elucidated only in the past few decades.[45-49] The current understanding of the basis of their effectiveness, often referred to as the *double gate theory,* may be simply explained as follows: Both pain-neutral touch sensations and nociceptive pain sensations reach conscious levels of the central nervous system (CNS) by transmission through the spinal cord. Each of these types of information travels in its own pathway or pathways dedicated principally to transmission of this particular type of information. Both types of information reach the brain through a second, generally polysynaptic and slower transmitting, pathway system that the two types of sensation share in common. If pain impulses flood the polysynaptic pathway, touch sensations are blocked from normal transmission and numbness of an extremity may result. On the other hand, if the common polysynaptic pathway is flooded with tactile or *pain-neutral* sensations, spontaneous pain impulses may be blocked from transmission. Acupuncture—both classic acupuncture done with needles only and electroacupuncture done by passing stimulating electric currents through the acupuncture needles—seems to produce analgesia in a manner similar, if not actually identical, to that of electrical transcutaneous neuro-stimulation (TNS). TNS employs cutaneous electrical stimulation, usually square wave pulses, at a frequency and intensity that elicit a local tingling or buzzing sensation. To be effective, this stimulation must be pain neutral, not painful. Studies that have compared TNS with acupuncture suggest that the mechanism by which both produce analgesia is similar if not identical, and that patients who respond to one technique are likely to respond to the other. The classic acupuncture lines and points have proven to be nonessential and in some instances perhaps even detrimental. Placement of needles or stimulating electrodes adjacent to, proximal to, or spanning the area of pain generally gives the best pain-relieving results (Fig. 5.7). Mechanical or electrical stimulation at remote points along classical acupuncture lines was less effective in at least one study, even though acupuncture brings with it a psychological mystique and personal contact that undoubtedly help to improve its effectiveness.[63] Other studies have shown that the best responders to acupuncture and TNS are those patients who are strongly suggestible. This does not imply

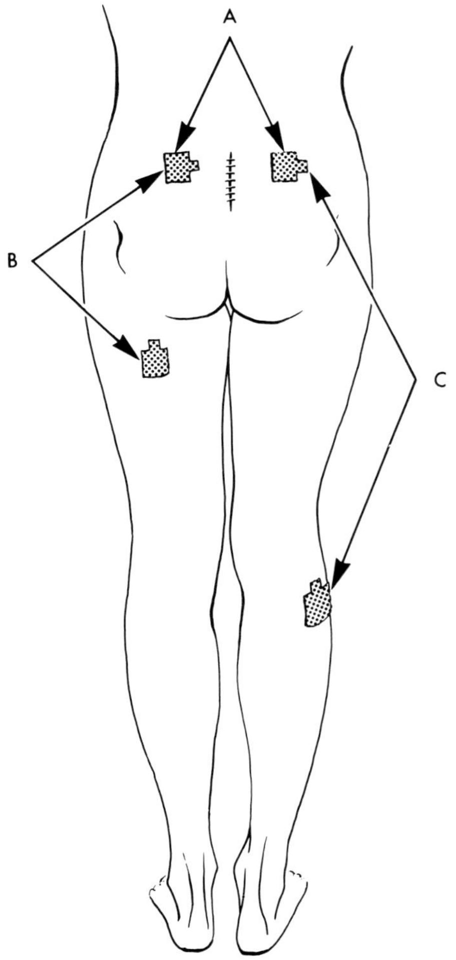

FIGURE 5.7. Transcutaneous neurostimulation (TNS) can be quite useful for failed back syndrome sufferers. Illustrated are the most frequent sites of successful application for the control of pain in the low back **(electrode pair A),** buttock pain **(electrode pair B),** and sciatic leg pain **(electrode pair C).**

that these techniques work through suggestion alone, but that they work best when supplemented by positive suggestion.

Acupressure and *moxibustion*, cutaneous stimulation by focal applications of pressure or heat, respectively, are variations on classical acupuncture that have some proponents. The first technique, acupressure, is rapidly gaining popularity in the United States. The second technique, moxibustion, remains popular primarily among Oriental peoples. This latter technique involves burning incense or medicinal herbs either directly on the skin or in small metal containers set on the patient's skin. The resulting small cutaneous burns, often symmetrically placed, can be puzzling to the uninitiated Occidental, who may incorrectly interpret them as evidence of child abuse or masochism.

TNS may be useful in both *chronic pain* and *postoperative or posttraumatic pain*.[64] Routine use of TNS postoperatively minimizes or eliminates patients' need for centrally depressive and potentially dangerous narcotics. Patients who have undergone restorative back surgery often can begin valuable activity and ambulation sooner than if they had to rely on pharmacologic therapy.

There are two major *disadvantages to acupuncture*. First, acupuncture entails penetration into, if not through, the skin. Numerous complications have been reported, including cellulitis, nerve injury, and even pneumothorax. The second drawback is that acupuncture must usually be performed by trained acupuncturists—specialists who are in relatively short supply and whose services add to the cost of the technique.

The major *complication of TNS* is skin irritation from the electrode placement sites. A variety of different electrode contact material is now available, including electrolyte moistened pads, electrolyte jellies, and solid gel pads. Rotating the contact points at the corners of an imaginary square on a daily basis will help to minimize this complication. It is recommended that TNS not be used in patients wearing cardiac pacemakers, but otherwise the technique seems relatively safe.

Both *acupuncture* and *TNS* have the *disadvantage* of being cumbersome, time-consuming, and expensive (if one includes the acupuncturist's fee or the cost of the stimulator device). The major attractiveness of both techniques is their relative safety, since they provide hypalgesia and pain relief without systemic medication. Unfortunately, neither technique is effective for all patients, and both provide a variable and essentially unpredictable degree of pain relief for different patients. Claims for the efficacy of both techniques vary widely. I have no personal experience with acupuncture, although acupuncturists claim success rates in the range of 60% to 90%. My experience with TNS has been primarily in the management of chronic pain, where my success rate has been 50% to 60% of patients achieving at least partial pain relief, but only half of these achieving pain relief sufficient to outweigh the nuisance value of continued application and use of the TNS device.

The *technique of TNS* use varies from clinic to clinic, depending in part on personnel availability. In some pain clinics, one or more paramedical or medical persons are assigned specifically to TNS therapy. These therapists are able to spend time with their patients both in introductory sessions and in daily therapy. This patient contact is likely to be quite valuable because of the positive-suggestion aspect alluded to earlier, and it undoubtedly improves results through more effective application of electrodes and stimulation parameters and encouragement of better patient compliance. When using TNS in an office setting, I have generally had patients use the device for one to three one-hour sessions at weekly intervals prior to continuing its use at home, initially on a loan basis. During the one-hour session, the patient is seen two or more times and likely skin sites are mapped—generally proximal to the pain or straddling the pain along a dermatomal or peripheral nerve distribution (Fig. 4.4). Stimulus parameters of frequency, amperage (or power output), and pulse width (if this variable is included in the particular device in use) are altered to deliver into the patient the maximum input that remains pain neutral and does not cause local muscle contraction. It is unclear how much difference changing these various parameters makes to the effectiveness of therapy, so long as the two basic considerations of pain neutrality and avoidance of muscle spasm are observed. Some therapists feel that patients who would otherwise not achieve pain relief can do so by careful manipulation of stimulus parameters, but my personal experience has not supported this contention.

The optimum *time duration of TNS* varies widely from patient to patient. It is best to continue TNS for periods of at least 30 to 60 minutes, since the pain-relieving effect often develops gradually. Once good pain control has been achieved, the device should be turned off during the test period to assess the duration of pain relief. Most commonly, pain relief persists beyond the period of actual stimulus application, although a few patients find it necessary to use continuous stimulation. The duration of pain relief beyond stimulus application varies from a few minutes to several days. In a few cases of mine, patients have found it necessary to use the stimulator only one hour weekly to obtain lasting benefit. With continued use, some patients experience progressive improvement in pain relief with progressive prolongation of the poststimulation amelioration of pain. Others find that the effectiveness gradually wanes. In some cases, this is undoubtedly related to a waning enthusiasm for the bother and nuisance of using the device, but in other patients this seems to be a real or physiologic phenomenon. Why this occurs is unknown, but it could be related to habituation in the brain opiate-receptor system.

Systemic Pharmacologic Therapy

During the decades in which I have dealt with patients with the failed back syndrome, I have discovered the area of systemic pharmacologic therapy to be both the *most abused* and the *most underused* of the therapeutic approaches available for the management of these patients. The abuse that I have encountered has primarily centered around injudicious and excessive use of narcotics, inappropriate withholding of narcotics, and illogical prescribing of muscle-relaxing medications. The area of underuse that I encounter with disturbing frequency involves systemic anti-inflammatory drugs and antineuralgia drugs. The other class of medications considered in this section is psychotropic pharmaceuticals.

Anti-Inflammatory Drugs

At least a score of systemic anti-inflammatory drugs are currently commercially available in the United States. This plethora of drugs attests both to the importance of these compounds and to the considerable patient idiosyncrasies encountered in their use. *Acetyl salicylate*, or *aspirin*, remains the basic standard against which most other anti-inflammatory drugs are compared. This remarkable drug was the first major anti-inflammatory drug to become commercially available and remains one of the most valuable. For optimum anti-inflammatory effectiveness, higher doses than are customarily used for aspirin's analgesic or antipyretic effects must be used. For an average adult, 3 g or 4 g daily in divided doses is generally required. As is true with most of the anti-inflammatory drugs, dosage must be carefully and individually tailored to balance side effects and effectiveness. Aspirin is a gastrointestinal irritant and prolongs blood clotting by interfering with platelet function. As a result, gastrointestinal bleeding is always a potentially serious complication, and patients should be cautioned about bloody or tarry stools and should be observed clinically for evidence of anemia or seriously impaired blood coagulation. Gastric irritation is perhaps the single major limiting feature in the use of aspirin. It can be minimized by having patients take aspirin with or before meals, with milk or antacids, or even with a large glass of water. Enteric-coated aspirin dissolves in the small intestine and thus bypasses direct gastric acidification. This does not prevent intestinal upset in all patients, but it is quite helpful for many. When aspirin is taken on an around-the-clock basis for its anti-inflammatory effect, the delayed absorption with enteric coating is not a problem.

A variety of *nonsteroidal anti-inflammatory drugs* now compete with aspirin in the pharmaceutical marketplace (see Table 5.1). Many of these drugs are said to have a diminished likelihood of causing gastrointestinal irritation and bleeding when compared to aspirin, but all of them are poorly tolerated by some patients. Some offer the advantage of longer duration of action, even once-a-day dosing, and one preparation is available for parenteral (intramuscular) administration.

Adrenal corticosteroids remain the most potent of the anti-inflammatory drugs. Among these, prednisone, dexamethasone, and methylprednisolone are probably the most popular. All of the adrenal corticosteroids have multiple, extremely potent effects and are potentially quite dangerous for long-term high-dose usage. Included among their potential side effects are iatrogenic Cushing syndrome, disturbance of other hormonal systems, fluid retention, hypertension, muscle weakness, osteoporosis,

TABLE 5.1. Nonsteroidal anti-inflammatory drugs.

Class	Chemical name	Brand name	Average dose
Salicylates	Acetylsalicylic acid	Aspirin	900 mg/4–6h
	Salicylsalicylic acid	Disalcid/Monogesic	1,500 mg q12h
	Sodium or potassium salicylate	Pabalate	600 mg/q4h
	Chlorine magnesium salicylate	Trilisate	1,500 mg/q12h
	Diflunisal	Dolobid	500–1,000 mg/q12h
Pyrazoles	Phenylbutazone	Butazolidin	100 mg/q6h
Acetic acids	Indomethacin	Indocin	50 mg/q8h
	Tolmetin sodium	Tolectin	100–400 mg/q6h
	Sulindac	Clinoril	200 mg/q12h
Propionic acids	Ibuprofen	Motrin	400–800 mg/q6h
	Naproxen	Naproxyn	275–550 mg/q12h
	Fenoprofen	Nalfon	300–600 mg/q6h
	Flurbiprofen	Ansaid	100 mg/q6–8h
	Ketoprofen	Orudis	50 mg/q6–8h
Oxicams	Piroxicam	Feldene	20 mg/q24h
Fenamates	Meclofenamate	Meclomen	100 mg/q6–8h

and psychiatric disturbances. When used on a long-term basis, the potential side effects of these drugs must be monitored extremely closely, and dosages must be strictly minimized. An every-other-day dosage schedule is often recommended to limit the suppression of endogenous hormone production. Although chronic use is dangerous and therefore of limited usefulness in failed back syndrome sufferers, local depository injections and short-course therapy are extremely useful. Local depository injections are discussed in detail later. These have the benefit of providing high local drug concentrations with limited systemic exposure. Short-course, high-dose, systemic steroid therapy was advocated in a report published by British clinicians several years ago.[65] These authors reported spectacular long-term relief of lumbago and sciatica in ambulatory patients treated with dexamethasone, beginning with 64 mg per day and tapering over one or two weeks. Unfortunately, my success rate in applying this therapy on American patients has been far more modest. My experience in several dozen patients includes more nonresponders than responders, but does include several examples of rapid and lasting success. I continue to use this form of therapy in otherwise healthy patients with acute or subacute episodes of lumbago, sciatica, or both who have limited and relatively stable neurologic deficits, usually combining pharmaceutical therapy with bed rest therapy. Of the available adrenal corticosteroid preparations, I prefer either dexamethasone (Decadron) or methylprednisolone (Medrol) for failed back syndrome sufferers. These two drugs seem to have a reduced incidence of psychologic complications and seem to cause less severe fluid retention than some of the other corticosteroids.

In the opening paragraph of this section I singled out anti-inflammatory pharmacotherapy as one of the most effective, yet most *underused, of the noninvasive therapies* available for the management of failed back syndrome patients. It is discouraging repeatedly to evaluate patients who have suffered for months or years without a trial of anti-inflammatory therapy and who then respond dramatically to this relatively simple therapeutic measure. One recent patient, who was able to return to heavy farm labor for the first time in two years within two months after anti-inflammatory therapy with ibuprofen was instituted, told me, “I had almost lost faith in doctors, but you have now restored my faith!” With characteristic modesty and exemplary honesty I pointed out to him that his dramatic improvement had been produced not by me but by a simple bottle of pills.

But which patients are *candidates for anti-inflammatory drug therapy?* I have achieved the best results in patients with chronic aching backs, especially those who exhibit the *double-peak* characteristic of *arthritis-like* pain. Patients who suffer principally from sciatica, especially sciatica with a burning or tingling quality suggesting neuralgic pain, are more likely to benefit from anti-neuralgia therapy (which will be discussed later)—

but occasionally they may achieve significant benefit from anti-inflammatory therapy.

I advise anti-inflammatory drug therapy for nearly every systemically healthy patient I see with *chronic lumbago* that has not responded to enforced inactivity or enforced activity or that has responded only transiently to these therapies. In prescribing anti-inflammatory drugs, one must be cognizant of their significant *analgesic property.* The physician who prescribes these drugs must be certain that they are not merely masking a potentially dangerous malignancy. He must also be aware of any potentially surgically correctable problem in order to determine how long to continue drug therapy—especially marginally effective therapy. At a minimum, I review lumbosacral spine radiographs, CT scans, or MRI scans in addition to taking a careful history and doing a physical examination before recommending anti-inflammatory drug therapy. The analgesic effect of these drugs can be a valuable asset when anti-inflammatory drug therapy is *combined with enforced activity therapy,* enabling patients to tolerate therapeutic activity more easily and for longer periods.

A history of currently or recently active peptic ulcer disease with gastrointestinal bleeding is a strong *contraindication* to anti-inflammatory drug therapy. Rarely, however, I recommend such therapy to patients who have experienced considerable gastrointestinal symptoms if they have proven to be refractory to a variety of other noninvasive and invasive therapies. In these patients, it is particularly important to minimize the side-effect risks with a regular intake of antacids and even with concomitant therapy using belladonna alkaloids (Donnatal), cimetidine (Tagamet), ranitidine (Zantac), or sucralfate (Carafate).

Anti-inflammatory drug therapy is complicated by the large number of available drugs and by the considerable *differences in patient response* to therapy (see Table 5.1). It is easy for neurosurgeons and orthopedic surgeons to become more interested in surgery than in drug therapy and therefore to be reluctant to spend the necessary time with patients to work through an effective anti-inflammatory drug program. Rheumatologists, internists, clinical pharmacologists, and family practitioners can perform this role admirably but should have a sufficient understanding of the complexities of back disease to know when to abandon anti-inflammatory therapy in favor of more invasive or surgical therapy. The differences in patient response to anti-inflammatory drugs appear both in the side effects they have and in therapeutic effectiveness. Dyspepsia with epigastric distress is by far the most commonly encountered side effect with all of the anti-inflammatory drugs, yet in a given patient this side effect may be prominent with one anti-inflammatory drug and not with another. On the other hand, a second patient may find exactly the reverse, tolerating the first drug but not the second. Therapeutic effectiveness varies with proper drug dosage as well as proper drug selection. Ideally, an anti-inflammatory drug should be found for each patient that will provide maximum effectiveness and minimum side effects. A lack of effectiveness for a given drug cannot be assumed on the basis of recommended drug doses only. The rate of degradation of the nonsteroidal anti-inflammatory drugs is enzymatically limited, and blood levels rise sharply once sufficient dosage is given to saturate the body enzyme systems. At this level, small increases in drug dosage may produce large improvements in effectiveness or sudden increases in side effects. But until this break-point level is reached, one cannot assume that the drug is ineffective—even though this level may not be reached for a given patient until drug dosage is considerably above the recommended dosage.

Duration of therapy with anti-inflammatory drug therapy is also quite important. I caution my patients that if the drug seems to bring relief, this means it should be continued, not that it is no longer necessary. In other words, patients who have suffered for many months with a chronic painful condition are unlikely to be cured in a short period of time, especially since many of them harbor persistent degenerative processes that will continue to plague them for many years, if not for the rest of their lives. I have encountered a tendency among some practitioners to prescribe anti-inflammatory drugs in short courses of two or three weeks and not to continue this therapy even though beneficial effects are beginning to be felt. I recommend continuation for a minimum of two to three weeks and allow at least four to six weeks before maximum improvement is assessed. If the anti-inflammatory therapy brings useful improvement with acceptable side effects and little risk, I have no objection to patients continuing this medication for months or even years—although they require continued medical supervision throughout this period to guard against occult gastrointestinal bleeding, impaired blood coagulation, hepatic disturbance, or other potential side effects of long-term usage.

Antineuralgia Drugs

Antineuralgia drugs are principally effective for patients with sciatica or with radiating pains of a burning, tingling, or lancinating quality that suggest nerve origin (see Table 5.2). Most useful among the neuralgia drugs are some of the anticonvulsant drugs. However, I have found some success with specific vitamin therapy, one centrally acting muscle relaxant, and anti-inflammatory and psychotropic drugs.

Phenytoin (Dilantin) and *carbamazepine (Tegretol)* are the most widely employed anticonvulsant drugs that have significant antineuralgia effectiveness. Their use is widely known in the treatment of tic douloureux and painful multiple sclerosis (MS), but their effectiveness in treating chronic sciatica is often overlooked. Phenytoin may cause allergic skin rashes or ataxia at higher blood levels. Carbamazepine is perhaps a more effective antineuralgia drug than phenytoin but causes nausea or dizziness with elevated blood levels and rarely may cause acute or chronic leukopenia. Both drugs initially have long half-lives in the body, although carbamazepine stimulates an increase in body enzymes over a few weeks of use, so that its half-life falls to as short as six to eight hours. This means that when drug therapy is first initiated, clinical effectiveness is apt to be delayed until a sufficient blood level is gradually reached. This also means considerable latitude can be tolerated in dosage schedules, especially with phenytoin. Some patients prefer a b.i.d. (twice daily) or even a once daily dosage rather than the more customary t.i.d. (thrice daily), q.i.d. (four times daily), or q6h (every six hours) schedules. The long half-life also means that toxic blood levels can gradually develop with prolonged use, resulting in late onset of ataxia, dizziness, somnolence, or confusion as dose-dependent phenomena. The slow onset of effectiveness can be speeded up by giving loading doses of phenytoin, but this is poorly tolerated with carbamazepine. In fact, when carbamazepine is administered it is usually best to begin with a very small dose and to increase the dose gradually over several weeks. This slow schedule minimizes the side effects of dizziness and nausea that may interfere with abrupt initiation of high-dose treatment schedules.

Clonazepam (Klonopin) is another anticonvulsant that has some benefit as an antineuralgic drug. This drug tends to cause drowsiness, at least initially. Habituation often develops, so that the drug's effectiveness wanes after a period of months. I find it useful for patients with acute crises of sciatica, and I use it especially in patients who are intolerant of or allergic to both phenytoin (Dilantin) and carbamazepine (Tegretol). The usual dosage is 0.5 mg to 2 mg q.i.d. or q6h.

Baclofen (Lioresal) is a centrally active muscle relaxer and antispasticity drug that inhibits both monosynaptic and polysynaptic spinal reflexes and that is an analog of gamma-aminobutyric acid

TABLE 5.2 Drugs useful for neuralgic pain.

Generic name	Brand name	Usual dose	Secondary effects
Diphenylhydantoin	Dilantin	100 mg t.i.d. or b.i.d. or 200 mg b.i.d.	Mildly sedating, frequent allergic rash
Carbamazepine	Tegretol	200 mg b.i.d. to q.i.d.	Rare suppression of white blood count
Clonazepam	Klonopin	0.5 to 2 mg b.i.d. to q.i.d. or only q.h.s.	Sedating
Baclofen	Lioresal	10 to 20 mg t.i.d. or q.i.d.	Muscle weakness at higher doses
Thiamine HCL	Vitamin B_1	100 mg b.i.d. to q.i.d.	Uncertain effectiveness
Amitriptyline	Elavil	10 to 50 mg q.h.s.	Sedating or depersonalizing
Trazodone	Desyril	50 to 100 mg q.h.s.	Sedating or depersonalizing
Haloperidol	Haldol	0.5 to 2 mg q.h.s.	Sedating or depersonalizing

(GABA), an inhibitory neurotransmitter. In addition to its muscle-relaxing and antispasticity actions, it has been demonstrated to have an ameliorating effect on trigeminal neuralgia and on spinal pain. When used chronically in doses of 10 mg to 20 mg q6h it can provide considerable relief for sciatic pain and seems to have an additive effect with phenytoin or carbamazepine.

The scientific validity for using *vitamin therapy for neuralgic pain* is extremely tenuous. I have the distinct impression that this therapy provides a useful adjunct to anticonvulsant medications and have encountered several patients who have obtained striking relief of neuralgic pains with vitamin therapy only. There is little proven scientific confirmation of such an antineuralgic effect, but I have no objection to using an effective placebo if that placebo is safe and perhaps even beneficial dietetically. I rely principally on thiamine hydrochloride (vitamin B_1) 200 mg to 400 mg daily, with a full awareness that at these dosage levels a considerable amount of the vitamin is excreted unchanged in the urine. It has been clearly shown that normal nervous tissue is heavily biochemically dependent on thiamine and that damaged and regenerating nervous tissue requires larger than normal amounts of this vitamin. Nicotinic acid has a less secure place in the biochemistry of nervous tissue, but at dosages of 50 mg b.i.d. or t.i.d., it acts as a mild peripheral vasodilator. The mild flushing that patients experience certainly adds to its placebo effectiveness, and perhaps the improved circulation to injured areas offers some direct therapeutic benefit.

Anti-inflammatory drugs and *psychotropic drugs* may also benefit patients with neuralgic pains. These drugs are discussed elsewhere. The anti-inflammatory drugs may have a direct ameliorating effect on inflamed or injured nerves, may provide a secondary benefit by reducing perineural inflammation, or may simply act through their significant nonspecific analgesic effect. Many of the psychotropic drugs have been shown to have an effect on central transmission of pain impulses and certainly offer indirect effects on neuralgic pain through psychic amelioration.

Muscle-Relaxing Drugs

Muscle-relaxing medications are frequently prescribed improperly. Patients with predominantly leg or sciatic pain almost never achieve significant relief from these drugs; patients with combined back and leg pain only occasionally obtain relief from these drugs; and patients with predominantly low back pain obtain relief from these drugs only if muscle tightness or spasm is an integral part of their disorder. To prescribe drugs aimed at muscle relaxation when pain originates from an injured nerve is illogical, yet such prescriptions are frequently written by well-meaning practitioners. If a scheme of symptomatic classification is used, such as that propounded in earlier chapters, most errors in prescribing muscle-relaxing medication can be avoided. Nonetheless, even in the category of patients with predominantly low back pain, accurate prescribing requires a sufficiently careful physical examination and a sufficiently accurate diagnosis to determine whether pain of muscle origin is present as a primary or secondary basis for the patient's discomfort.

Among the available muscle-relaxing medications (see Table 5.3), I prefer *methocarbamol (Robaxin), cyclobenzaprine (Flexeril)* or *orphenadrine citrate plus acetaminophen (Parafon Forte),* reserving *diazepam (Valium)* for special circumstances. I am fully aware that the effectiveness of methocarbamol as a pure muscle relaxant has been seriously challenged, yet I find it extremely helpful clinically. Methocarbamol seems to have a minor tranquilizing effect and seems to produce muscle relaxation principally by a depressant action at a spinal or central level. It is not a major tranquilizer and causes little sedation. For patients who tolerate aspirin well, Robaxisal, a combination of methocarbamol and aspirin, is often useful; it combines in a readily available single tablet the analgesic and anti-inflammatory effects of salicylate and methocarbamol's muscle relaxation. Orphenadrine offers the advantage of a longer duration of action but seems similar in effectiveness to methocarbamol. Orphenadrine is combined with acetaminophen as Parafon Forte, a compound that supplements the primary muscle-relaxing effect with a mild analgesic effect. The analgesic additive may be a muscle relaxant, since it helps limit secondary protective muscle tightness in response to pain. Cyclobenzaprine produces muscle relaxation peripherally with minimal central muscle-relaxing effect. It is chemically related to the tricyclic antidepressants (such as amitriptyline and imipramine) and thus can be dangerous if used concomitantly

TABLE 5.3 Commonly employed muscle-relaxing medications.

Generic name	Brand name	Relative muscle-relaxing potency*	Relative sedating effect*
Baclofen	Lioresal	+++	+
Carisoprodol	Soma	+	++
Chlordiazepoxide	Librium	++	+++
Chlorzoxazone	Parafon, Spasgesic	+	++
Cyclopenzaprine	Flexeril	++	++
Dantrolene	Dantrium	+++	+
Diazepam	Valium	++	+++
Meprobamate	Equanil, Miltown	++	++
Metaxalone	Skelaxin	+	++
Methocarbamol	Robaxin	+	++
Quinine sulfate	Quinamm	+	+

*Scale of + to +++ based on clinical observations.

with monoamine oxidase inhibitors such as isocarboxazid (Marplan), phenelzine (Nardil), or tranylcypromamine (Parnate). It not uncommonly causes drowsiness, dizziness, or dry mouth. *Baclofen (Lioresal)* was discussed earlier as an antineuralgia drug because of its spinal inhibitory action, but it is marketed primarily as a muscle-relaxing and antispasticity drug. Thus it can be used either chronically for its antineuralgia effect or acutely for its muscle-relaxing effect. *Diazepam* is unquestionably a good muscle relaxant, but its tranquilizing properties cause me to limit its use to special circumstances. For ambulatory patients or patients whom one is attempting to motivate to return to a program of enforced activity, the tranquilization and impairment of motivation diazepam produces may be undesirable. Diazepam can also severely aggravate or primarily induce emotional depression, and its long-term use in failed back syndrome sufferers is fraught with the danger of precipitating a serious psychiatric deterioration. On the other hand, when patients are being treated with enforced inactivity, diazepam is often the drug of choice. Enforced inactivity is usually carried out over a relatively restricted period of time and is easier to carry out with a somewhat tranquilized patient. Supplementing enforced inactivity therapy with diazepam achieves both muscle relaxation and tranquilization. *Dantrolene sodium (Dantrium)* is an extremely potent, peripherally acting muscle relaxer that is rarely used in the treatment of patients with failed back syndrome. Dantrolene is so potent that muscle relaxation can produce muscle weakness. It is occasionally useful in patients with acute crises of severe, visible, and palpable muscle spasms that do not rapidly relax with other muscle relaxers and topical supplements.

Analgesic Drugs

Analgesics or anodynes continue to be one of the *most abused classes of medicines* in current general use. Abuse through excessive use, with or without addiction, is widely recognized, especially in our drug-conscious modern society. On the other hand, I frequently encounter abuses in the opposite direction: a *failure to prescribe* adequate amounts of pain-relieving medications. This latter abuse is particularly prevalent in the early postoperative period. Many physicians, especially young physicians more attuned to the pill-popping propensity of our present generation, are admirably aware of the potentials of drug dependency and drug addiction attendant upon the use of opioids and other analgesics. They do not always understand, however, that improperly withholding opioids during the early postoperative period may in fact increase rather than decrease the risk of subsequent drug addiction. Pain is an undesirable and distressing phenomenon in our human existence. The postoperative pain that follows lumbar surgery is often distressing indeed. If patients with severe acute postoperative pain are denied adequate relief in the early postoperative course, they quickly learn to fear their pain and dread its return. As a result, they tend to request anodynes increasingly more regularly and more stridently as the surgeon attempts to withdraw the relief they need too soon. I do not condone the long-term use of opioids, and in general I feel that it is extremely unwise to send patients home on strong or frequent opioids. Instead, I advocate adequate opioid or nonopioid analgesics during the postoperative period when pain is reasonably expected to be severe, continuing this beyond the first week if painful complications (such as wound infection) develop. Most opioids lose their effectiveness in less than four hours, so having medication available on an every-three-hour basis is important in this early limited period. When the patient spontaneously begins to request opioids less frequently, the dose can gradually be reduced and the suggestion can be made to the patient that he consider intermittent substitution of oral medications to space out the parenteral opioid. The oral medications may be either less potent opioids or nonnarcotic analgesics, but care must be taken in combining opioids with mixed opiate agonist-antagonist analgesics. Opioids act on the CNS to reduce the patient's emotional reaction to pain, but actually neither block the transmission of pain impulses nor reduce the initiation of pain impulses at the site of tissue damage or inflammation. As a result, oral preparations containing salicylates or acetaminophen are often more effective than parenteral opioids alone. A reduction in opioid intake can usually be facilitated by judicious supplementation with other appropriate medications: muscle-relaxing drugs for painful muscle spasms, anti-neuralgia drugs for burning dysesthetic sciatica, and anti-inflammatory drugs if acute pain persists longer than expected in the absence of complications.

Pain-relieving drugs can be grouped in two main categories: *nonnarcotics and opioids*. This categorization does not include drugs that produce their pain-relieving effect secondarily, such as anti-neuralgia drugs, anti-inflammatory drugs, and antibiotics. Several of the anti-inflammatory drugs also have a significant pain-relieving capability, perhaps related to their ability to interfere with prostaglandin metabolism. These drugs, including aspirin and ibuprofen (Motrin), often synergize quite effectively with opioids, and for some types of pain of inflammatory origin they may be even more effective than opioids. Nearly all anti-inflammatory drugs have the potential for causing stomach distress, a reaction that can be minimized by ingesting the drug with meals, antacids, or a large glass of water.

Acetaminophen (Tylenol) shares with aspirin an antipyretic effect and the ability to synergize usefully with opioids, but it has no appreciable anti-inflammatory effect. The major attractiveness of acetaminophen is its limited risk of causing stomach distress. However, large doses or prolonged heavy intake can lead to serious hepatic difficulties. *Mefenamic acid (Ponstel)* is also a prostaglandin inhibitor and an analgesic and anti-inflammatory drug of mild potency, but it is popular primarily for menstrual cramps. *Ethoheptazine* is similar in potency to *propoxyphene (Darvon),* but has been less popular. This preparation comes combined with aspirin as *Zactirin.*

Several nonnarcotic analgesics have both pain-relieving and opiate-antagonist properties. The *mixed opiate agonist-antagonist drugs* do not synergize well with opioids and, in fact, may precipitate acute opiate withdrawal symptoms when administered to patients who are physically dependent on opioids. *Propoxyphene (Darvon)* is a widely employed drug of this class. It is available in oral preparation either alone or compounded with aspirin or acetaminophen. Considerable controversy has developed in recent years because of the drug's widespread use, its proven potential for abuse, and its mild addictive potential. When taken in conjunction with barbiturates or alcohol, dangerous CNS depression may result, and deaths have been reported. Several studies have also challenged the effectiveness of propoxyphene. These studies challenge whether its pain-relieving effect is any more potent than aspirin, or whether it is even as potent as aspirin.

Pentazocine (Talwin or Talacen) is said to be more potent as an analgesic than the above-mentioned drugs; another advantage is that it can be administered parenterally as well as orally. Some patients are unable to tolerate pentazocine because of agitation, confusion, or even disorientation. *Nalbuphine (Nubaine) and butorphanol (Stadol)* are potent opiate agonist-antagonist drugs. At the present time, they are available as parenteral solutions only. They are said to have a pain-relieving potency nearly as great as morphine and to cause little respiratory depression.

The most commonly employed *opioids* are *codeine, oxycodone, hydrocodone, meperidine (Demerol), morphine,* and *hydromorphine (Dilaudid)*—listed roughly in order of increasing potency. Codeine may be given parenterally or orally. It synergizes well with aspirin or acetaminophen and is often compounded with these drugs. *Oxycodone* is an oral preparation that comes compounded with aspirin (Percodan) or with acetaminophen (Percocet or Tylox). These two formulations are extremely popular and are often rather freely dispensed despite their serious addicting potential. Hydrocodone is most commonly compounded with acetaminophen (Vicodan) and may have a slightly lower addiction potential than oxycodone. *Meperidine (Demerol)* is most commonly administered parenterally. It is generally well-tolerated, produces less of a euphoric effect than morphine, but may cause severe, prolonged confusion and agitation. It may be given orally, but its extremely high addicting potential is a major liability. I feel that there are few, if any, indications for allowing patients to take meperidine except while hospitalized. Certainly no patient should be allowed to take potent opioids at home unless he has convincingly demonstrated to the physician or surgeon that he has a good likelihood of avoiding addiction through conscientious, intermittent, and intelligent self-administration. *Morphine* is an extremely potent analgesic and has strong psychic effects. It is most commonly administered in parenteral form, but recently an oral controlled-release (12-hour) formulation (MS Contin) has gained popularity for the treatment of chronic pain. Its pain-relieving effectiveness has been attributed at least in part to its psychic effects, with this effect being likened to a form of chemical lobotomy. This psychic effect makes morphine a particularly useful agent when pain is combined with agitation, severe anxiety, or dread of the condition causing pain (such as terminal cancer). On a per milligram basis, *hydromorphine (Dilaudid)* is the most potent opioid in general use. Although the potency of its psychic effect is less than that of morphine, it is approximately equal in analgesic effectiveness, in causing respiratory depression, and in its addicting potential. *Methadone (Dolophine)* is used chiefly in narcotic withdrawal and maintenance programs, but may on rare occasions be useful for the failed back syndrome patient. Methadone has a morphinelike action but causes less severe physical dependency and a more protracted, but less severe, withdrawal syndrome. Its long duration of action (36 to 48 hours) differs markedly from the other commonly used opioids, though its pain-relieving effect seems to be of considerably shorter duration (4 to 8 hours) than its central depressant effect. Frequent administration can lead to a cumulative depressant effect and dangerous oversedation or respiratory depression. It may, on rare occasions, be useful for the patient with chronic pain who cannot be weaned from opioids and for whom no other pain-relieving therapy proves to be effective.

Physical and psychologic addiction is a potentially serious complication of narcotic use that is well-recognized by physicians and patients alike, even though the reason for the relative frequency of addiction is not always clearly appreciated. The emotional "high" or sense of pleasure and euphoria that narcotics bring may be minimal or even absent in patients who take narcotics for severe pain. As a result, chronic pain sufferers are less likely to continue to request narcotics for their psychic effects than casual or "street" users. As discussed earlier, psychologic dependence can certainly occur if patients learn to fear and dread their pain and learn to look forward to narcotic medication for the relief of pain. Physical dependency occurs with prolonged narcotic intake in all classes of users, patients included. Perhaps surprising to many practitioners, however, is the fact that the withdrawal symptoms experienced by patients who have used narcotics chronically and in large doses for severe pain are often surprisingly mild if those patients are abruptly relieved of their pain by an operative procedure.

What makes opioids so dangerous for chronic use in pain sufferers is their *stimulating effect on pain,* a feature of opioid pharmacology that is not widely appreciated. Opioids have a dual effect on the nervous system—both a depressing effect and a stimulating effect. When morphine is given to a cat, for example, the stimulating effect predominates, and wild and uncontrolled behavior ensues. In humans, this stimulating effect is overpowered by a CNS suppressing effect. Current pharmacology has explained this in terms of polypeptide or endogenous opiate biochemistry in the CNS. The practical result is that with increasing use of opioids, the more prolonged CNS stimulating effect becomes progressively more pronounced. As a result, when the short-term CNS depressing and pain-relieving effect wears off, after three hours or so, the patient actually experiences increased pain. This can represent an augmentation of his organic pain or, in extreme instances, the pain can be entirely a manifestation of *opioid withdrawal.* Thus, the longer a patient takes opioids, the less likely it is he will be able to stop taking them because of the pain generated by their *withdrawal.* Many patients have seen depictions of street junkies being withdrawn from narcotics. This kind of withdrawal can be extremely unpleasant, not merely because of the associated diarrhea, jittery nerves, tremulousness, and anxiety, but because of real and severe pain. This type of withdrawal reaction can be acutely precipitated by giving the patient drugs that are *opiate antagonists* (such as naloxone or Narcan) or mixed opiate agonist-antagonists (such as propoxyphene or Darvon, and nalbuphine or Nubaine). Many patients who have taken opioids chronically report that they are "allergic to" or "had a reaction to" propoxyphene or other nonnarcotic anodynes. When such a history is obtained, one must weigh it carefully to assess whether this is indicative of opiate addiction and precipitation of opiate withdrawal symptoms by the opiate antagonist component of these drugs.

Around-the-clock dosage of opioids at intervals of every three hours (or less frequently if methadone is used) is advocated in hospices for the terminally ill and in certain pain clinic settings that deal with patients in chronic pain. The rationale is an attempt to limit the psychologic dependence on opioids by limiting rebound opiate withdrawal pain and the dread that it precipitates. For chronic pain patients, minimizing the dread of pain can make it easier to begin a program of gradual reduction in opioid dosage and ultimately the substitution of nonnarcotic pain medications. This approach is fraught with difficulty and must be carried out with a cooperative and understanding patient who is receiving full psychologic support and support of other curative or at least pain-relieving therapies. During this period of opioid withdrawal, the side effects of physical dependency that occur can be ameliorated with other medications: *belladonna alkaloids (Donnatal)* or *kaolin with pectin (Kaopectate)* to control stomach cramps and diarrhea, and *tranquilizers, beta-adrenergic blockers* (such as propranolol or Inderal), *alpha-adrenergic stimulants* (such as clonidine HCl or Catapres), or *clonazepam (Klonopin)* to control anxiety, tremulousness, and pain. The ideal supportive therapy for this period of opiate withdrawal is, of course, the elimination of pain through effective restorative or ablative therapy.

The plethora of pain-relieving drugs currently marketed in the United States has been criticized by pharmacologic purists and has recently been under scrutiny by the U.S. Food and Drug Administration. The list of available preparations includes many *composite drugs,* and it is these drugs that have come under special attack. Pharmacologic purists point out that few of these combinations are based on quantifiably beneficial drug-drug interactions and that there is little scientifically valid data to suggest that these multidrug combinations are any more effective than their basic ingredients alone. The potential for a greater number and greater variety of side effects with multiple drug combinations has been pointed out. The rationale is that patients who really need only the major component drug should not be unnecessarily exposed to the other drugs present in composite preparations; patients who require multiple drugs can achieve the same effect by taking multiple pills.

After years of dealing with pain sufferers, many of whom have suffered chronically and who have been exposed to a variety of pain-relieving medications previously, I disagree strongly with the contention that multiple drug combinations should be eliminated from the marketplace or their availability severely curbed. I have little experience dealing with rats or other laboratory animals subjected to experimentally induced pain, but I do know that nearly all studies that I have read comparing various analgesic medications report that at least a significant minority of patients achieve pain relief with nearly all of the drugs that have been tested. Humans respond unpredictably to pain-relieving medications. Over the years, I have encountered numerous patients who have obtained excellent and useful pain relief from one of the nonnarcotic drug combinations, even though they have not previously obtained pain relief with a series of other drugs. Whether this represents a true idiosyncratic response or a placebo response does not alter the fact that these patients have been able to resume a more normal, useful, and fulfilling life with the aid of these relatively safe medications than they had previously been able to achieve with other available preparations. Every practicing physician is also acutely aware of the major problem of patient compliance when using any form of pharmacotherapy. A series of drugs conveniently formulated in a single pill or capsule is much more likely to be ingested, and more likely to be ingested in correct dosage, by the average patient than if that patient were required to take the same multiple ingredients in a series of separate pills or capsules.

The *placebo effect* is a potent one that has misled many clinicians and investigators. Recent evidence suggests that placebo medications may actually alter the brain-stem opiate polypeptide systems that mediate pain. If this observation is correct, this means that placebo medications alter not only a patient's psyche but also his actual pain perception. The placebo response is of course strongly influenced by patient suggestibility and by the patient's trust in his clinician. In most series, approximately one third of patients exhibit some pain-relieving response to placebo administration and approximately two thirds do not. Especially in view of the brain polypeptide observations, one must be careful not to assume that a patient's pain is not real just because he responds favorably to placebo administration. This suggests that the patient may be more responsive to positive suggestion and may be more trusting of his physician, but the pain relief brought by the placebo may be very real indeed.

There are two major general risks in placebo administration. First, the nurses who administer the placebo medication tend to assume, correctly or incorrectly, that the clinician has concluded that his patient's pain is not real and that the patient is a "crock" or psychologic sufferer. Second, placebo effectiveness is proportional to the patient's trust in his physician, but the discovery that he has been given "phony" medication may cause serious inroads on this trust and may have a significant deleterious effect on future therapeutic efforts.

Psychotropic Drugs

Antidepressants and *tranquilizers* are often useful in the management of patients with the failed back syndrome. Pain and suffering are subjective assessments and are therefore exquisitely subject to modification by psychic factors. The development of effective pharmacotherapy has been one of the great medical advances of our generation. This has largely eliminated the use of lobotomies as psychotherapy and has sharply reduced the need for psychiatric hospital beds.

Patients who have suffered for months or years with pain or disability are almost certain to exhibit some degree of *emotional depression*. Even if their pain is organic, its prolonged continuation and the severe disruption of personal life and productivity that it causes are certain to generate a secondary or reactive depression. Primary or preexisting depression renders a person who develops a painful and disabling illness less likely to be able to deal with that illness. Chronic disability may result from symptoms that would not be disabling to an emotionally healthy patient.

Anxiety is another potent and common psychologic force in failed back syndrome sufferers. Worries over livelihood, masculine or feminine image, or sexual performance, as well as fear and dread of pain all contribute to emotional tension or anxiety. As is true with depression, an anxiety-prone personality may have preceded the back difficulty or a newly developed anxiety can severely hamper recovery and prolong suffering and disability.

The abuse of psychotropic drugs has also been severe and frequent by both physicians and patients. It is easy for the physician to prescribe tranquilizers when he does not understand the patient's disease. This certainly is easier than attempting to understand a patient's psychodynamics or taking sufficient time to give that patient the emotional support and simple psychotherapy that is needed. Patients also find it easier to "pop pills" than to face the harsh reality of a disabling disease. Accepting the responsibility for an active role in one's recovery or rehabilitative process is essential but is emotionally demanding. This unpleasant drain on a patient's psychic energy can too easily be shirked when the handy cop-out of tranquilizers sings its siren song in nearly every popular magazine and at many social gatherings. Tranquilizers can have a significant detrimental effect on physical and intellectual performance in the workplace and at home. Equally important is their disruptive effect on the motivation to continue a rehabilitative or restorative program. When used wisely to control disabling and destructive anxiety, depression, or both, and to help control pain in association with these disorders, psychotropic drugs can be extremely beneficial. When abused by patient or physician they can produce the proverbial pimple on the posterior of progress and can be a serious detriment to therapy.

The list of available *psychotropic drugs* grows longer every year. *Diazepam (Valium)* was mentioned earlier because it possesses useful muscle-relaxing properties in addition to its tranquilizing properties. I will not attempt to sort through the list of available tranquilizers, since these drugs are employed ubiquitously in medical practice and most practitioners are already familiar with their own favorites. Among the antidepressants, I have relied most heavily on *imipramine (Tofranil), desipramine (Pertofrane),* and *amitriptyline (Elavil).* As discussed earlier, these drugs seem to have some effectiveness in ameliorating pain nonspecifically and pain of neuralgic origin specificially. Amitriptyline also seems to have some slowing effect on the central transmission of pain impulses.

Intravenous Lidocaine Therapy

Intravenous infusions of lidocaine, or other local anesthetics, offer the possibility of sustained and at times cumulative benefit.[66] Outpatient infusions of 1 to 5 mg/kg provide relief of diffuse musculoskeletal, neuralgic, or deafferentation pain for about half of the patients treated, but with relief lasting more than a week in about one fourth of the responders. The mechanism of the prolonged benefit is unknown, but might be due to desensitization of central or peripheral pain neurons to chemical neurotransmitters.

Psychological Therapy

The importance of psychological difficulties in patients with the failed back syndrome is discussed in detail under psychogenic factors in Chapter 3 and has been referred to frequently throughout other sections of this text. Psychiatric ramifications are an important element of every case of failed back syndrome and must be addressed at every level of therapy.[67] I feel it is useful to consider *three echelons or gradations of approach* to these psychologic problems, whether they bear a cause or effect relationship to the major disease. *Office psychotherapy* should be a part of every contact between clinician and patient. A greater commitment of time and effort is required if a patient is to enter into one of the *anxiety and pain-relieving therapies* that I designate as *psychosomatic psychotherapy.* Embarking upon *formal psychotherapy* requires an acceptance by the patient. This form of therapy is extremely beneficial for preexisting or "reactive" psychologic manifestations with disturbances of personality or interpersonal relationships. Unfortunately, formal psychotherapy is of limited effectiveness in the management of pain per se.

Office Psychotherapy

Office psychotherapy, as I define it, does not entail formal psychotherapeutic methodology and does not require extensive psychiatric training. As already stated, some degree of psychologic reaction or preexisting psychopathology is present in almost every patient who suffers from the failed back syndrome. Furthermore, the suffering caused by pain is a psychologic phenomenon. As such, its severity is dramatically influenced by psychologic stress, depression, and anxiety.

Although many physicians view their role in society with an element of self-reverence, not all physicians are aware of the potential impact of their words on their patients. The *physician's words,* once loosed upon the patient, can have dramatic and sometimes unexpected impact. A casually selected word or phrase may be misconstrued by the patient as a pronouncement of doom, futility, rejection, or damnation to eternal suffering. This interpretation, or misinterpretation, of the physician's words may have serious destructive psychologic impact on the patient's pain, confidence in his physician, and motivation toward recovery. On the other hand, seemingly minor aspects of the physician's role during contact with the patient can bestow significant beneficial effects. An attitude of *careful attention* to the patient's historical recounting not only aids the physician in arriving at a correct diagnosis and selection of appropriate therapy, but may also buoy the patient with hope and confidence—and may help considerably to reduce the patient's pain and anxiety. Similar benefits can derive from careful discussion with the patient to explain the physician's detailed assessment of the patient's problem, the potential therapeutic measures that are available, and the physician's rationale for recommending a specific diagnostic or therapeutic choice from among the available alternatives. As stated earlier, it is always more beneficial to state to a patient that "nothing needs to be done" than to state that "nothing can be done." A Pollyannaish optimism or an overly cheerful encouragement that does not take into account the patient's anxieties is not likely to be beneficial. This kind of *inappropriate reaction to a problem* that has brought severe distress and disruption to a patient's life is usually not well accepted and may erode the patient's confidence in the physician. It is often true that the patient must learn to live with the problem, but this need not be expounded to the patient as a pronouncement of doom. The message will be just as realistic but better accepted and less destructive if it is expressed in supportive language. The patient should be made to feel that although he indeed must learn to live with the problem, he need not face the prospect of such a living hell totally alone and without support. Facing a continuing, anguished nightmare of existence will be somewhat easier if the patient is made to realize that he can continue to call upon the physician for physical, pharmacologic, and emotional support.

The physician should always be keenly conscious of the fact that there is no such thing as *purely organic or purely nonorganic pain*. The physician must always be conscious of the ever-present cyclic interaction involving tissue injury, pain, and psychological reaction or predisposition. Pain can lead to actual tissue injury just as certainly as emotional distress can lead to real pain. All persons who experience pain experience an emotional reaction to that pain. In most patients the emotional reaction to pain is appropriate and nondestructive, but in some patients the emotional reaction is maladaptive and can be detrimental to the patient's well-being and recovery. Sorting out the relative importance and etiologic significance of physical and psychological factors is rarely easy—even for trained psychiatrists and psychologists. Every health care worker should be aware of the dual, yet intertwined, roles of "psyche" and "soma" in the failed back syndrome and of the universal cyclic interaction between pain and emotions.

The physician must be able to *communicate* these concepts to patients, stressing the interaction of psyche and soma. This must be done to *educate* the patient about the importance of the intertwined duality of the pain experience. Communicating these concepts is important in reassuring the patient that the physician is attempting to help him by dealing with psychological as well as physical factors, so that the patient does not feel that the physician is simply rejecting him. This communication must be done in a fashion that is meaningful to the patient. The use of polysyllabic medical jargon usually results in noncommunication. Even simply phrased statements often must be repeated and rephrased before the anxious and distracted patient can grasp and retain the concept. Patients who suffer from chronic pain often hold themselves in low esteem, feeling that they are worthless to themselves, to others, and to society. Consequently, they are often so distracted that they experience difficulty in comprehending concepts, and they are often poorly motivated to undertake physical or psychologic therapy.

Careful preparation of the patient through effective communication is extremely important if the physician concludes that *formal psychotherapeutic referral* is necessary. Effective psychotherapy requires patient understanding and cooperation. Abrupt referral of a patient to a psychiatrist or psychologist can easily be destructive to therapeutic efforts, rather than constructive, if the patient misconstrues this referral as rejection or punishment.

Referring patients to a *back specialist in a distant city* may be severely destructive psychologically if the referring physician has in mind not consultation but dumping an unwanted patient. Effective psychological support and continued monitoring for potential psychological deterioration can rarely be provided by a specialist in a distant city, and rejection by a trusted physician may be more psychologically destructive than the physician realizes.

Physicians and other health care workers who deal with failed back syndrome patients should be aware of the importance of *psychosexual factors* in this disease process.[68] Altered perceptions of body image, limitation of sexual activity and sexual gratification, and the impact of these difficulties on *intimacy* can be devastating consequences in any relationship. Men may become *impotent* because of neurologic damage or pain, with psychologic predisposition adding a major additional factor in many instances. Men with a background of childhood insecurity or poor work motivation seem especially likely to become impotent, perhaps as the result of a weak masculine self-image. Either partner may experience pain during intercourse, which is technically called *dyspareunia*. Impotence and dyspareunia are serious and psychosocially destructive problems that patients are often hesitant to discuss with their physicians. Conversely, not all physicians are comfortable discussing matters of human sexuality and thus fail to inquire about problems in this important area or fail to discuss such problems frankly with their patients when they are verbalized. For men, simply ventilating frustrations and fears about impotence may be therapeutic. If there is no evidence of neurologic damage, reassuring patients of the primary importance of psychological factors and pain in human impotence can be reassuring if this is phrased in terms of intact functional sex mechanisms that are merely transiently impaired by pain or disease. The woman partner can play an important role in male impotence if she better understands the situation. She can try to control her own frustrations, can take a more active role in lovemaking, and can assist in timing sex relations when the patient is most relaxed and least uncomfortable. Pain during intercourse may often be aided materially by alterations in sexual techniques. A small lumbar support, such as a rolled bath towel or small pillow, can lessen back pain in women. Positions other than the traditional missionary position (face to face, man on top) can at times be helpful. A technique sometimes advocated for the second and third trimesters of pregnancy may be useful for patients with low back disease. In this technique, both partners lie on their sides and the male achieves vaginal intromission from a position behind his female partner, supplementing this, if desired by both partners, with manual clitoral stimulation. Simply timing pain- and anxiety-relieving medications to provide maximum benefit at the time of lovemaking can also be significantly useful.

The *role of the office nurse* in office psychotherapy should also be maximized. Many patients who are intimidated by discussing psychologic problems with the physician feel more relaxed discussing these problems with the office nurse. This is perhaps particularly true with female patients being treated by female nurses and male physicians. Patients frequently have access to the office nurse while they are waiting for the physician. These waiting periods can be uncomfortable and anxiety-generating and can be put to good use by interaction with a receptive and supportive office nurse. The nurse may take some active role in simple directive psychotherapy but should certainly communicate to the physician what she has learned of the patient's psychological problems.

One must always keep in mind that *suicide* is a well-recognized complication of the failed back syndrome. In the last two decades, I have dealt with five patients who have committed suicide and about a half dozen others who were unsuccessful. The thoughtful practitioner should learn to recognize potentially suicidal depression and ideation and should react therapeutically to even seemingly casual expressions of suicidal intent. The emotional support and simple psychotherapy given during routine office contacts may be sufficient to deter the patient from attempting to seek a final solution to his problem. If a patient is felt to be possibly suicidal, experts in suicide prevention urge that the patient be confronted with the specific query, "Are you considering doing away with yourself?" If the answer is at all affirmative, the second question should be, "How do you plan to do it?" The person who has contemplated both deed and method should be considered a real suicide risk. If the danger of suicide seems imminent, it should be recognized during the office contact and more definitive psychotherapy should be arranged. The following case report illustrates this risk, as do the cases reported on pages 220 and 228:

Case 7

This 43-year-old carpenter injured his back and left leg when a scaffold collapsed in 1975. He sustained extensive fractures of his left ankle and direct injury to the superficial peroneal nerve, causing burning pain in his foot. Foot pain was largely relieved by local neurectomy in 1976, but low back pain radiating into left buttock and posterior thigh gradually increased over a two-year period. Radiographs of the lumbosacral spine showed asymmetry of the left L4-L5 facet.

In May 1977, diagnostic anesthetization of the left L5-Sl facet initially gave dramatic improvement in pain and limitation of back motion. Before the injection, he could barely forward bend to touch his knees, but immediately following the injection he could forward bend to touch his toes painlessly. A repeat facet anesthetization one month later, with intrafacet methylprednisolone acetate (Depo-Medrol) injection gave much less convincing improvement and no pain relief beyond the first hour or so. A protracted trial of various anti-inflammatory drugs gave partial and temporary improvement only. A lumbar myelogram in December 1977 showed only blunting of the left S1 nerve root pouch. Lumbar discography was clearly abnormal at L5-S1 with large central filling, posterior extravasation, and reproduction of the patient's back and left buttock pain.

He was treated with a back corset and an episode of hospital bed rest without significant improvement in back and left buttock/posterior thigh pain. He was extremely proud of his physique and male image and enthusiastically attempted a program of enforced activity. Unfortunately, back pain persisted and began to interfere with his sex life. He remained disabled for work but busied himself with community projects and his gun collection.

After considerable discussion of alternative therapies, he underwent laminectomy in September 1978 with excision of a moderately bulging disc at L5-S1 on the left side and placement of a modified interbody bone fusion. After wearing a chair-back steel brace for three months he seemed considerably improved. Unfortunately, back pain with radiation into left buttock and posterior thigh gradually recurred as he attempted to become increasingly active. A series of bilateral L5-S1 facet anesthetizations and steroid injections in the fall of 1979 continued to give partial, temporary relief but no lasting relief. A radio-frequency facet neurectomy in October 1980 produced no lasting benefit.

The possible advisability of further surgery, including posterior spine fusion, was discussed on several occasions, but the patient was reluctant to consider further surgical intervention. In January 1981, repeat myelography showed no obvious abnormality. Discography was again normal at L4-L5. Discography at L5-S1 disclosed postoperative changes with moderate but not severe pain at the time of injection. Intradiscal methylprednisolone was injected. He failed to return for his next follow-up visit. In a telephone call his wife reported that he had become increasingly despondent and completely impotent. She reported that he had begun using pain-relieving drugs excessively over the past several months and that he had taken his life with one of the guns from his collection.

Psychosomatic Psychotherapy

Psychosomatic psychotherapy is a term I use to characterize a series of therapeutic modalities that apply psychologic or intellectual techniques toward a solution of physical as well as psychologic problems. Included in this category of therapy are hypnotherapy, biofeedback, transcendental meditation, and yoga.

Hypnotherapy can be a valuable adjunct for pain control for the patient who is susceptible to hypnotism. Hypnotism seems to be an extreme form of suggestibility, and not all patients are suggestible enough to benefit from it. A mistrust of or lack of confidence in the therapist can seriously hinder this form of therapy. At its most effective, hypnotherapy can be used as a general anesthetic, and I have performed some limited operative procedures on hypnotized patients. Direct hypnotic suggestions that pain will be absent have relatively limited usefulness. For the patient with true organic pain, the therapeutic suggestion is rarely strong enough to eliminate the pain for very long. On the other hand, if the pain is principally psychologic in origin, simply suggesting its absence will not eliminate the root cause, and either recurrent pain or some other form of disability will quickly resurface. Hypnotherapy may be helpful in teaching patients to relax and in teaching them to respond less vigorously to their pain. The application of both of these approaches can lead to significant reduction in use of anodynes and psychotropic drugs.

Biofeedback is a process that trains patients to modify their body processes such as heart rate and skin temperature. Obviously, simply slowing the heart or respiratory rate or reducing body temperature will have little beneficial effect on pain. However, the biofeedback process may be extended in an effort to help patients to relax physically and mentally. Curbing a physical or emotional response to a painful stimulus can usefully reduce the patient's pain and improve his performance.

Transcendental meditation (TM) is a less scientific and more ancient approach with many of the same goals as biofeedback. While not relying on electronics, practitioners of TM may also learn to modify their body processes and may extend this skill to a reduction in pain awareness and a reduction in responsiveness to a painful stimulus.

Yoga espouses many of the same physical, emotional, and spiritual goals as TM. Yoga couples the introspective intellectual techniques with a physical program of graded limbering and relaxing exercises and postures. This may be particularly beneficial for failed back syndrome sufferers because it combines a gentle method of enforced activity therapy with the psychologic and psychosomatic therapy.

All four of these psychosomatic therapies should be undertaken cautiously, especially hypnotherapy and yoga, because of the possibilities of psychologic and physical injury. In the hands of cautious and experienced therapists, they are for the most part quite safe. Although they are time-consuming, it may be time well spent for the chronic sufferer.

Formal Psychotherapy

Formal psychotherapy is certainly indicated for patients who are overtly or potentially suicidal. It is also indicated for patients with severe and disabling anxiety or depression who are willing to accept the premise that psychologic mechanisms are a major determinant of their disability. Patients with chronic pain personalities (see the discussion of psychogenic factors in Chapter 3) and patients with anxiety-prone or depression-prone personalities predating their back disease offer several therapeutic challenges to the psychotherapist. Attempting to alter basic personality structures may be time-consuming and frustrating. To be successful, this requires extensive patient cooperation and sufficient patient intelligence to permit adequate insight and grasp of psychologic principles. The personality of recurrent and chronic pain is often particularly impenetrable to formal psychotherapy. These patients typically have insulated themselves thoroughly with defense mechanisms, have been poorly able to form interpersonal relationships, and have led strongly job-oriented lives with little room for diversion, mutual emotional support, and emotional expression. But total personality restructuring need not be the sole goal of formal psychotherapy. Many patients will benefit significantly from a more limited development of insight into their perceptions of and responses to their illness. Patients must be willing to accept the psychiatrist's therapy and to participate actively in the therapeutic process. They must realize that a reduction in their pain is a laudable but secondary goal of psychotherapy and that its primary goal is to improve their ability to live with, or in spite of, their continued physical disability and pain. At the other extreme of the psychopathologic spectrum, patients with severe and refractory depression might be candidates for electroconvulsive shock therapy (ECT). When severe depression is combined with a painful failed back syndrome, ECT can occasionally provide a valuable source of relief of pain and suffering.

Chronic Pain Centers

Chronic pain centers, especially those that operate on an inpatient basis, usually include psychosomatic psychotherapy as an integral part of their therapeutic programs. Although some centers employ one or more of the formal techniques just discussed, others employ a looser amalgam of physical and psychologic therapies. This begins with a carefully graded physical therapy program for enforced activity therapy. Physical therapy is closely and personally supervised by therapists who are supportive and attentive but gently demanding of the patient's active participation. Added to this psychologically supportive physical program is more formal psychiatric therapy to generate improved insight and control. This accounts for much of the unique success that chronic pain centers enjoy. Many centers stress to their patients that their major role is not the elimination of pain, since patients are usually sent to pain clinics only after elimination of pain has been proven to be an unattainable goal. Many patients experience less pain after a period of pain clinic confinement, but even more patients find that they have improved primarily in their ability to enjoy life and resume productivity in spite of their pain. Occupational therapists and physical therapists can be of great assistance in achieving these latter goals by training patients in the use of alternative muscle groups and alternative techniques of performing the activities of daily living at home and at work. The group-therapy aspect of inpatient pain clinics also contributes to their usefulness. Patients discover firsthand that they are not alone in their disease and suffering, and they can observe others who are gradually able to resume a more normal and rewarding life in spite of similar disease.

The main *drawback of the pain clinic approach* is its cost. Four to eight weeks of confinement with intensive therapy can be expensive indeed, and not all third-party payers are sufficiently convinced of the effectiveness of such therapy to make them eager to accept responsibility for its cost. A lack of patient acceptance of an inpatient pain clinic experience can also be a drawback, but can be signally improved if the referring physician properly prepares the patient in advance about the true goals of the clinic and about the heavy emphasis placed on psychosomatic or formal psychotherapeutic approaches.

The *effectiveness of pain clinic therapy* must be evaluated in terms of immediate response and recidivism. Quantitative measures of short-term effectiveness include a reduction in intake of pain medication, a prolongation of hours of useful activity, and an improvement in the percentage of patients able to return to work at home or on the job. The reported effectiveness of pain clinic therapy in terms of short-term results varies widely and depends in part on the parameter of measurement chosen by the reporting institution. Third-party payors are more likely to look closely at the recidivism rate, since a short-term improvement is of only limited value if it is not maintained. Patients who return to work for only brief periods soon begin to draw compensation again from insurance carriers. This more limited long-term effectiveness should provide a sobering check on referral of patients to these often beneficial institutions. Furthermore, patients who are openly resistant to psychologic manipulation are likely to receive much less benefit from an inpatient pain clinic confinement, and their referral to such a facility should be viewed with skepticism and pessimism.

If there is reasonable hope of *actually relieving pain* through other methods with acceptable risk, these methods should be suggested before pain clinic referral. I do not think that a specific endpoint of *irreversibility* can be placed on disability. That is, I do not believe it is valid to say that a person who has not returned to work in two or three years after his first back operation is unlikely to ever return to work and therefore should be referred to a chronic pain center to learn to live with it. There is no doubt that the more prolonged a person's disability, the more intractable his medical condition is likely to be and the more suspect his true motivation to return to work is. But patients who remain disabled simply because the true organic basis of their disorder has not been determined and an appropriate and effective therapeutic program has not been tailored for their needs have not been given a fair chance to recover. Even though the statistical chance of recovery to gainful employment grows dimmer with passing months, those patients encountered by a therapist who have not been given a fair chance to recover deserve vigorous and persistent therapeutic effort.

6

Needle Therapy

When noninvasive therapies fail to provide adequate relief in a reasonable period of time, the possibility of usefully escalating therapeutic efforts to *invasive therapy* must be considered. Before exploring any form of open surgical invasive therapy, I first carefully survey the therapeutic potential of the variety of needle procedures that are available to that patient (i.e., procedures that involve introducing needles into the patient's body to produce a therapeutic benefit). For some specific diagnostic conditions, specific needle procedures are the therapeutic procedure of choice, even outweighing noninvasive therapy in some situations, such as the patient with severe trigger points. In my opinion, needle procedures are performed far too infrequently in the treatment of the failed back syndrome. I grant that many needle procedures provide relief for only a few weeks or months, but during this period many patients are able to resume more normal activity, even gainful employment. Furthermore, needle therapy can frequently be repeated with cumulative or at least repeated benefit for the patient. Thus, needle procedures enjoy an important advantage over open surgical procedures, which cannot feasibly be repeated (except at prolonged intervals) because of their greater cost to the patient, including cost in terms of risk, time required for recovery, and money.

Therapeutic needle procedures fall into *three major technical categories: injection of restorative or corrective agents* (adrenal corticosteroids, saline, and possibly phenol), *injection of destructive or neuroablative agents* (phenol, alcohol, and hypertonic saline), or *radiofrequency (RF) electrothermal heat lesions*. Logic dictates that the restorative injections are generally preferable over the other two techniques, both of which produce tissue destruction. Whenever possible, restoration of function is preferable to merely masking the problem by destructive interruption of transmission of pain impulses from the abnormal area to those areas in the brain where they reach consciousness. The restorative injections are limited in two ways: (1) their power to restore and (2) the longevity of their benefit. Nonetheless, for some patients these procedures may bring relief that is indeed dramatic. Often, if a single injection does not give sufficiently long-lasting relief, a series of injections may suffice to restore the patient to a long-lasting state of improved functioning—so long as the complications and undesirable effects of these injections do not outweigh the benefit they produce. The destructive procedures in general carry greater risk of unwanted side effects. Sensory loss in undesirable areas, weakness, autonomic disturbances, and increased pain may all result.

Over the past two decades, I have acquired a sobering appreciation of the body's remarkable capacity for getting through to consciousness the normally vitally *important messages about pain*. As one begins to learn peripheral and central *neuroanatomy,* one tends to draw an analogy between the sensory portion of the nervous system and a telephone network. Unfortunately for the pain sufferer and his neurosurgeon—although fortunately for the survival of biological organisms—information about pain seems to spread from the periphery to the brain with the persistence and convoluted complexity of transmitted gossip rather than as precisely transmitted telephone messages. Interrupting the pathways that should transmit pain impulses from a given area all too frequently or too soon fails, as alternative pathways through overlapping nerves or alternative central connections come into play. This conception of pain transmission has generated in me a certain awe about the organization of the human body and a keen awareness of my limitations as a neurosurgeon in attempting to relieve pain through ablative or destructive methods.

Corticosteroid and Anesthetic Injections of Local Tender Areas

Some of the best and most predictable results from needle therapy in the failed back syndrome come from this category of injection therapy. Several types of structures may give rise to *local tender areas* as a result of a number of different etiologies. All have in common the facts that they cause pain spontaneously or upon motion, that they are focally tender to compression, and that at least temporary relief can be obtained from local anesthetization. As a general rule, the more focal the tender area is, the more likely an injection is to produce a good result. Another characteristic of these locally tender foci is that they usually respond poorly, if at all, to bed rest therapy or systemic anti-inflammatory drug therapy. Indeed, for most patients with these locally tender foci, injection therapy offers by far the best chance of relief. The pain generated by these foci not uncommonly radiates some distance away. Radiation into buttock, posterior thigh, or upper lumbar region from foci in the lumbar area or posterior pelvis is quite common. A similar radiation of pain is usually produced by firm compression at the epicenter of the tender focus and by initial injection into the focus. Focal anesthetization with short-acting or longer-acting anesthetic drugs is usually performed at the time of corticosteroid injection to confirm the focal nature of the tenderness and pain, as well as for humanitarian purposes.

Trigger points are by far the most common of the palpably tender foci that are amenable to corticosteroid injection therapy (see page 21). In failed back syndrome patients, 70% of *periosteal trigger points* are found over the posterior iliac spine at the site of the periosteal attachment of the conjunction of lumbodorsal and gluteal muscles.[49] Other periosteal trigger point sites occur more laterally along the posterior iliac crest, over the sacrum or sacroiliac joints, or along the interspinous ligaments. *Muscular trigger points* occur most commonly as painful and tender loci in lumbar paraspinal or gluteal muscles. The term *fasciitis* is a controversial one, as discussed earlier (see page 21). This term is often used to describe more diffuse areas of tenderness that occur not infrequently in the lumbar, sacral, or gluteal region. The diffuse nature of the tenderness seen with these conditions makes them unsuitable for local injection therapy. These areas are more apt to respond to local topical therapy, systemic anti-inflammatory drugs, and a program of gentle but persistent enforced activity and exercise. Focal, painful tender areas may occasionally be discovered over the *sacroiliac joints* unilaterally or occasionally bilaterally. The tenderness in these conditions may well arise from the *sacral ligaments* rather than from the joints themselves. This is important, since injection into the joints is technically difficult, but injection into ligaments and ligamentous attachments along the sacral side of the sacroiliac junction is technically much simpler.

A classic and not uncommon site of focal tenderness and disabling pain is the *ischiogluteal bursa* overlying the ischial tuberosity. As described earlier (see page 22), this classical "pain in the arse" causes focal tenderness at the site where the buttocks come in contact with a chair, severely impairing normal sitting.[22] Its presence may be suspected both by the history and by observing a prominent "one cheek sign," with the patient sitting on only one buttock cheek. Once this condition has been confirmed by palpation over the ischial tuberosity, local injection therapy can often bring dramatic relief of pain. *Coccydynia* results in a tender and painful tailbone (see page 56). This focally tender disorder most commonly follows local trauma and is most severely symptomatic when the patient attempts to sit or defecate or with intromission during intercourse in female patients. Most cases of coccydynia heal with time and avoidance of reinjury, but occasionally injection into and adjacent to the sacrococcygeal joint with long-acting corticosteroids can bring gratifying relief and foreshortening of the recovery period.

In Chapter 3, reference was made to the fact that *local diagnostic anesthetic injections* may at times provide prolonged pain relief, presumably by interrupting pain cycles. A more specific form of *local anesthetic injection therapy* entails the injection of local anesthetics into focally tender areas of chronically spastic *fixed muscle spasms* of lumbar paraspinal or gluteal muscles. These *muscular trigger points* may at times persist for many days or weeks as areas of extreme tenderness and pain, despite vigorous local therapy with heat, liniments, and massage and vigorous systemic therapy with muscle relaxers, anti-inflammatory drugs, and anodynes. Topical cold applications represent one attempt to induce local analgesia. For the more refractory sites, local infiltration with anesthetic agents is at times warranted. One must weigh the temporary muscle relaxation and pain relief that these anesthetics bring against the additional tissue injury produced by needle insertion. A small diameter needle and a combination of short- and long-acting anesthetics is most desirable. I have generally refrained from using even dilute solutions of phenol or carbolic acid in these situations for fear of inducing muscle harm, although some therapists feel that solutions of 0.25% to 0.5% produce little tissue damage and may give pain relief lasting for several weeks. To perform such injections, the area of maximum muscle tenderness and tightness is identified by palpation, and systematic injection of local anesthetics is carried out throughout the area of tender tumescence.

Corticosteroid injections into local tender areas may be done with either short-acting or long-acting preparations. In my practice, I rarely employ the short-acting preparations, since most patients who suffer from the failed back syndrome have long-standing conditions that seem to respond best to long-acting depository corticosteroid preparations. I have occasionally used *triamicinolone acetonide (Aristocort or Kenalog)* or *beta methasone (Celestone),* but I have an unsubstantiated impression that results are less predictable with these agents than with *methylprednisolone acetate (Depo-Medrol),* with which I am more familiar. In a review of my patients injected between 1979 and 1984 with corticosteroids for painful and locally tender periosteal trigger points, 57% of 125 injections brought total or excellent improvement lasting an average of 4.5 months.[49] Although 26% brought *no* useful improvement, 15% brought improvement lasting greater than 6 months.

The *risks of local depository corticosteroid injections* are relatively small. In over two decades of use, I have not encountered a patient who has developed an abscess at the injection site. Infection remains a possibility with any injection therapy, especially therapy that involves corticosteroids, since these agents inhibit the body's defenses against infection. On rare occasions, patients develop increased local pain and tenderness that persists for several days or even a few weeks. The phenomenon of allergy to cortisone shots is described and could be the basis for these unpleasant responses. Presumably, such a relatively short-lived reaction would be mobilized against some labile ingredient in the preparation, since the synthetic adrenal corticosteroid itself persists for ten days or more and the "inert" carrier may persist as white flecks in the tissues for many weeks. Repeated injections into the same site at frequent intervals may cause dangerous softening of local tendons and ligaments. Tendon rupture following repeated corticosteroid injections has been reported, although I know of no documented instance of local tissue injury when depository corticosteroids have been injected at a frequency of no more than six- to eight-week intervals. Systemic hormonal effects are usually mild or are not noticeable at all to the patient. Occasionally, patients will notice some fluid retention or aggravation of symptoms from peptic ulcer disease, and some women will notice transient menstrual irregularity. Diabetic patients should be cautioned to check their urine sugars carefully for several weeks following injection, although significant disturbances in glucose metabolism are rarely seen.

After local depository corticosteroid injections, *beneficial effects* are usually delayed in onset. Patients should be cautioned that local pain and tenderness will return once the local anesthesia has worn off and that the area may be more sore than usual for a few days. During this interval, local applications of cold and, later, heat may be beneficial. Most patients report that beneficial effects become obvious three to five days following injection, although I have observed a range of two to seven days. The duration of beneficial effects is extremely variable. Certainly not all patients obtain relief, even temporarily. Those who do obtain relief may notice this relief only for as long as the corticosteroid remains active (i.e., ten to fourteen days following injection). At the other extreme, some patients find that a single injection gives permanent relief or relief lasting at least a year. A large number of patients fall in between, with the most common response being pain relief lasting from four to eight weeks.

If pain relief lasting at least three weeks is not obtained, I generally do not recommend *repeat injection therapy.* The exception is the occasional patient whose clinical picture is strikingly suggestive of a focal process that should respond to local corticosteroid therapy and who has obtained excellent pain relief from local anesthetization. Patients who obtain relief of intermediate duration from a single injection are certainly candidates for repeat injection. Repetitive corticosteroid injections into a given site may cause a dangerous weakening of local tendons or an increase in susceptibility to infection. For patients needing more frequent or prolonged series of injections, consideration should be given to supplanting corticosteroid injections with prolotherapy injections (see the following section). As a result, I have generally insisted on a six-week interval between injections and prefer not to give more than four injections in any given year. Not uncommonly, repeated injections will give a cumulative benefit, so second and third injections are clearly indicated even though repetitions beyond this number are approached with more skepticism. Patients who obtain excellent relief for several months following injection—relief that permits them to enjoy a distinct functional improvement during this period—should certainly be given the benefit of this often extremely gratifying therapy. That more surgeons and other physicians are not aware of the potential benefits of this form of therapy is distressing. This therapeutic limitation was brought forcibly to mind by a patient who came to my office on the Eastern Coast of the United States while on business. After telephoning his neurosurgeon in his home state on the West Coast, this practical businessman entered the office with the pronouncement, "My trigger point flared up again and before we go any further I want to know if you inject trigger points." When I replied affirmatively, he expressed great relief, stating that he had seen numerous physicians in both his state and mine who refused to consider this form of therapy, even though he had received benefit over a period of several years from a series of three or four such injections. When I examined the patient I agreed that he suffered from a classic trigger point, and subsequent transcontinental follow-up confirmed that the steroid injection I gave him had again brought lasting relief. (Other cases are presented on pages 163, 205 and 220.)

Prolotherapy

The technique of *prolotherapy* is not widely known among neurosurgeons and orthopedists, even though a national Prolotherapy Society exists and holds annual meetings. Prolotherapy consists of local injection into painful and tender areas, usually ligamentous structures, of a solution that most commonly contains a combination of phenol (carbolic acid), glycerol, and bupivacaine (Marcaine).[69-72] Some publications suggest that this technique is effective because it strengthens local ligamentous structures, thereby making them less subject to injury and painful strain.[69,72] The proof for this assertion is inconclusive, but this understanding of how the method works influences the way in which it is applied by individual practitioners. Therapists who believe that prolotherapy's effectiveness is due to its tissue-strengthening properties recommend frequent injections, once or even twice weekly. An alternative explanation for the effectiveness of prolotherapy is based on an appreciation that phenol is a powerful neurolytic agent, and dilute solutions seem to inactivate small-diameter pain fibers more than large-diameter touch or motor fibers. My experience has been that many patients obtain pain relief lasting four to eight weeks following a single phenol injection. Accordingly, if the effectiveness of prolotherapy is due to its neurolytic effect, frequent injections are not necessary for the vast majority of patients.

I have employed prolotherapy for more than two decades. I use this injection therapy for *focally painful and tender local areas* such as trigger points and occasionally for more diffuse fasciitis. I have generally employed prolotherapy in patients who have obtained excellent temporary relief from local anesthetization and who have failed to obtain lasting relief from several local injections of depository adrenal corticosteroids. For these patients, prolotherapy injections at intervals of six to twelve weeks often bring dramatic relief of pain and improvement in functioning. In the review of my patients injected between 1979 and 1984 for painful and tender local periosteal trigger points (discussed in the previous section), 42% of 108 injections of phenolic prolotherapy brought excellent or total pain relief lasting an average of 2.4 months.[49] Poor or no relief was obtained following 31% of injections, but 7% produced relief lasting 6 months or more. Although these results are not as good as those obtained with corticosteroid injections, nearly all patients were offered prolotherapy if they obtained only temporary relief from corticosteroid injections or no relief from corticosteroids despite having obtained excellent short-lasting relief following local anesthetization. The following case illustrates the usefulness of prolotherapy in a patient with a failed back syndrome (other cases are presented on pages 163 and 165):

Case 8

This 34-year-old office manager with a strong family history of low back disease began experiencing episodes of low back pain while in her teens. She was followed by an orthopedic surgeon for a number of years and exhibited gradually increasing symptomatology. During this period, she was treated with anodynes, exercises, and several brief periods of bed rest. In April 1976, she was hospitalized by her orthopedist with a particularly severe and persistent episode of nonradiating low back pain. Lumbar myelogram was normal. Neurosurgical consultation confirmed neurologic normalcy but limitation of back motion by severe pain. Lumbar discography was normal at L3-L4 and L4-L5. Injection at L5-S1 of 2 ml of 76% diatrizoate meglumide and sodium (Renografin 76) elicited severe back pain. Radiographs showed posterior midline protrusion but not free extravasation. Intradiscal methylprednisolone (Depo-Medrol) and continued bed rest brought gradual improvement, permitting hospital discharge and return to work.

In the fall of 1976, another severe episode of nonradiating back pain occurred. Two diagnostic facet nerve blocks at L4-L5 and L5-S1 produced only slight reduction in pain. Repeat intradiscal injection of 80 mg of methylprednisolone (1 ml) by way of a posterior approach initially seemed to bring relief. Unfortunately, relief rapidly faded over the course of one month. Repeat myelogram performed six weeks later demonstrated a moderate anterior and bilateral defect at L5-S1 with a suspicious blunting of the L5 nerve root. Following myelography, laminectomy was performed at L4-L5 with normal findings. At L5-S1, a bulging midline disc protrusion was discovered and excised. This was followed by a posterior fusion performed by the patient's orthopedic surgeon.

Six months following surgery, she was able to return to her office managerial duties, and she has remained employed full time ever since. Within a year following surgery, she developed recurrent local pain and tenderness, with trigger points over both posterior iliac spinous processes. Local anesthetization and injection of methylprednisolone brought dramatic relief lasting two months. Two additional injections of methylprednisolone at ten-week intervals likewise gave six to nine weeks of excellent pain relief. Because of the persistent recurrence of local pain and tenderness prolotherapy injections were begun in 1978. Injections of 3 ml to 5 ml of prolotherapy solution at each tender site have been repeated at two- to four-month intervals over the subsequent three years. Throughout this period, the patient has remained fully employed. She has usually required opiate medications for the first few days following each prolotherapy injection, then obtains excellent pain relief lasting six to ten weeks following each injection, requiring only occasional muscle-relaxing and anti-inflammatory medications.

I consider prolotherapy to be *contraindicated* in (1) trigger points lying within muscle bodies, (2) ischiogluteal or other bursae, or (3) kissing pseudarthroses in situations in which the injected prolotherapy solution might reach the epidural space. Phenol does have some sclerosing properties, and it seems unwise to risk muscle damage or creation of intrabursal adhesions. Epidural injection of phenol carries some risk of impaired nerve functioning for weeks or months and creation of epidural adhesions—although both of these risks seem quite small with the dilute phenol solutions employed in prolotherapy. Inadvertent intrathecal injection of various sclerosing agents has been reported to cause disastrous neurologic complications—even death—and must be carefully avoided.

The *solution used for prolotherapy* should be constituted just prior to injection. I usually employ a 1% solution of phenol in 0.5% bupivacaine (Marcaine) with 20% glycerol. Each injection rarely exceeds 7.5 ml for injection of a single focus or 10 ml for injection of two foci. The area for prolotherapy inoculation is injected with lidocaine (Xylocaine) immediately prior to introduction of the prolotherapy solution, since this solution is painful when delivered into unanesthetized tissues. A 1% solution can easily be formulated by mixing 1 ml of 5% phenol in anhydrous glycerol (see the discussion of facet nerve injections and intrathecal injections in this chapter) with 4 ml of 0.5% bupivacaine without epinephrine. This solution is injected into the epicenter of the painful area and around the margins of the painful area. Since many of these tender areas lie in periosteum adjacent to bone, this involves injection along the body edge as well as a short distance away from the bone in the involved tendinous or ligamentous structures.

A special form of *phenol injection therapy,* not officially designated as prolotherapy, involves the use of phenol in oil injected as a sclerosing agent into painful *herniations of fat* through the fascial aponeurosis in the lumbosacral paraspinal region (see pages 22 and 55). I have rarely found convincing evidence for such fat herniations, have usually treated them with local anesthetic or steroid injections, and have no personal experience with the use of phenol in oil as a sclerosing solution—but the technique sounds logical if fat herniations can be reasonably and accurately confirmed. The solution recommended for this type of injection is 5% phenol in a mixture of almond oil, dextrose, and ethanolamine, with a series of four to six injections repeated as necessary at intervals of ten to fourteen days. Not only is phenol an important neurolytic agent, but this combination of agents should also cause local sclerosis, which may well succeed in causing sufficient local fibrosis to prevent further herniation through this thin fascial layer. One should be exceedingly careful not to inject deeply enough to injure paraspinal nerves, and I would even be concerned about injections deep enough to enter and damage paraspinal muscles. I cannot say from personal experience whether such a series of injections consistently gives lasting relief or whether it causes a new area of local pain for at least some recipients.

Intradiscal Injections

Intradiscal injections generally employ one of *two classes of compounds.* The first are injections designed to *reduce in bulk the nuclear portion of the disc.* Included in this category are the enzymes chymopapain, collagenase, and certain specific polypeptides. The second class of compounds are *anti-inflammatory drugs.* Both short-acting and depository preparations of adrenalcorticosteroids have been reported to be effective in this form of treatment. Intradiscal injection of nuclear-reducing solutions is generally employed in interspaces not previously operated upon. Injection of enzymes into previously operated spaces has been occasionally reported, but generally is felt to be relatively contraindicated for fear of epidural extravasation with the potential of dural or nerve root injury. Adrenal corticosteroids, on the other hand, can be used effectively in patients with previously operated interspaces as well as in those with unoperated interspaces.

Enzymes and Polypeptides

Intradiscal injection of enzymes is available to neurosurgeons and orthopedists but has declined greatly in popularity since it was first released for general use. Intradiscal injections of chymopapain were administered to over 17,000 patients in the United States over the decade following its introduction in 1968 in a series of nonblinded and often poorly controlled clinical studies.[73-75] From these studies it was reported that overall 68% of the patients achieved marked improvement, 15% achieved slight improvement, and 17% were unimproved. Approximately 3% of patients receiving chymopapain injections developed allergic or hypersensitivity reactions. These were occasionally severe, and several deaths resulted. Subsequently, a smaller study, only 105 patients, was reported that raised serious questions about the effectiveness of chymopapain relative to its safety.[76] This was a randomized, blinded study in which patients received an injection of either chymopapain or simply a "carrier" solution (cysteine, edetate, and iothalamate: the CEI solution). In this study, no statistical difference was reported between the short-term or long-term results achieved with patients in either group. Although both short-term and long-term results were slightly better with chymopapain, 50% of those who received only CEI solution achieved good results as compared with 59% achieving similar results with chymopapain. An obvious difference, however, was the rarity of allergic reactions or other complications in those patients who received only the CEI solution. This study has been criticized because of the small number of patients involved, but nonetheless it raised sufficient questions about chymopapain that the U.S. Food and Drug Administration withdrew the compound entirely from use in the United States.

During the 1980s, two large *double-blind* studies were carried out with different chymopapain preparations in the United States, leading to the eventual release of the drug for general use.[11,12] Both studies included patients with sciatica greater than lumbago, since smaller studies had shown only about a 50% improvement in the number of patients with predominantly lumbago—essentially the same as that achieved with placebo. The definitions of successful outcome were different in the two large studies, but in both groups the number of patients achieving a productive functional status without the need for narcotics was approximately 65% to 70%. Less than 1% of patients developed severe allergic reactions, and after standardization of treatment for those reactions no deaths were reported beyond the early investigative phases. After the release of the drug, however, a flurry of reports appeared documenting severe central nervous system complications with paraplegia, coma, or subarachnoid hemorrhage occurring shortly after chymopapain injection. There was considerable speculation that this represented inadvertent subarachnoid injection of the material, and laboratory and clinical data suggested that the toxicity probably was increased if water-soluable iodinated contrast materials were injected intradiscally as part of the same procedure. Perhaps because of the improving technical ability of those doing chymopapain discolysis, the drug's manufacturers reported a rapid reduction in the number of reported major complications over the next few years. *Increased back pain* following chymopapain discolysis has been reported to occur in one fourth to one third of patients injected and to persist for at least six weeks in perhaps in 10% or 15%. This has been considered not to be a complication of the procedure but one of its inherent properties.[11]

Chymopapain discolysis is used for *disc ruptures that have not previously been operated upon and that do not include free fragments in the spinal canal;* it is also effective for the relief of sciatica but not lumbago. Chymopapain discolysis is not advisable in discs that have been previously injected with chymopapain, for fear of severe allergic reaction. Overall, chymopapain discolysis is of relatively little benefit for the failed back syndrome sufferer, except for the patient whose original disc rupture was inadvertently overlooked during the first operation or who develops a new disc rupture at a previously untreated interspace.

The technique of chymopapain discolysis is essentially the same as that used for discography. Although the manufacturer cautions against performing contrast discography at the time of enzyme discolysis, contrast discography confirms proper placement of the needle into the nuclear portion of the disc, and some clinicians feel that greater safety is provided by allowing confirmation that materials injected into the disc space do *not* reach the subarachnoid space. The procedure is carried out in a fully equipped operating room or special procedure room under local anesthesia but with full anesthesia on standby and all the necessary medications and equipment available if needed for immediate resuscitation in the event of a life-threatening allergic reaction. Preliminary serum or skin testing can detect in advance many patients who seem to be severely allergic.

Even though chymopapain discolysis is of limited importance in the management of failed back patients, *the careful study it received* is of considerable importance to all patients suffering disorders of the lower back. An international series of five double-blind studies compared chymopapain injection to several different types of placebo intradiscal injections. It is important and well-known that all of these studies showed some beneficial effect from chymopapain, despite its risk and limitations. Equally important, but less often discussed, is the fact that each of these series showed that approximately half of those patients injected with a placebo also obtained relief of their sciatica. In each of these studies, patients were selected for chymopapain discolysis only if they fulfilled what the study designers considered to be the accepted criteria for the diagnosis of lumbar disc rupture causing sciatica unresponsive to conventional nonoperative therapy and if symptoms were severe enough and diagnosed with sufficient certainty to make them candidates for open surgical resection. The fact that half of these patients who were considered to be suitable candidates for either open surgery or chymopapain needle surgery were relieved by placebo injection raises strong doubts about our understanding of the pathophysiology of lumbar disc rupture and of the adequacy of what many consider to be accepted nonoperative therapy.

Intradiscal injections of *collagenase,* another *enzyme,* have received less extensive clinical evaluation.[77] Collagenase is said to be a more logical choice for enzyme therapy of the intervertebral disc because of the high collagen content of the nucleus pulposus. Experimental and clinical studies of this compound have been considerably more limited than studies of chymopapain, and the relative efficacy and safety of this form of therapy remain largely unknown. Collagenase is not presently available for general clinical use for intradiscal therapy in the United States.

A specific polypeptide, *trylasol,* has enjoyed some popularity in Europe as an intradiscal injection agent for therapy of lumbar disc disease.[78] This compound was chosen because of its apparent safety when injected into humans and because its ion-binding properties are thought to help reduce the bulk of the nucleus pulposus through inspissation or compaction of its molecular structure. Clinical trials have been conducted in several hundred patients with back pain, leg pain, or both. Most of these patients were selected because they did not have excruciatingly severe pain or severe or progressing neurologic deficits. In keeping with this clinical picture, most of the patients were found on myelography to have relatively small and usually centrally placed disc bulges. About 40% of injected patients obtained transient improvement, but only 25% obtained good improvement lasting at least a few months. Of those patients who did obtain some relief, approximately two thirds maintained their relief for at least six months. The only untoward reactions that were observed were post–lumbar puncture (LP) headaches, attributed to the transdural approach to disc injection that was used in this series.

Intradiscal Corticosteroids

Intradiscal corticosteroid injections were pioneered by Feffer.[79] In 1969 he reported a four- to ten-year follow-up study of 244 patients who had received injections into two or more discs of solutions containing hydrocortisone. He studied previously unoperated patients who suffered back pain, leg pain, or both. Some of his patients had objective evidence of neurologic loss as well. He reported that 67% experienced a remission of pain either immediately or within 48 hours. Over the next three years, the percentage of good responses fell to 47% of the total group, but good responders sustained lasting improvement. He concluded that intradiscal hydrocortisone injections were most beneficial for older patients with predominantly subacute back pain and with x-ray evidence of limited degenerative changes. The attractiveness of intradiscal steroids was further enhanced when Graham compared intradiscal chymopapain with intradiscal hydrocortisone in a double-blind study employing 20 patients. He concluded that chymopapain was not significantly superior to hydrocortisone.[80]

My results with intradiscal corticosteroid injections were reported in 1980.[81] I employed methylprednisolone acetate (Depo-Medrol), rather than hydrocortisone, in a series of 29 patients with low back disease. A total of 42 intradiscal injections were made. Overall, 52% of the injections gave relief for a minimum of one month and 33% for at least three months. Through the use of repeated injections, 21% of the patients obtained relief lasting six months to several years. The patients selected for this study were those with essentially normal myelograms and chronic pain that did not respond to nonoperative therapy. Discography was abnormal in all but two patients, both of whom had abnormalities on plain radiographs. Results were distinctly better in patients who received injections of 80 mg in 1 ml of methylprednisolone rather than 40 mg in 1 ml; 48% versus 33% obtaining relief for more than three months. Twelve injections were given to eight patients who had undergone previous lumbar disc surgery, and in this group 23% of injections gave improvement lasting at least three months. The only complications in this series were several instances of *post-LP headache* following transdural discography and occasional minor *menstrual irregularities in young women.*

I have found intradiscal corticosteroid injections to be extremely beneficial for severe and persistent back pain *following intervertebral disc infection* or *aseptic disc space inflammation or discitis.* Bacterial infections of the disc space must be treated vigorously with systemic antibiotics in sufficient dosage and for a sufficiently long duration (generally four to eight weeks) to ensure eradication of the bacterial infection. For many patients, eradicating the infection and providing external stabilization through bracing suffice to reduce back pain sufficiently to permit a return to normal activity (see page 66). I have encountered patients whose back pain remained intolerably severe despite an absence of or complete clearing of infection and who have responded nicely to intradiscal corticosteroid injection therapy. In each instance, the patient had received a prolonged and adequate course of appropriate systemic antibiotic therapy if disc space cultures confirmed, or clinical presentation strongly suggested, disc space infection; each was afebrile, and in each patient the white blood count (WBC) had returned to normal or near normal. All of these patients showed radiographic or computerized tomographic (CT) evidence of disc space sclerosis or destruction that had stabilized over an interval of at least several weeks and abnormally increased uptake on isotope bone and joint scans. The patients with aseptic discitis presented with severe and persistent lumbago, elevated sedimentation rate despite normal WBC, no fever, and sclerotic changes on radiographs or CT scans with markedly increased uptake on isotope scans. Prior to undertaking intradiscal corticosteroid therapy, I performed diagnostic aspiration of the involved disc space in each patient. Even with acute disc space infection, aspiration of pus is rarely possible. Accordingly, it is my practice to barbotage into the disc space 1 ml to 3 ml of preservative-free normal saline. I then send for culture the volume of saline that I can recover following barbotage, as well as cultures of the tip of the discogram needle stylet. The effectiveness of intradiscal steroid therapy in this condition is demonstrated by the following case (Fig. 6.1):

Case 9

This 68-year-old man underwent excision of an L4-L5 degenerated disc at another hospital in February 1981. He did well until he developed pneumococcal pneumonia in May 1981. Since that episode, he complained of increasing low back discomfort. In September 1981, he was discovered to have an elevated sedimentation rate but normal peripheral white count and no fever. Radiographs of the lumbosacral spine showed beginning destruction around the disc space at L4-L5. He was treated at his original hospital with one month of intravenous cephalosporin antibiotics, with eventual normalization of the sedimentation rate. However, excruciatingly severe back pain persisted.

He was transferred to the University of Massachusetts Medical Center in October 1981, complaining of intolerably severe low back pain that was poorly controlled with meperidine (Demerol) 100 mg to 150 mg every three to four hours. Radiographs showed severe destruction at the L4-L5 interspace. These changes had apparently been stable over the preceding two weeks, including one week off antibiotics. White count and sedimentation rate were normal. There was marked tenderness to palpation and percussion over the lower lumbar spine and severe limitation of all lower back and hip motions. Needle aspiration of the L4-L5 interspace with saline barbotage failed to yield viable bacteria, but intradiscal injection of lidocaine (Xylocaine) gave dramatic and almost complete relief of back pain lasting several hours. Three days later, the L4-L5 interspace was again needled and again cultures were negative for bacterial growth. One milliliter each of 1% lidocaine and 0.5% bupivacaine (Marcaine) again brought almost total and immediate relief of pain. One milliliter (80 mg) of methylprednisolone acetate (Depo-Medrol) was injected intradiscally. Some pain recurred by the following morning, but within three days back pain had again almost completely faded away. When seen in follow-up one and two months later, he was fully ambulatory and required only acetaminophen twice a day for pain relief.

Four months after the first injection, low back pain again increased in severity sufficiently to require opiates and analgesics. Plain radiographs showed no further destructive changes, and repeat intradiscal methylprednisolone injection again provided dramatic pain relief for the 15-month duration of follow-up.

Facet Nerve and Joint Injections

One of the more promising developments in the understanding and management of diseases of the lower back has been the concept of the *facet joint* as a major contributor to these diseases (see the discussions of low back pain in Chapter 3 and of invasive radiologic studies in Chapter 4). Increased interest has been directed toward specific therapy of the facet joints because there is increased recognition that disorders of the facet joint can and frequently do produce back and posterior thigh pain. Clinical interest in the facet joint was heightened by the reports of Reese, of Australia, in which he claimed dramatic success in relieving back pain problems with surgical section of the facet nerves.[82] His open surgical procedure (see the discussion of facet neurectomy in Chapter 7) never gained wide popularity, but this concept produced increased interest in a series of needle procedures aimed at the facet joints. These procedures fall into two major categories: *facet nerve interruption* or *neurectomy* and *intrafacet steroid injections.*[83]

Two needle techniques currently enjoy a growing popularity for therapeutic *facet nerve interruption* or *neurectomy.* The methodologically simpler of these two techniques, called *phenol facet neurectomy,* involves injection of a phenol solution under radiographic control into the vicinity of the superior and inferior nerves to each involved facet. This technique does not require any specialized equipment other than that necessary for routine radiography. The major limitations of this technique are that the phenol may track proximally along the facet

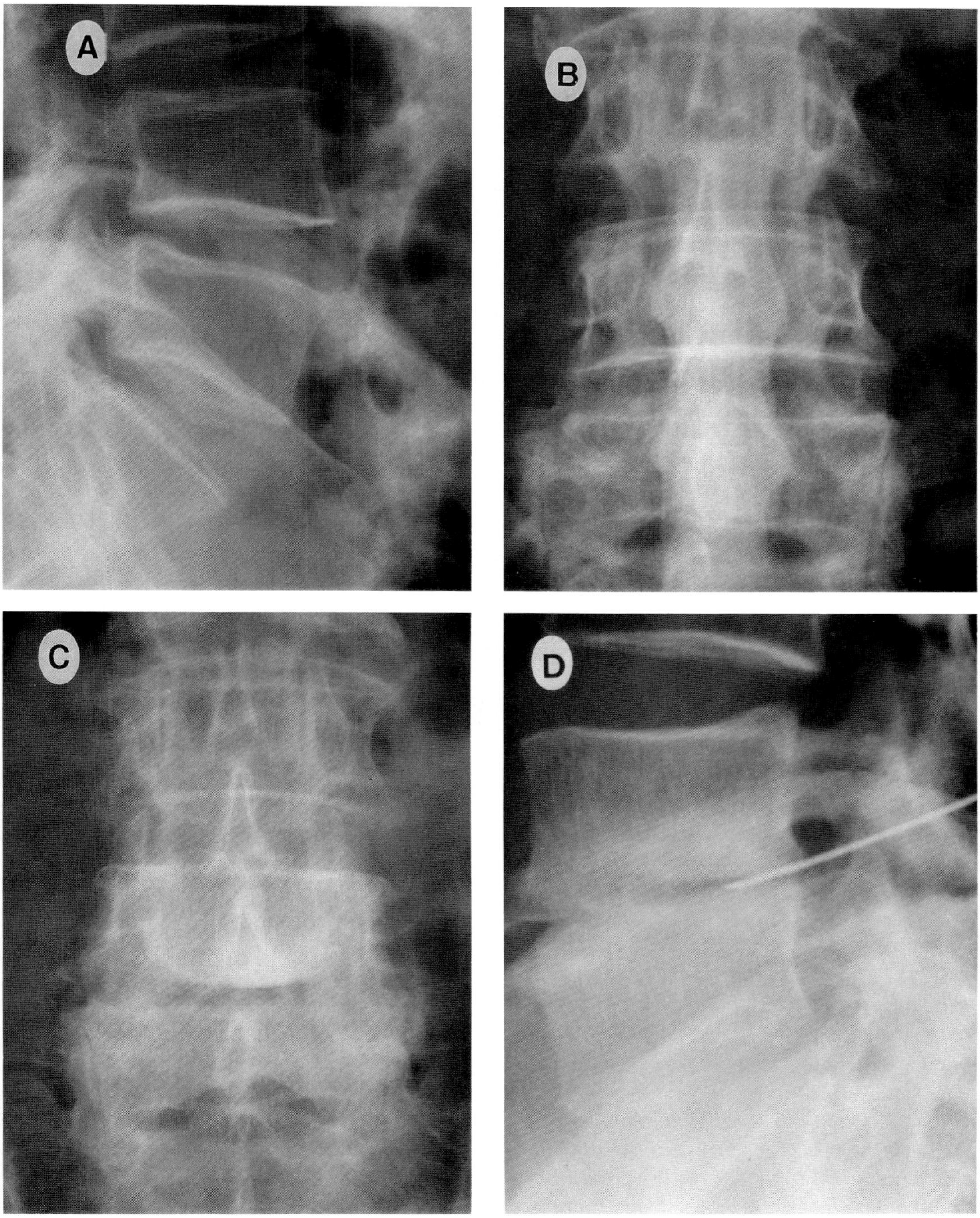

FIGURE 6.1. Intradiscal steroids can dramatically relieve back pain following disc space sepsis. **A and B:** These radiographs, of the patient discussed as Case 9, were taken early in the course of his sepsis, at a time when he was experiencing severe back pain accompanied by low-grade fever and leukocytosis. At this stage there was little, if any, detectable bone destruction. **C and D:** These radiographs were taken after prolonged antibiotic therapy had cleared the active infection, but at a time when the patient continued to be completely incapacitated by severe low back pain. Note the intradiscal needle used to aspirate and barbotage the interspace prior to steroid injection.

nerve branch to cause some denervation of the parent nerve root, causing undesirable sensory loss in the leg, and that local scarring may block access of the phenol to the facet nerves. Motor weakness is a much less common problem, and weakness that develops rarely lasts for long, even if the phenol is injected quite close to the nerve root. This is in contradistinction to alcohol injection. Alcohol injected close to a nerve root may cause severe and long-lasting involvement of both motor and sensory functions.

The second of these two techniques is *radiofrequency (RF)* or *electrothermal facet neurectomy.*[84,85] This procedure is more cumbersome than phenol facet neurectomy because it requires the use of an RF lesion-generating machine and special electrodes in addition to radiographic equipment. The lesions that are produced are extremely precise, and nerve root injury should never occur if careful radiographs are taken and if electrical stimulation is done prior to lesioning. On the other hand, this extreme precision can be a liability, since there seems to be some anatomical variability in the course taken by the superior and inferior facet nerves, and localizing facet nerves precisely is difficult. Electrical stimulation prior to lesioning is helpful if it reproduces the pattern of the patient's pain, although even this does not guarantee that the lesion will ablate the sensory nerve. It is difficult, if not impossible, to test reliably to determine whether adequate nerve ablation has been achieved. If a patient obtains dramatic pain relief and increased range of motion following lesioning, one can assume that adequate denervation was achieved. However, these nerve branches do not reach the cutaneous surface to permit easy testing of denervation, and a failure to relieve patients of all or even most of their pain may be caused not by inadequate lesioning, but by pain deriving from other structures in the back.

Intrafacet steroid injection offers the attractive possibility of restoring function to diseased facet joints. Intraarticular corticosteroid injections are often beneficial for painful inflammatory processes affecting other joints. At times, such injections give long-lasting or even permanent relief. The application of intraarticular injections to the facet joint has not yet gained wide popularity. Patients whose facet joints seem clinically to be the major source of their back pain, and who have obtained considerable relief from temporary facet anesthetization, are potential candidates for this procedure (Fig. 6.2). Facet neurectomy alone cannot be expected to provide denervation of the facet joint for more than a few months. If, however, a patient obtains excellent pain relief for many weeks following facet denervation, I strongly consider intrafacet steroid injections with phenol facet neurectomy. I do this in an effort to provide the patient with rapid onset of pain relief that will hopefully permit fuller mobilization and more rapid healing of the injected facet joint.

Before undertaking therapeutic facet needle procedures, *diagnostic facet anesthetizations* are necessary to ensure a reasonable chance of successful amelioration of the patient's distress and to ensure that the patient's pain is indeed arising from the presumably abnormal facet (see the discussion of diagnostic facet injections in Chapter 4). Many patients exhibit facet abnormalities on radiography but experience no pain from these presumably abnormal joints. In contrast, some patients, especially those who have undergone previous disc excision with interspace collapse, may experience severe facet pain but show little detectable change in the facet joints on plain radiographs or CT scans.

The *techniques* of *facet neurectomy* and *intrafacet steroid injection* begin with a similar approach to the abnormal and painful facet, and the technique for both of these therapeutic injections is essentially the same as that used for diagnostic facet injections. Skin wheals are raised 6 cm to 8 cm lateral to the midline, depending on the patient's corpulence. If multiple levels are to be treated, it is often preferable to insert a lumbar puncture needle or RF electrode needle at the level of each common facet nerve branch (i.e., halfway between each of two adjacent diseased facets and at the superior and inferior margin of the upper and lower facet, respectively). If a single facet is to be treated, often a single skin wheal will suffice, with movement of the needle or electrode to permit treatment of both superior and inferior facet nerves. Most commonly, facets are treated bilaterally, but occasionally patients with asymmetric facets and unilateral facet pain will benefit from unilateral facet therapy. Fluoroscopy and permanent confirmatory radiographs are most helpful during this procedure. During needle insertion and at the time of final needle placement, radiographic confirmation should be obtained in posteroanterior, lateral, and oblique projections—the latter to visualize the facet joint directly. In the posteroanterior view, the tips of the spinal puncture

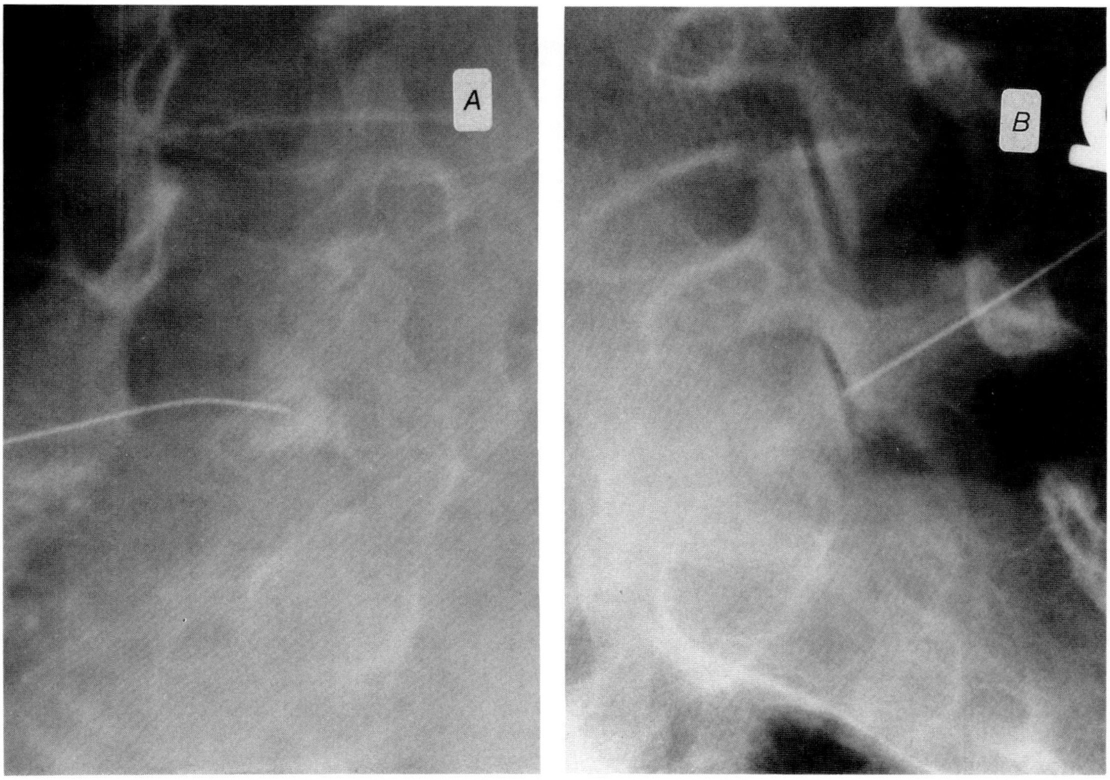

FIGURE 6.2. Intrafacet injections of steroids are of likely, but unconfirmed, benefit in treatment of lower back pain secondary to facet syndromes. **A and B:** These radiographs document intrafacet injections in two patients with radiographically abnormal facets, both of whom obtained pain relief following facet nerve anesthetization and both of whom achieved extended periods of pain relief with a combination of intrafacet steroid injection and facet nerve phenol injection. Radiograph A is from Case 5.

needles or the midportion of the active tip of the RF electrode needle should be positioned between adjacent facets at the point of the narrowest spinal width—in the oblique view, at the rostral and caudal ends of the target facets; in the lateral view, 3 mm or 4 mm dorsal to the dorsal rim of the intervertebral foramen.

Once the spinal puncture injection needles or the RF needle electrode is in place, *facet neurectomy* can be accomplished. Immediately prior to neurectomy, I inject 1 ml of lidocaine (Xylocaine) at the selected site, both as a diagnostic test to ensure the safety of the nearby nerve root and as a means to control the pain that is otherwise associated with facet neurectomy. Chemical facet neurectomy is accomplished by injecting 0.5 ml to 0.75 ml of 5% anhydrous phenol in glycerol or 0.5 ml of 10% anhydrous phenol in glycerol at each site of proposed facet nerve interruption. Electrothermal RF facet neurectomy is preceded not only by local anesthetic injection but also by two electrical tests (Fig. 6.3). As the first test, a stimulating current (generally 1 millisecond pulses, 100 Hertz, and 0.5 to 3 volts) is applied, preferably prior to final local anesthetization. If the stimulation reproduces the patient's customary back and posterior thigh pain, this may be considered prognostic of a good outcome. On the other hand, if electrical stimulation causes pain distally in the sciatic distribution or motor movements in the leg, improper needle placement is confirmed. Once a local anesthetic has been injected, reproduction of the patient's pain by local stimulation is less likely to be observed. Furthermore, if local anesthetization causes interruption of function of the adjacent nerve root, subsequent thermal lesioning must be carried out with great caution, if at all, because of the increased risk of inadvertent nerve root damage. The second test is done when electrothermal lesioning begins. Local tissue temperature in the vicinity of the facet nerve

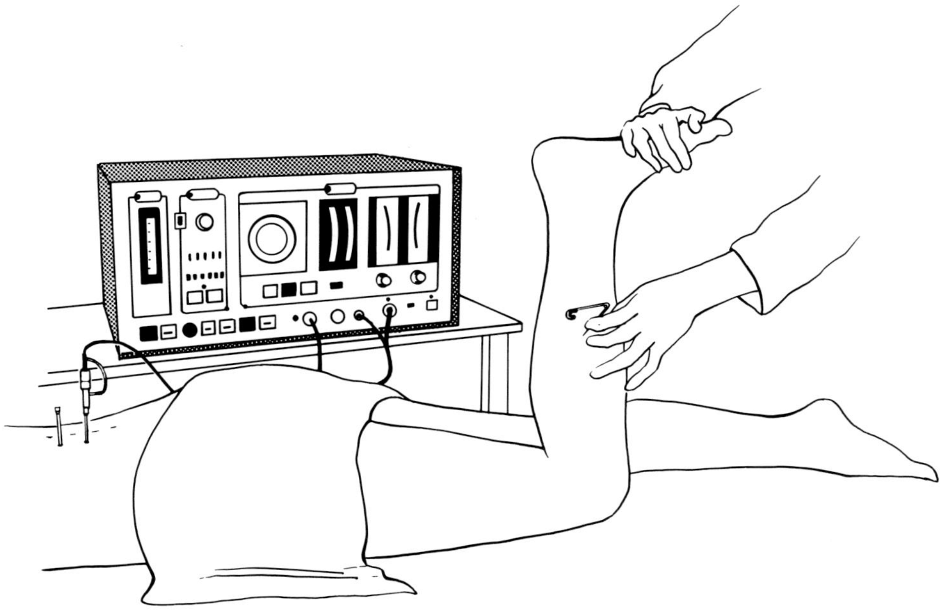

FIGURE 6.3. Radiofrequency (RF) electrothermal lesioning of facet nerves permits reversible testing of lesioning. Raising the temperature to 50 degrees Celsius produces physiologic blockade of nerve transmission without tissue damage. The patient can then be tested for evidence of interruption of sciatic nerve root functioning, which would be an unintended and unwanted addition to facet nerve interruption.

is raised into the range of 45 to 50 degrees centigrade long enough to permit testing of motor and sensory functions in the lower extremity. At this temperature, neurologic functioning is reversibly interrupted without permanent lesioning. Once safety from nerve root injury has been documented, the electrode tip temperature can be raised to 90 to 95 degrees centigrade and held at this temperature for two to three minutes. I have generally employed either a 7 mm or 10 mm exposed electrode tip, depending on the patient's bulk.

Corticosteroid injections directly into facet joints are done with a 22-gauge spinal needle, using an almost identical approach as that described for facet neurectomy. The patient is turned to the oblique position under the fluoroscope to visualize the cleft of the facet joint. The spinal needle is manipulated with the aid of fluoroscopic guidance until the tip enters the facet joint. Entry into the facet joint can be confirmed by intraarticular injection of 0.25 ml to 0.75 ml of radiographic, water-soluble contrast medium, but this is usually not necessary. In my practice, I employ almost exclusively the concentrated preparation of methylprednisolone acetate (Depo-Medrol), 80 mg per ml, since this drug remains active at the injection site for ten days to two weeks. Others prefer to inject dexamethasone (Decadron); although this drug remains active for only several days, its use obviates the injection of the inert carrier present in methylprednisolone into the facet joints. Usually no more than 0.25 ml to 0.5 ml of the drug can be injected. Additional amounts of the drug may be injected just outside of the facet joint.

The *results of facet neurectomy* are difficult to determine precisely from the medical literature. Published reports are often poorly controlled, patient selection often varies widely, and conclusions regarding efficacy are frequently conflicting. Some surgeons have used facet neurectomy for nearly any patient with predominantly back pain. In contrast, I have limited the use of this technique to patients with lumbago radiating into, but not strongly below, buttock and posterior thigh unilaterally or bilaterally, whose pain is aggravated more by hyperextending than by flexing the back and who have demonstrated good temporary relief from facet anesthetization. Most of these patients demonstrate abnormality of their facets on radiography, CT scan, and/or isotope bone and joint scan. In a brief review of a personal series of 20 RF or phenol facet neurectomies, three patients obtained no lasting relief. One of these was the only patient to suffer exclusively low back pain without extension to the buttock and posterior thigh, one was the only patient to suffer exclusively sciatic pain, and one obtained only equivocal relief from diagnostic facet anesthetization. Six patients obtained fair relief, defined as 25% to 50% relief lasting at least one month. Ten patients obtained good to excellent relief, defined as greater than 50% pain reduction lasting a minimum of two months; three of these patients experienced relief greater than 75% lasting longer than three months. All ten of these patients were treated with phenol rather than radio frequency. As discussed under facet neurectomy in Chapter 7, facet nerves are extremely short nerves, and even complete interruption of these nerves will be followed by regeneration within a few months in nearly every patient. This period of pain relief may be sufficiently valuable to patients to justify repeated facet nerve interruptions. In some patients, the pain relief and improved range of back motion brought by facet nerve interruption may permit that patient to successfully undertake a program of enforced activity, which may in turn produce lasting benefit. The following case history illustrates the usefulness of facet neurectomy (other cases are presented on pages 102 and 140):

Case 10

This 56-year-old businesswoman had suffered intermittently for a decade with nagging right lower backaches. Following relatively minor lifting, she developed severe pain in her right lower back, buttock, and posterior thigh (but not below the knee) that failed to remit despite two weeks of bed rest at home. Examination at that time was said to have disclosed some lumbar tenderness, no neurologic abnormality, but "straight leg raising positive 40 degrees on the right"—with the patient recalling that this seemed to elicit back pain but not sciatic pain. A myelogram showed no abnormality. She was treated with muscle relaxants, anodynes, and further bed rest without improvement. Two months after the onset of severe pain, laminectomy was performed with excision of a slightly bulging L5-S1 intervertebral disc.

This surgery failed to provide relief, although she continued to be able to work in a limited fashion for the next two years. When first examined at the University of Massachusetts Medical Center, she still complained of right lower back, buttock, and posterior thigh pain that was aggravated by activity. Examination showed tenderness to deep palpation over the L5 right paraspinous area, with back motion (especially hyperextension) limited by pain at this site. Straight leg raising to 50 degrees caused back pain without sciatica. Radiographs disclosed dramatic sclerosis of the right L5-S1 facet, which was congenitally malrotated.

Phenol facet neurectomy was coupled with intrafacet steroid injection, confirming a symptomatic facet syndrome. Facet injections were repeated ten weeks later after she had obtained eight weeks of sufficient pain relief that she had gone dancing with her husband for the first time in over two years. Ten weeks after the second injection, she noted some return of discomfort but felt that this was not sufficiently severe to warrant reinjection.

The literature on steroid injections is quite limited, and reliable *quantification of efficacy* is not yet possible. However, intraarticular and intrabursal steroid injections are well-acknowledged as effective therapy for painful afflictions at other sites in the body. My current impression is that intrafacet steroid injections are likely to be most beneficial for the patient with back and posterior thigh pain of a type consistent with a facet syndrome, with lumbago aggravated especially by hyperextending the back, and with radiographs, CT scans, or isotope scans documenting degenerative changes in one or two facet joints in the area of clinical suspicion.

The most common immediate or short-term *complication of facet* neurectomy is that of local back pain caused by the chemical or thermal lesion. This pain is rarely very severe, especially if facet nerve denervation has been successfully accomplished. The most serious potential complication is lumbar or sacral nerve root injury. This complication is avoidable during RF facet neurectomy. If electrical stimulation prior to lesioning elicits sciatic sensory radiation or motor phenomena, the needle electrode should be withdrawn to a safe position. RF lesioning should be performed only with caution in a patient who develops sciatic nerve root anesthesia following local anesthetization prior to lesion making, since the ability to test reliably by electrical stimulation or reversible thermal blockade may be lost. Some risk of nerve root injury is inherent in the technique of phenol facet neurectomy because of the inability to control the spread of the phenol solution once it is injected into body tissues. This risk can best be minimized by careful radiographic control. As yet, I have not encountered any instance of infection in or around the facet joint following any of the facet needle procedures. The major long-term risk of neurectomy is the weakening of back muscles. The recurrent nerve branches that innervate the facet joints also innervate the interspinous muscles. Denervating these muscles is certain to lead to atrophy and secondary weakening of the back structure. The importance of this side effect is unclear, since the complexity of these patients' clinical problems makes it nearly impossible to evaluate any possible delayed ill effects attributable solely to local muscle atrophy.

A special application of facet neurectomy is encountered in patients with *painful pseudarthroses* of lumbosacral fusions. The same recurrent nerve branches that normally innervate facets and interspinous muscles innervate the fusion graft site. As discussed under fusion problems in Chapter 3, fusion pseudarthroses are not necessarily painful. However, if pain originating from a pseudarthrosis can be documented by local anesthetization, more long-term relief can be obtained by facet neurectomy (Fig. 6.4). The exact path of regrowth of these nerves is unpredictable, although generally lesioning close to a documented pseudarthrosis and more proximally along the expected course of the nerve should yield optimum results. Phenol normally gives a wider area of neural interruption than RF lesioning, but in the dense scarring that usually surrounds a spinal fusion this wider dissemination may be sharply curtailed. The more limited lesion obtained with the RF technique can be partially compensated for by making a series of adjacent lesions in the suspect area—although the multiple lesions are in themselves likely to induce significant short-term back pain.

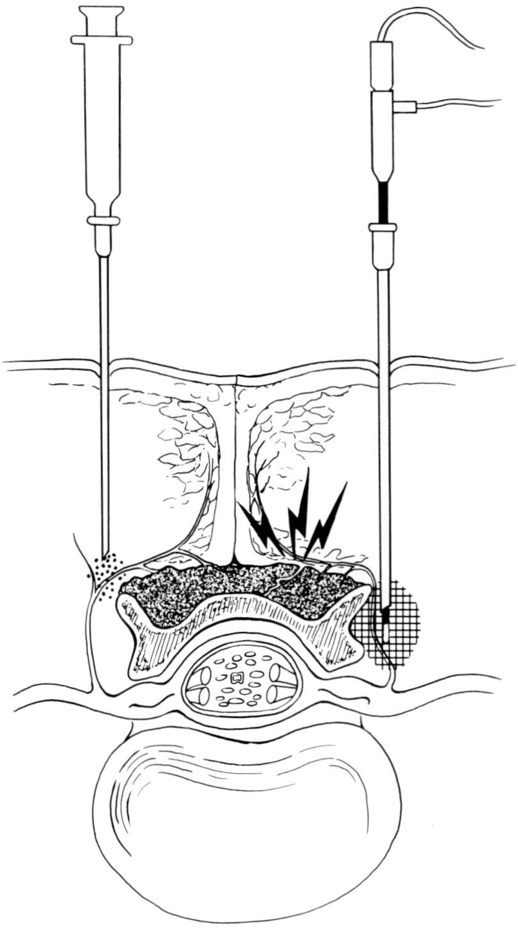

FIGURE 6.4. Facet nerve lesioning may be beneficial for patients with symptomatic pseudarthrosis. Recurrent facet nerves eventually innervate the fusion bone and transmit pain from the pseudarthrosis site. These nerves may be destroyed by phenol injection (left, stippling) or RF lesioning (right, cross hatching).

Sacroiliac Joint Injections

Pain arising from the sacroiliac (SI) joint can often be relieved for long periods by corticosteroid injections into the SI joint or adjacent joint capsule. *SI joint pain* is usually perceived over the lower back, buttock, and posterior thigh. The pain may spread across the lower back but rarely spreads below the knee. There may be tenderness to local pressure over the SI joint, especially if inflammation arises principally from the joint capsule, but it is often difficult to determine whether localized tenderness and pain of this type actually arises more from periosteal trigger points than from the joint capsule itself. Pain is usually triggered by the extremes of straight leg raising, but also by the extremes of bent leg raising and specifically when the examiner manually stresses the SI joint by twisting the patient's pelvis or by forcefully cross-adducting the flexed hip. Radiographs rarely disclose focal degenerative changes, but isotope bone and joint scans may be focally abnormal. Confirmation can be obtained by injecting the joint with anesthetic agents, usually mixed with a radiographic contrast medium to ensure that the injection reaches the intraarticular space.

The technique of SI joint injection is essentially the same as that described for diagnostic SI joint injections on page 105. For patients with tenderness along the SI joint capsule to manual palpation, a technique can be employed similar to that used for periosteal trigger point injections, as described on page 99.

The major *complication of SI injection* is that of infection, since corticosteroids lower tissue resistance to infection in the area of local high concentration. The *limitations of SI injection* are related first to the imprecision by which this diagnosis can be confirmed as the patient's principal source of pain and not just a single contributing factor, and second to the limitation common to all intraarticular steroid injections, which is their limited ability to provide lasting pain relief. Whether instraarticular steroids hasten joint degeneration is a topic of considerable discussion but with little conclusive evidence.

Epidural Injections

Diagnostic paraspinal and epidural injections, as discussed in Chapter 4, may be extremely beneficial in planning specific therapy, especially for patients who suffer predominantly leg pain as a part of their failed back syndrome. On rare occasions these diagnostic injections, especially injections into the epidural space, may provide long-lasting pain relief. In situations of documented or suspected *epidural adhesions,* diagnostic injections that help to disrupt these adhesions may become therapeutic injections, though quantified proof of efficacy is not available. With this goal in mind, the volume of anesthetic injected just prior to injection of other active agents into the epidural space is often specifically tailored in the hope of causing some disruption of adhesions. Injections into the lateral epidural space around nerve roots will cause nerve root anesthetization with volumes as small as 0.25 ml, but injecting volumes of 1 ml or 2 ml of anesthetic may help to disrupt adhesions in this area. Similarly, epidural injections over the dorsum of the thecal sac may produce adequate analgesics or anesthesia with volumes as small as 3 ml to 5 ml. Injecting volumes as large as 10 ml or 15 ml may help to disrupt adhesions in this area.

A specific and often valuable form of epidural therapeutic injection can be accomplished with the aid of *epidural catheters* placed in the dorsal epidural space, in or slightly rostral to the spinal area of maximum pain (Fig. 6.5). Anesthetic injection through these dorsally placed catheters results in more widespread sensory interruption than is achieved with lateral epidural or paraspinal injections. As a result, epidural catheters may be employed beneficially for the therapy of back pain as well as sciatic pain. Once in place, percutaneous catheters may be left in place for periods of up to several weeks. Catheters may also be permanently implanted, attached to a mechanical pump or reservoir system; this technique is discussed as a surgical technique in Chapter 7. Percutaneous epidural catheters may be used for repeated injections of anesthetics or morphine. Injections of small doses of

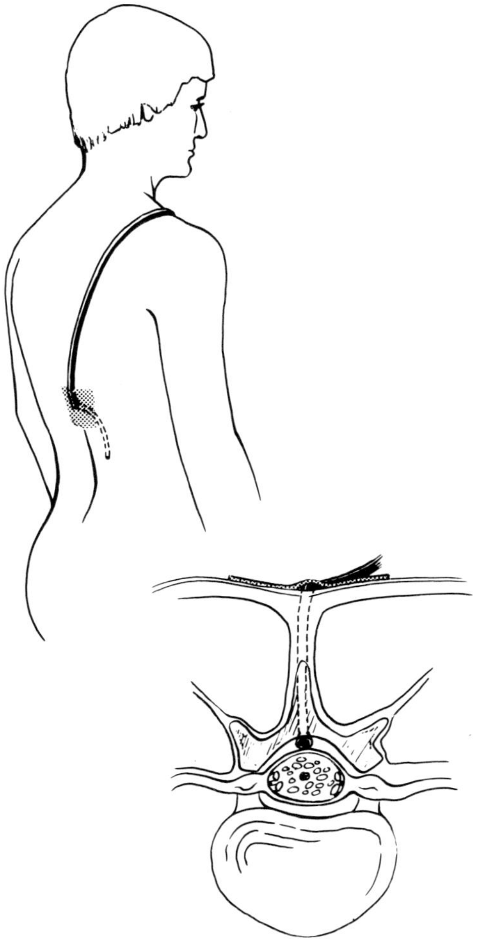

FIGURE 6.5. Epidural catheters may be placed in the thoracic or lumbar region for repeated use over days or weeks. Strict asepsis must be maintained at the catheter exit site and at the site of injection. The catheter lies in the epidural space at the level of painful abnormality or rostral thereto.

epidural morphine (3 mg to 8 mg) can bring dramatic pain relief without sensory loss or motor impairment and with a result that lasts 10 to 15 hours.[86] The morphine is usually diluted in 5 ml to 10 ml of normal saline to ensure better distribution throughout the epidural space. Presumably, the morphine is effective by penetrating the dura to interact with the opiate receptor systems of the spinal cord. Bupivacaine (Marcaine) can also be injected with these catheters. Doses of 5 ml to 10 ml of 0.25% to 0.5% often will produce hypalgesia without motor impairment and will often bring pain relief lasting from 6 to 10 hours.

Epidural injections of morphine or bupivacaine at 8- to 12-hour intervals can be *therapeutic in two important ways*. First, this technique is useful in *detoxifying patients* from drug addiction and dependence on large doses of systemic medications. If adequate local pain relief is achieved, systemic narcotics and potent tranquilizers can often be terminated. If this is done abruptly, the withdrawal reaction can be psychologically helpful in convincing the patient of the danger of such medication. Often patients discover that once they are free of their painful dependence on narcotics (see page 135), the total amount of pain they experience is actually less than it was during their period of narcotic addiction and can actually be better controlled with nonnarcotic analgesics than with large doses of narcotics. Second, this technique is useful to *permit a program of enforced activity* in a patient whose pain previously precluded such therapy. For some patients, pain relief coupled with active physical therapy over a period of two to three weeks can bring dramatic physical and psychologic improvement. This often results in a significant decrease in pain and significant improvement in the patient's tolerance of the pain that persists following termination of epidural injections.

Lasting relief of back and leg pain can at times be obtained from *epidural steroid injections*.[87-89] Patients who suffer predominantly from leg pain often obtain striking benefit from lateral, periradicular epidural steroid injections placed alongside the affected nerve root within the bony spinal canal. This is especially likely to be beneficial if diagnostic injection of anesthetics at this same site has brought good temporary pain relief. Such periradicular injections, performed with radiographic control, often provide relief of sciatica when midline epidural injections do not, presumably because local adhesions at the lateral operative site bar access of the steroid to the area from which symptoms arise. For the patient with pain predominantly in the low back, or back pain with bilateral leg pain, a midline dorsal epidural injection is more likely to be beneficial than a unilateral lateral injection. I have found such injections to be particularly useful for acute flare-ups of pain following minor or major trauma in failed back syndrome patients who had been relatively pain free prior to their injuries. Presumably in these patients chronic epidural adhesions have been present but asymptomatic until the time of reinjury. At that time, the injury probably caused irritation and inflammation in the nerve roots or more diffusely throughout the lumbar area. Adrenal corticosteroid injection probably does little to alter the status of the chronic adhesions but is most likely to be effective in reducing the inflammatory reaction to trauma. Epidural steroid injections may be beneficial in patients with chronic pain if the pain is secondary to chronic irritation by constricting adhesions, overlying pseudarthrosis, or lateral recess stenosis with nerve root swelling due to a combination of irritation and compression. In patients with presumed epidural inflammation due to adhesions, coupling epidural steroid injections with large-volume injections of saline or local anesthetic in an effort to break up adhesions should be contemplated. For those patients with chronic mechanical compression of nerve roots, it is doubtful that the epidural steroid injection in any way lessens the degree of extradural compression. On the other hand, the steroid in high local concentration may significantly reduce the bulk of swollen and inflamed nerve roots. The result is to free these nerve roots from compression by reducing their bulk rather than by expanding the space in which they are forced to exist. This mechanism is identical to that observed with cervical spondylotic disc disease in which nonoperative therapy is often strikingly successful in relieving radicular pain even though the severe bony changes themselves are not altered by cervical immobilization or anti-inflammatory therapy.

The major *risk of epidural injections* of all types is that of *infection*. This is particularly a problem with indwelling catheters and must be guarded against with meticulous skin care and aseptic technique at the time of each injection. Even with acute needle placements for single-injection epidural therapy, sepsis remains a recognized risk. The epidural abscess that results usually produces excruciatingly severe back pain with or without sciatic pain and may rapidly lead to neurologic deficit or even a cauda equina syndrome. If this complication occurs, it is important to recognize it early. One must then undertake early surgical evacuation of the abscess and administer appropriate antibiotics based on cultures and sensitivities obtained from bacteriologic study of the abscess contents.

Nerve root injury is a less likely complication that may follow epidural injections, especially injections placed laterally perineurally. These injections should always be performed under local anesthesia to check for the possibility of such damage. However, needle placement may require anesthetization in the vicinity of the nerve root and needle placement must be close to the nerve to be beneficial. If significant sciatic pain is encountered during needle placement, subsequent diagnostic or therapeutic injections should be made incrementally and cautiously, examining the patient between injections for evidence of loss of nerve root function. If anesthetic injections are a part of therapy, a loss of function should result; in these circumstances, some risk of nerve root injury is unavoidable.

Inadvertent *subdural or subarachnoid puncture* is another potential source of complications with attempted epidural injections. Anesthetic agents, especially in large volumes, injected within the thecal sac usually produce much more profound motor and sensory blockade than epidural injections. Spinal anesthesia that ascends to high thoracic or cervical regions can cause serious respiratory problems. Inadvertent spinal anesthesia limited to the lumbar or low thoracic region is less likely to be life-threatening but can necessitate several hours of unplanned hospital observation when epidural injections are done on an outpatient basis. Inadvertent intrathecal injections can also have unexpected and serious consequences if the thecal space is obliterated by adhesive arachnoiditis at the site of injection. Injections into and between nerve roots trapped by arachnoidal thickening may be extremely painful. Furthermore, these injections can cause temporary or permanent neurologic impairment, especially with larger volume injections. Epidural injections should not cause post-LP headaches, but inadvertent penetration of the dura and arachnoid, with or without intrathecal injection, may subject the patient to the risk of this unpleasant side effect.

Placement of epidural catheters brings with it an additional specific risk of complication. These catheters are usually soft plastic or rubber tubes that are passed into the epidural space through metal needles, usually a side-hole Touhey needle. During such a catheter placement, even a very limited retraction of the catheter back into the needle can cause shearing off of the catheter tip within the patient. This retained foreign body may or may not form a nidus for increased epidural adhesions but certainly poses an added malpractice risk for the surgeon or the anesthesiologist who performs the procedure.

The following brief case reports illustrate the usefulness of the two major versions of epidural injection:

Case 11

This 38-year-old homemaker underwent excision of an L4-L5 disc at another hospital in 1978 for complaints of back and left leg pain. Initially, postoperatively she improved, although she was never pain free. Over subsequent months, back and radiating sciatic left leg pain gradually increased in severity. Two myelograms showed no abnormality, and she failed to respond to bracing, bed rest, physical therapy, and muscle-relaxing medications. She was seen at the University of Massachusetts Medical Center 2 1/2 years later complaining of back and left sciatic pain. Range of back motion was severely limited, and straight leg raising to 40 degrees caused radiating leg pain. There was slight hypalgesia over the anterior left shin and dorsal foot, but the neurologic examination was otherwise normal. A trial of anti-inflammatory and antineuralgia medications gave partial relief only. Three-level lumbar contrast discography was normal at L3-L4 and L5-S1. At L4-L5, excruciatingly severe pain followed injection, even though there was no posterior extravasation of dye. Intradiscal injection of an anesthetic brought immediate relief of back pain, and intradiscal methylprednisolone (Depo-Medrol) rapidly gave lasting relief of this component of her pain.

Sciatic pain persisted. Five days following disc injection, a 22-gauge LP needle was placed fluoroscopically in the left epidural space at L4-L5, adjacent to the L5 nerve root, and 0.5 ml of 1% lidocaine (Xylocaine) was injected. This produced analgesia in the anterior left shin and dorsomedial foot and gave prompt and total relief of sciatic pain. One millimeter (40 mg) of methylprednisolone was injected prior to withdrawal of the needle. Within five days, sciatic pain had faded and disappeared. Following this procedure, the patient was completely able to discontinue narcotics after having required 60 mg to 120 mg of codeine every four hours over the preceding year. Eight weeks later, increased back pain resulted after she slipped while climbing onto the cabin of a sailboat, but leg pain remained totally relieved. A repeat intradiscal injection once again relieved her back pain.

Case 12

This massively obese 32-year-old homemaker developed severe sciatica following a fall. Myelography disclosed a small defect at L4-L5 and L5-S1 on the right. In 1976 she underwent excision of both discs at a local hospital. Sciatica persisted and necessitated a large intake of narcotic medication.

She came under my care two years later. Two separate diagnostic epidural nerve root blocks at L4-L5 and L5-S1 on the right seemed to give her relief of pain. Epidural methylprednisolone acetate (Depo-Medrol) injection brought no lasting relief. In 1979, sensory rhizotomies were performed at L5 and S1 nerve roots. This allowed her to become free of significant narcotic intake, but she continued to complain of right sciatica and low back pain. Management was complicated by a hysterical personality with episodes of hysterical paralysis and hemisensory loss. She ambulated with a cane with exaggerated posture but did gradually lose 50 pounds.

In 1981, she developed a sudden onset of excruciatingly severe back pain immediately after washing her kitchen floor. Pains became progressively more severe despite bed rest at home supplemented by local heat, norphenadine (Norflex), and dihydrocodinone-aspirin compound (Percodan). She was hospitalized at the University of Massachusetts Medical Center with a painful "fixed" muscle spasm. She was treated for ten days with complete bed rest and intravenous (later oral) methocarbamol (Robaxin) coupled with ibuprofen (Motrin), local heat, and back liniments. Pain seemed to improve somewhat, but she tended to lie completely motionless in bed, despite repeated urging to increase her activity. After ten days of bed rest an epidural catheter was placed in the lumbar midline by Dr. Robert Burney of the Pain Control Unit. Twice daily injections of 5 mg of morphine in 10 ml of normal saline gave her complete relief of pain. With considerable urging she became progressively more ambulatory and discontinued Percodan altogether. After a ten-day course of epidural morphine injections, 80 mg of betamethsone (Aristocort) was injected epidurally and the catheter was withdrawn. Some rebound pain ensued, but she was able to remain active without narcotics and was discharged five days later. Six months later she remained symptomatic but was able to be active in caring for her home and her ailing husband.

Intrathecal Injections

Needle therapy of failed back syndrome disorders using intrathecal injections employs either restorative or destructive, neuroablative solutions. Restorative injections are designed to restore function or reduce pain and disability without causing sensory loss or other neurologic deficits.

Restorative Injections

The chemical agents used for *restorative intrathecal injections* are *anesthetics and adrenal corticosteroids*. The most commonly employed anesthetics are lidocaine (Xylocaine) and tetracaine (Pontocaine). Because anesthetic injections intrathecally are not reliable as restorative injections, they are usually injected principally for diagnostic purposes or as an anesthetic to permit forced stretching of localized adhesions. The choice of agent and the volume and concentration of the agent used are thus determined more by these other considerations than by a principal concern for their potential restorative effectiveness. At times, however, the injection of anesthetic agents alone can interrupt a cycle of pain and bring long-lasting relief from suffering. In practice, this lasting benefit is much less commonly seen following single intrathecal injection than following repeated injections through an epidural catheter, but it should be kept in mind that such lasting effects can occasionally occur. Consequently, it is frequently beneficial to allow an interval of days or even weeks to elapse between diagnostic anesthetic injections and later destructive, neuroablative injections. If during this interval the patient enjoys sustained pain relief, neuroablative injections may be avoided, and perhaps intrathecal steroid injections may be tried in hopes of abolishing residual or recurrent discomfort.

The use of *intrathecal corticosteroid injections* is particularly controversial.[49,90-94] Published medical literature documents significant complications following such injections. Most of the severe neurologic complications have occurred in patients with potentially progressive disorders such as multiple sclerosis, and nearly all have followed multiple injections, injections of extremely large volumes of Depo-Medrol, or injections at short intervals. There is, however, considerable and strong published support for the efficacy of intrathecal corticosteroids for relieving painful disorders of the low back. This published literature is considerably complicated, however, by a series of publications on the use of intrathecal corticosteroids in the treatment of multiple sclerosis, with most of these treatments involving multiple injections.

Except for the few septic complications, the *reported neurologic complications* most often affected the thoracic spinal cord at a distance from the site of injection, even though it has been documented that corticosteroid injected into the subarachnoid space concentrates in the lumbar theca. The identification of the corticosteroid as the causative agent for these neurologic complications has been based exclusively on circumstantial evidence. The published literature involving *corticosteroid subarachnoid injections in experimental animals* is also confusing.[95] A number of investigators emphasize the apparent beneficial effect of intrathecal injections, some emphasize an induced pleocytosis and a possible increased risk of arachnoiditis, but none have been able to reproduce the type of neurologic complications impugned to be a complication in human use. The risk of intrathecal reaction or production of arachnoiditis seems to be aggravated by concomitant injection of corticosteroids with blood or nonwater-soluble contrast agents.

Overall, a considerable literature and clinical experience attest to the *therapeutic benefit of intrathecal corticosteroid injections,* which may provide long-term symptomatic relief or may facilitate and make possible forced activity restorative therapy. Several authors have commented that intrathecal corticosteroid injections are at times beneficial when epidural corticosteroid injections have failed. My experience has been that intrathecal corticosteroid injections may at times be the only treatment that can bring intermediate or long-term relief in patients suffering intractably from the pain of *lumbar adhesive arachnoiditis.* The practitioner must be aware that the manufacturer of methylprednisolone acetate (Depo-Medrol) has specifically advised against its intrathecal use because of the potential for risk, but its potential risk seems clearly to be smaller than that of repeated surgical intervention. Furthermore, the manufacturer's recommendation carries no legal weight in proscribing any drug therapy, as clearly enunciated by the Legal Department of the American Medical Association, other than a particular burden of informed consent.[96] Intrathecal corticosteroids may be used freely for an individual and specifically informed patient if pain relief is a valid goal for that patient.

I have reviewed *my own experience with intrathecal corticosteroid injections* given during the period from 1979 to 1987.[49] One hundred eight intrathecal injections of methylprednisolone acetate (Depo-Medrol), 80 mg per ml, were given in the treatment of 35 patients with painful low back disorders with median follow-ups of three years nine months. Pain relief was excellent (more than one month of almost total relief or more than four months of useful partial relief) in 62% of injections and poor in 30%. Twenty-nine of these patients had undergone previous back surgery, and 100 injections produced excellent relief in 63% of these patients, poor relief in 27%. If pain relief was experienced, it lasted more than one year in 10% of injections and six to twelve months in 22%. Ten patients were documented as having extensive adhesive arachnoiditis of Type II or Type III, all but one following prior back surgery; fifty-nine intrathecal injections provided excellent relief in 74% and poor relief in only 18%. Eight patients who obtained only poor relief underwent subsequent "salvage" surgery with four good outcomes; two others committed suicide. No patient in this series experienced significant complications. Nine patients underwent myelography following intrathecal treatment, and none of their myelograms demonstrated significant changes. Intrathecal therapy frequently brought pain relief in patients who had not responded to epidural steroids.

Intrathecal restorative injections are most useful for patients who suffer *pain predominantly in their backs or simultaneously in their backs and both legs.* Patients with *adhesive arachnoiditis* seem to respond well to such injections. As discussed on page 160, pain may develop or exacerbate in the presence of fixed and unchanging scarring if *trauma or excessive activity* induces nerve irritation and local swelling within the nerves. In these instances, long-lasting pain relief may occasionally follow intrathecal adrenal corticosteroid therapy given alone or in combination with systemic antineuralgia therapy and perhaps systemic anti-inflammatory therapy. An illustrative case report follows:

Case 13

This 44-year-old homemaker had an L4-L5 disc rupture excised with bilateral posterior spine fusion of L4 to sacrum in 1974, after a protracted bout with lower back and right leg pain. Postoperative recovery was incomplete despite her attempts to remain active. Myelogram in 1976 disclosed focal nerve root blunting at L4-L5 on the right. Needle therapy failed to give lasting relief even though anesthetization of the L5 nerve root brought temporary excellent pain relief. That same year the fusion was fenestrated and L5 root surgical sensory rhizotomy was performed. After this, the patient noted marked improvement in leg pain, but bilateral posterior iliac pain continued. Focal tenderness was present over the right posterior iliac spine and over the left bone donor site. Multiple injections of these local tender areas with anesthetics, steroids, and later with prolotherapy solution repeatedly brought intervals of pain relief lasting six to ten weeks. Interestingly, each time the left bone donor site was anesthetized she noted immediate relief of pain medial to her left knee. In 1978, the tender area at the left bone donor site was resected *en bloc*. Microscopic analysis disclosed multiple small neuromata. Following this, sciatic and back pain remained at a low level with the aid of hydantoin (Dilantin), ibuprofen (Motrin), and sulindac (Clinoril). She was able to space the rightsided posterior iliac prolotherapy injections in intervals of three to six months.

In 1980 and 1981, both back and right leg pain gradually increased in severity, markedly limiting her activities at home and socially. A single intrathecal injection of 80 mg (1 ml) of methylprednisolone acetate (Depo-Medrol) brought her "the best relief in years!" Her response at this time was, "Why didn't you do this years ago?" Pain relief over the next nine months remained sufficiently valuable so that she was able to resume dating for the first time since her husband's death two years before.

Intrathecal restorative injections of steroids may also be beneficial for patients with lower back and bilateral leg pain of other etiologies. This is true of patients with *epidural scarring* or *diffuse epidural inflammation* who have not responded to epidural injections or who are not candidates for epidural injections because of obliteration of the epidural space. Occasionally, patients with *unilateral sciatica* secondary to acute or chronic nerve root injury, nerve root compression by scar, or lateral recess stenosis may benefit nicely from intrathecal steroid injections. These patients are usually subjected initially to two stages of lateral epidural injections: first diagnostic anesthetic injections then therapeutic injections. If satisfactory anesthetization cannot be achieved because of the density of epidural scar or because of overlying fusion bone, intrathecal injections as near as possible to the site of emergence of the inflamed nerve root may be beneficial.

Corticosteroids are the most useful restorative agents for intrathecal injections. Although several forms have been reported by others to have been used intrathecally, I have generally preferred *methylprednisolone acetate (Depo-Medrol)* in the stronger concentration of 80 mg per ml. Because methylprednisolone comes with an inert carrier substance that is slow to clear from the subarachnoid space and that may have deleterious side effects, I have chosen this concentration in an effort to minimize the amount of this inert carrier agent that must be injected with the corticosteroid while still obtaining the benefit of the long-acting, slow-release nature of this methylprednisolone preparation. I have generally injected only 1 ml of this solution at each treatment. In addition, I rarely if ever give a second intrathecal steroid injection less than two months following the first injection and generally do not give more than three intrathecal injections in a 12-month period.

The *technique of intrathecal restorative injections* is essentially that of lumbar puncture or spinal anesthesia (see pages 88 and 108). I have performed both anesthetic and corticosteroid intrathecal injections on an outpatient or day surgery basis. Patients are not allowed to drive home. They are instructed to remain recumbent in the vehicle en route home and to spend the remainder of that day and night more or less in bed. All patients are instructed to use these simple remedies if symptoms of post-LP headache occur: bed rest, hydration, and simple analgesics containing caffeine. All patients are also instructed to report severe or persistent headaches and any unexpected neurologic symptoms or unusual pain.

The chief *complication* of restorative intrathecal injections is *LP headaches*. This type of headache and its specific therapy have been described in detail earlier (see page 87). Post-LP headaches may in fact occur more frequently following intrathecal steroid injections than following simple lumbar punctures because of the corticosteroids. Since these agents have a potent anti-inflammatory effect and a mild retarding effect on wound healing, they may slow the closure of the needle puncture site in the thecal sac. This persistent opening in the thecal sac is the source of the internal spinal fluid leak that causes this uncomfortable and posturally triggered form of headache.

Infection is the most dangerous complication that may follow intrathecal steroid injections. Again, the anti-inflammatory effectiveness of these agents may facilitate the establishment of an infection. Indeed, both bacterial and fungal infections have been reported following intrathecal corticosteroid injections. *Chemical meningitis* is largely preventable with careful technique and clean equipment. Injection through needles or with syringes contaminated by antiseptic solutions or inadvertent injection of such solutions can have serious consequences, but should be avoidable. The *initiation of or aggravation of arachnoiditis* is a potential complication of intrathecal restorative injections. The uncertainty of the cause of arachnoiditis was discussed under adhesive arachnoiditis in Chapter 3. Arachnoiditis has been diagnosed clinically following the injection of anesthetic agents, myelographic contrast agents, and chemical irritants as well as having been confirmed as a spontaneously occurring disease entity. The few clinical reports of severe arachnoiditis in association with intrathecal corticosteroid injections have all been in patients with complex spinal disorders, all of whom underwent multiple needle procedures, including multiple corticosteroid injections. As yet, I have not encountered any proof through personal experience or through the medical literature of arachnoiditis being caused or severely aggravated by single or widely spaced multiple injections of adrenal corticosteroids.

Destructive or Neuroablative Injections

Subarachnoid injection of *destructive neurolytic agents* is occasionally indicated in patients with protracted pain secondary to a failed back syndrome. Since these injections are designed to interrupt nervous tissue functioning in a prolonged or semipermanent way, they should not be used in patients with prolonged pain until restorative or corrective therapies have proven to be ineffective. The deliberate interruption of nervous tissue functioning and the subsequent loss of sensation and motion that results are serious steps to undertake. To undertake these steps without reasonable assurance of their effectiveness would not be medically sound and would be unfair to the patient. As a result, this form of injection should rarely, if ever, be undertaken until preliminary diagnostic injections have been performed and have given reasonable assurance that the proposed neurolytic injection has an acceptable likelihood of providing the pain relief that the patient and his physician seek.

The most commonly employed *neurolytic agents* used for subarachnoid injection are phenol and alcohol. Injections of iced or hypertonic saline enjoyed a brief popularity but are rarely used now. Subarachnoid injection of phenol (carbolic acid) for pain relief was pioneered in England. The use of these agents to perform *chemical sensory rhizotomy* was introduced in the United States principally by my former teacher, Dr. James C. White.[97] Following the introduction of this technique at Massachusetts General Hospital, the number of surgical cordotomies performed for pain relief declined sharply. Subarachnoid phenol injections produce selective sensory interruption. Higher concentration, larger volumes, or longer applications of phenol can cause motor weakness, but sensory loss appears earlier with solutions of standard concentration (5% phenol in anhydrous glycerol or 7.5% phenol in iophendylate). It has been assumed that this differential clinical effect is based on a greater sensitivity of the unmyelinated or lightly myelinated pain fibers, with the heavily myelinated motor and touch fibers being better protected. Histologic evidence, however, challenges this assumption, since the observed pattern is one of maximum damage circumferentially and superficially in each affected nerve root without obvious differential destruction of small fibers more than large fibers. A brief clinical report illustrates the usefulness of intrathecal phenol rhizotomy in a failed back syndrome patient:

Case 14

This 21-year-old hospital employee injured her back in 1969 while lifting. This led to persistent right sciatica and low back pain that failed to improve with prolonged nonoperative therapy. Myelogram showed no obvious defect, but sciatica persisted. In 1970, she underwent laminectomy at L4-L5 and L5-S1 and discectomy at L5-S1 on the right, but with only transient improvement. Repeat myelogram five months later remained normal. Epidural diagnostic nerve blocks with steroid confirmed that her sciatic pain still seemed to arise from the S1 nerve root. Symptoms persisted despite protracted pharmacologic, enforced activity, and enforced inactivity therapies.

In 1974, repeat myelogram was normal and discogram was abnormal only at L5-S1, although disc injection at this level caused severe back and leg pain. Epidural lidocaine (Xylocaine) and methylprednisolone acetate (Depo-Medrol) gave no lasting relief. Repeat laminectomy was performed with lysis of moderately dense epidural scar around the S1 nerve root. She improved for several months following this procedure, but again back and leg pain recurred. In 1975, repeat epidural surgical neurolysis and posterolateral fusion were performed with lasting improvement in back pain.

Sciatica persisted and in 1977 repeat epidural lidocaine and methylprednisolone failed to give lasting relief. Subsequent myelogram was normal except for some enlargement of the S1 nerve root pouch at the operative site. Intrathecal tetracaine (Pontocaine) diagnostic spinal block gave excellent temporary relief with the anesthetization of L5 and part of S1 roots. This was followed by phenol sensory rhizotomy, which produced good sensory loss in the L5 and S1 distribution. Subsequent to this, sciatica was much improved and she was able to discontinue regular narcotics.

Over subsequent years, lumbar trigger points developed and were controlled with local injections of methylprednisolone and prolotherapy. Sciatica returned 16 months following phenol rhizotomy, and repeat phenol rhizotomy was performed in 1978 after repeat myelography demonstrated persistent patency of the lumbar thecal sac. This procedure restored the sensory loss in her leg and gave her an additional 12 months of excellent improvement in sciatica. A third phenol sensory rhizotomy was performed in 1980. Despite using larger doses, complete analgesia could not be obtained in the L5 and S1 nerve root distribution, even though mild weakness of dorsiflexion and plantar flexion of the ankle transiently appeared. Relief of sciatica was significant but incomplete. She continued to require nonnarcotic analgesics several times weekly but remained active as a homemaker and mother.

Intrathecal, subarachnoid injections of *absolute ethyl alcohol* have been in use longer than injections of phenol. However, alcohol injections have a less selective effect on sensory fibers and a greater likelihood of causing loss of motor and autonomic functions. As a result, absolute alcohol is now less commonly used than intrathecal phenol, especially for the common disorders that plague failed back syndrome sufferers.

Subarachnoid injections of *iced or hypertonic saline* for relief of pain and spasticity enjoyed brief popularity. These injections produce a transient interruption of pain sensation and reflex arcs that rarely lasts more than a few days or weeks. The injections are extremely painful and usually necessitate general anesthesia. Iced normotonic saline solutions will cause some neurolytic effect if sufficient thermal injury is created, and some amelioration of pain has been reported from subarachnoid barbotage with room-temperature saline. The best effects with this approach have been reported through the use of hypertonic saline solutions. Presumably, these solutions cause a neurolytic effect through the production of osmotic injuries in nerve roots. In my limited experience with these techniques in patients with the failed back syndrome, I have not found them to be significantly beneficial.

The *technique* of performing a *subarachnoid phenol sensory rhizotomy* begins with lumbar puncture. Some surgeons are willing to perform this procedure on an outpatient basis, but I have insisted on at least overnight hospitalization because of the possibility of urinary retention, initial motor weakness, or painful reaction to the procedure. The procedure must be done on a bed or a tabletop that can be tilted to raise the patient's head and shoulders higher than his pelvis, or vice versa (Fig. 6.6). This can be accomplished with a tilting fluoroscopy table or quite adequately in a hospital bed. To use a hospital bed, the patient is positioned near the head of the bed and the head of the bed is elevated or lowered as needed. The ability to tip the patient's trunk up or down is vital to this procedure, since localization of the neurolytic phenol solution within the thecal sac is accomplished gravimetrically by having the solution flow to the nerve root exit pouch that has been selected for treatment. The patient is placed in the lateral position with the painful side down. His knees are bent upward, his head bent forward, and his back arched outward, as in the performance of a routine lumbar puncture. An added touch in patient positioning is said to aid in the differential interruption of sensory more than motor root fibers. This involves tilting the patient backwards 10 degrees during the performance of phenol sensory rhizotomy. The rationale for this maneuver is to layer the phenol solution more into the dorsal half of the thecal sac than into the ventral half, since sensory nerves lie dorsal to motor fibers within the sac.

The needle puncture should be placed at the site of suspected maximum nerve root involvement or as near to it as possible. Patients with previous posterior spinal fusions more commonly than not will experience pain originating from nerve roots protected from needle access by the fusion bone. In these instances the needle is placed adjacent to the rostral end of the fusion. In all patients it is important to have myelographic confirmation that the thecal sac is open to prevent unwanted and potentially dangerous pooling of phenol in unexpected places. Confirmation of subarachnoid placement of the

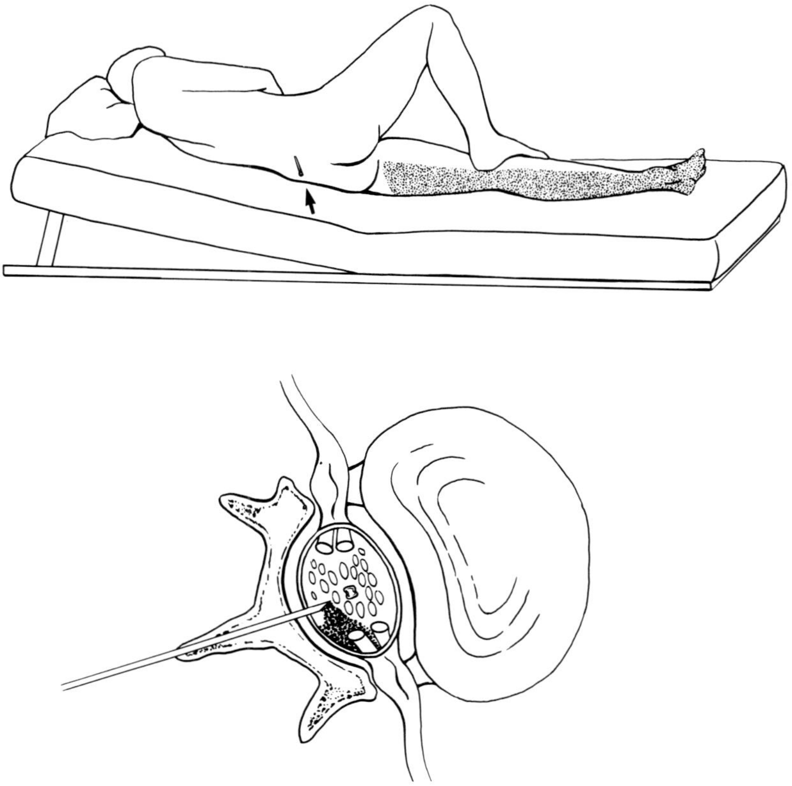

FIGURE 6.6. Phenol (chemical) sensory rhizotomy is done with the patient laterally recumbent on a tilting bed or table. Spinal puncture is done as close as possible to the site of maximum pain. The patient is positioned with the painful side down and with slight posterior rotation to provide maximum pooling of the hyperbaric phenol solution over sensory nerve rootlets. The extent and depth of sensory interruption is monitored by careful and repeated cutaneous sensory testing as incremental injections are made.

needle tip by free withdrawal of cerebrospinal fluid (CSF) is also extremely important, since subdural, extraarachnoidal injections may produce uncontrollable and undesirable effects. Also, because the phenol cannot easily penetrate through the arachnoid, an injection into the subdural space usually fails to induce adequate sensory interruption. The most commonly used phenol solution for lumbar subarachnoid sensory rhizotomy is a 5% solution in anhydrous glycerol. The glycerol is extremely hyperbaric and holds the phenol in the desired area. Solutions of 7.5% or 10% are occasionally used when penetration through scarred nerve roots is desirable, but these higher concentrations carry a greater risk of motor root injury.

The volume of phenol solution injected into the subarachnoid space should rarely exceed 1 ml. Injection should always begin with a tiny test dose, generally 0.05 ml. If the phenol solution has been contaminated with water or saline, that portion of the phenol that has been liberated from the glycerol or iophendylate (Pantopaque) may spread rapidly throughout the subarachnoid space, producing a spectacularly widespread neural interruption. If this occurs following only a test injection, the results are almost never lasting, but such widespread dissemination could be potentially disastrous following large-volume injections. Following the initial test injection, additional increments of phenol and glycerol are injected, generally in volumes of 0.1 ml to 0.2 ml.

Following each injection, the patient is carefully tested for the cutaneous loss of pinprick and later loss of touch perception that ensues one to three minutes following each injection. If sensory loss begins to appear at a cutaneous segmental level lower than the proposed target area, the patient's shoulders are lowered relative to the pelvis. Conversely, if sensory loss begins to appear at segmental levels rostral to the desired target area, the patient's shoulders are raised relative to the pelvis. Once proper localization is achieved by patient positioning, additional increments are given at approximately five-minute intervals, each time carefully testing sensory and motor functions between injections. The desired endpoint is that of analgesia or anesthesia in the desired sensory area with no more than slight weakness of dorsiflexion or plantar flexion. Weakness that develops at this stage of the test almost invariably clears within the first 24 hours, but heralds the need to discontinue further injections to prevent lasting motor weakness. When the desired depth and cutaneous distribution of sensory loss have been achieved, further injections are discontinued, but the patient is left in exactly the same lateral position for an additional 30 to 45 minutes. This is done to ensure complete resorption of the phenol and glycerol before shifting any residual active compound to unwanted areas within the thecal sac.

A 7.5% solution of *phenol in iophendylate (Pantopaque)* offers the advantage of fluoroscopic guidance in addition to cutaneous sensory monitoring during performance of phenol sensory rhizotomy. This is rarely necessary in the lumbar region but may be useful if thoracic sensory interruption is planned. For lumbar injections, cutaneous sensory localization is preferable to fluoroscopic guidance because it increases the accuracy of sensory interruption in the desired cutaneous area and it obviates the problem of residual iophendylate. Phenol is actually more soluble in iophendylate than it is in spinal fluid and so remains chemically active in iophendylate solution for at least several hours within the thecal sac. Iophendylate loaded with phenol must be completely removed from the subarachnoid space following sensory rhizotomy to avoid delayed neurolytic effects at other sensory levels that come in contact with the solution over subsequent hours or days.

Perhaps the greatest *limitation of subarachnoid phenol sensory rhizotomy* is a *failure to obtain adequate sensory loss and pain relief.* A failure of pain relief despite an adequately deep and properly distributed sensory loss is not a limitation of the procedure *per se,* since the procedure can do no more than interrupt sensory fibers. If this interruption fails to produce pain relief, it is not the procedure that has failed but the choice of the procedure that has failed. This, of course, does not necessarily imply that the choice of the procedure was faulty. Since much of what is undertaken in medicine is based on statistical probabilities of success, a certain percentage of failure is inherent. The limitation of this procedure comes when it proves impossible to induce adequate or lasting cutaneous sensory loss. This can be the result of phenol solutions that have lost their strength because of advanced age, but more commonly results from perineural scarring or arachnoidal thickening that prevents penetration of the chemical agent to the nerve root. In these instances, using stronger solutions or adding a potentiator, such as silver nitrate, may improve penetration, but may do so at the expense of concomitant motor weakness.

The second major *limitation of subarachnoid phenol sensory rhizotomy* is its *limited duration of action.* The induced sensory loss rarely persists for more than 12 to 18 months, and lasts considerably shorter periods of time if more cautious injections of lower volumes are performed. For some patients this duration of action is sufficient to permit healing of unstable or injured tissues and to permit the patient to follow a vigorous restorative program. For other patients pain will recur when sensory awareness returns or within weeks or months thereafter. For these patients repeated injections may be contemplated. It must be kept in mind that each injection causes some local scarring, so that subsequent injections are likely to require larger volumes or greater concentrations of phenol. These therefore carry an increased risk of leg or bladder weakness, while at the same time offering a reduced chance of satisfactory sensory interruption.

The chief *complication* of subarachnoid phenol sensory rhizotomy is *unwanted neurologic loss.* With lumbar or lumbosacral subarachnoid phenol injections, urinary incontinence or retention follows rhizotomy in 3% to 5% of patients with unilateral block and 5% to 10% of patients with bilateral block. The frequency with which motor weakness in the leg or foot is encountered increases with increasing concentration and volume of phenol solution injected. The risk is also significantly greater in the presence of arachnoidal scarring, which can cause pocketing of phenol around motor roots and chemical interruption of their fibers. Patients whose subarachnoid space is open and essentially normal myelographically and who receive injections of 5% phenol in anhydrous glycerol not exceeding 1 ml face an incidence of transient motor weakness of less than 1%. The production of barely detectable motor weakness may be used as one of the endpoints of phenol sensory rhizotomy, and this degree of motor loss almost invariably clears within 24 hours. When significant bladder and motor complications occur they are rarely permanent. I have not encountered a patient whose phenol-induced complication persisted for more than 12 to 18 months. A second complication of subarachnoid phenol sensory rhizotomy is related to the *chemical irritation* or *meningismus* that this acid compound causes. For 24 to 72 hours following the procedure some patients will complain of increased back pain, cramping leg pain, and stiff neck. Some even develop a headache and fever. Symptomatic therapy with rest, anodynes, and muscle relaxers usually suffices. The phenol solution itself is a potent bactericidal agent, so infection is rarely encountered.

Subarachnoid alcohol injections are performed with a technique similar to that used for subarachnoid phenol injections. The major difference in technique relates to the difference in specific gravity of the two compounds. Whereas phenol is hyperbaric relative to spinal fluid and therefore settles in the most dependent portion of the thecal sac, absolute alcohol is hypobaric relative to spinal fluid and rises to the highest part of the thecal sac. Great care must be taken during performance of alcohol subarachnoid injections to ensure that the patient's thoracic and cervical spines are lower than his lumbar spine to prevent inadvertent upward migration of the hypobaric alcohol. Unilateral intrathecal blocks of sciatic nerve roots are performed with the patient on his side with the painful side uppermost and with the table in a 10- to 15-degree Trendelenburg (head down) position. For patients with pain principally in the caudal or coccygeal regions, alcohol blocks are occasionally indicated. This procedure is performed with the patient in the knee-chest position or prone on a tilting table with a bolster under the pelvis and the table in 30-degree Trendelenburg position. A lumbar puncture is performed as close as feasible to the spinal level at which sensory denervation is planned. For patients with chronic, benign pain, amounts of absolute alcohol exceeding 1 ml or 1.5 ml are rarely indicated. This is usually injected in aliquots of 0.25 ml to 0.5 ml, with the result controlled by careful and repeated sensory and motor examination during the procedure.

The major *limitation* of subarachnoid alcohol injection is that this agent gives a less selective sensory interruption than phenol. As a result, autonomic disturbance and leg weakness are more likely to occur. The frequency and severity of this complication can be reduced if small amounts of alcohol are used, with careful motor and sensory examination being performed to permit cessation of the procedure at the first sign of motor weakness.

Epidural, Paraspinal, and Intrathecal Radiofrequency Nerve Root Procedures

An alternative method of sensory interruption of lumbar nerve roots for pain control is *radiofrequency (RF) electrothermal lesioning*. Small-diameter pain-conducting nerve fibers seem to be selectively damaged by heat lesioning, and it is possible to create nerve root lesions that principally interrupt sensory conduction rather than motor conduction. The technique is, however, somewhat *unpredictable* for two reasons. First, it is difficult to know when a physiologic thermal blockade of sensory nerve conduction has been converted to a lasting destruction of sensory fibers. Second, the margin of safety between sensory and motor interruption is at times small, and motor weakness may appear abruptly during the course of intended sensory lesioning. Nerve root interruption by this technique can be accomplished percutaneously, either paraspinally where the nerve root exits from the neuroforamen or epidurally at the point where the nerve root enters the neuroforamen. On rare occasions, such as with patients having dense arachnoiditis and epidural adhesions, this technique may be used by transdural contact with the target nerve root. Transdural RF lesioning is not recommended for patients with patent spinal canals, since a free flow of spinal fluid conducts heat away and makes it difficult to obtain adequate electrode tip temperatures. Furthermore, transdural electrode placement is likely to be less precise than the other placement sites in patients with patent canals because of the free mobility of the nerve roots within the spinal fluid.

The *technique* of RF electrothermal nerve root lesioning involves needle electrode placement at the desired sites in much the same fashion as described earlier (Fig. 6.7). Fluoroscopic guidance is required and confirmatory radiographs to document electrode placement should always be taken for future

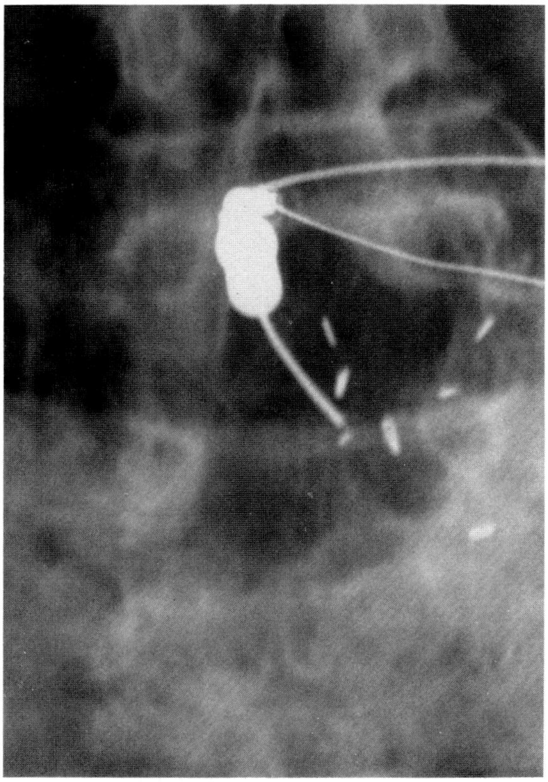

FIGURE 6.7. Radiofrequency (RF) lesioning of nerve roots may be carried out paraspinally, epidurally, or intradurally. Intradural lesioning is usually possible only in the presence of extensive arachnoiditis, because spinal fluid present in large volumes would rapidly conduct away added heat. RF lesioning has a differential effect, interrupting sensory transmission before motor transmission is damaged, but this effect is not always reliably predictable. This radiograph shows an RF probe tip placed adjacent to a painful S2 nerve root intradurally in a woman with severe lumbar arachnoiditis. L5 and S1 nerve roots had previously been surgically sectioned and the bulk of her residual pain had been documented to arise from this nerve root.

use and as an aid to planning additional procedures that might be required. Tip temperatures are raised to 50 degrees centigrade and are held at this temperature long enough to permit sensory testing to confirm the accuracy of electrode placement. Lesioning is likely to be quite painful and may require methohexital (Brevital) or narcoleptic anesthesia. Local anesthesia is much less desirable because anesthetization of the nerve roots precludes careful sensory and motor testing during performance of lesioning. If the patient is unable to tolerate diagnostic electrothermal blockade, electrical stimulation at low voltage and amplitude may suffice to confirm localization. An initial lesion is made with a tip temperature of 80 to 90 degrees centigrade for one minute. Following this the patient should retain full power but should exhibit hypalgesia in the appropriate area. Supplemental lesioning can then at times be carried out without additional anesthesia. Ideally, a three-minute lesion should be made to guarantee permanence, although this carries a significant risk of undesirable motor lesioning as well.

The major *risk of electrothermal nerve root lesioning* is inadvertent motor weakness. This risk can be minimized by careful testing and staged lesion-making as described above. Unfortunately, some patients will abruptly develop major motor loss during the course of lesioning, and this possibility should be carefully discussed with the patient prior to undertaking lesioning. The major *limitation of this technique* is failure to produce lasting sensory loss or pain relief. As discussed earlier, electrothermal blockade may cause interruption of nerve impulse transmission without nerve fiber destruction, and this may be impossible to distinguish clinically at the time of attempted lesioning. In my limited experience with this technique, I have found that even with extensive lesioning, often with some motor loss, sensory awareness not uncommonly returns within the first 24 hours, bringing with it a return of the patient's pain.

Lumbar Sympathectomy

Lumbar sympathectomy can be useful for those patients who suffer principally from *sympathetically mediated pain*. There is considerable debate over how many patients suffer from sympathetically mediated pain as their principal ailment and what proper term should be applied to their form of suffering. Clearly there is a wide spectrum of presentation with clinical features that include pain and hypersensitivity, dystrophic changes, circulatory changes and changes in cutaneous sweating. Terms such as *major* or *minor causalgia* and *reflex sympathetic dystrophy* are variously defined by various official groups and unofficial users of the terms, but it seems to me that the term reflex sympathetic dystrophy should be reserved for those patients who demonstrate overt dystrophic changes in their limbs.

Patients with failed back syndromes rarely present primarily with disorders of sweating or circulation, but these features may be secondary factors in a dysautonomic state producing sympathetically mediated pain. The most common clinical picture is one of constant diffuse burning pain in the extremity, with or without dystrophic changes. There is usually an associated and often striking hypersensitivity of the limb to touch, which triggers an extremely unpleasant or painful response. This can be so pronounced that even looking at a hand or other object approaching the affected limb can trigger actual pain. Trophic changes most commonly cause stiffness and degeneration of joints, but can also cause loss of skin thickness, hair, and nails. Skin may become blanched or blue if the limb is cold or on occasion may become reddened and slightly swollen if the limb is unusually warm. *Diagnostic sympathetic block* is essential in making the diagnosis of sympathetically mediated pain and is also important to perform since one or several anesthetic blocks often provides long-lasting pain relief, especially if the blocks are begun soon after the onset of dysautonomic symptoms. Before being offered sympathectomy patients should be given trials of calcium channel blocking agents (such as Nifedipine), propranolol, or dibenzaline. Simply reversing the dysautonomic component of reflex sympathetic dystrophy accomplishes only a portion of the therapy needed, since attention must still be directed to the dystrophic tissues, especially joints, and to the painful underlying condition that triggered the dysautonomia. Treatment with nonsteroidal anti-inflammatory drugs and aggressive physical restorative therapy are equally important components of treatment.

Percutaneous lumbar sympathectomy can be accomplished either by *injection of phenol* (or carbolic acid) or by *RF lesioning* of the lumbar sympathetic chain. These sympathetic ganglia lie just lateral to the ventral portion of the second, third, and fourth lumbar vertebral bodies in the retroperitoneal space. Open surgical sympathectomy will not be discussed, since this is well-described in neurosurgical and general surgical literature and is being supplanted largely in failed back patients by percutaneous techniques.

There is no clear consensus as to *how many lumbar sympathetic ganglia need to be interrupted* for a maximum effect. Both the open surgical literature and the experience of some who practice percutaneous techniques suggest that an optimum sympathectomy should include at least L2 and L3 ganglia, and many advocate including L4 as well. However, in at least one busy pain-management center lesions are made at only a single level, after which the patient begins an aggressive physical restorative program. The available literature suggests that more limited sympathectomy is likely to be associated with a much greater frequency of recurrence at shorter intervals than following the more extensive techniques.

Phenol or alcohol lumbar sympathectomy can be carried out through a single six-inch needle placed percutaneously from the paraspinal lumbar region to a point just lateral to the ventral portion of the L2 or L3 lumbar vertebral body. Placement of the needle tip in the retroperitoneal space is often confirmed by injection of a small amount of aqueous contrast material under fluoroscopic and radiographic control. The area is then injected with from 3 ml to 10 ml of lidocaine or bupivacaine while measurement of skin temperature and limb perfusion (measured with a plethysmograph) monitors the results of sympathetic interruption. If satisfactory sympathetic interruption is achieved, the area can be injected with 2 ml to 4 ml of 5% or 10% phenol in anhydrous glycerol or 5 ml to 10 ml of aqueous phenol or absolute alcohol. Pretreating the area with local anesthetics is important because the phenol or alcohol solutions are extremely irritating and painful.

RF lumbar sympathectomy is carried out by a similar approach, but either multiple needles or multiple placements of the same needle must be used if more than one ganglion is to be interrupted or if multiple lesions are to be made along the rostrocaudal extent of the ganglionic chain in an effort to completely destroy each ganglion. RF lesions can be made after placing a 0.5 ml to 1 ml anesthetic test injection, but it is preferable to make the lesions under neuroleptanalgesia without injection of local anesthetics, so that there is a greater likelihood that the sympathetic interruption that is observed results from electrolytic lesioning, not simply from local anesthetic that has tracked beyond the area of the electrolytic lesion.

The chief *complication of lumbar percutaneous sympathectomy* is painful or neuropathic damage to the lumbar (somatic) nerve plexus, causing increased pain in the leg or pelvis and possibly even weakness, sensory loss, or sphincter disturbance.

Compensatory hyperhidrosis, or abnormally increased sweating over the trunk or face, is rarely encountered with unilateral sympathetic lesions, but both this problem and male impotence can occur following bilateral lumbar sympathectomy. Extensive sympathectomy can lead to postural hypotension, though this is usually not disabling. Needle penetration of abdominal viscera or damage to ureters or retroperitoneal vessels should be avoidable with careful surgical technique.

One of the major *limitations of sympathectomy,* a limitation encountered in both upper limb and lower limb sympathectomies carried out for sympathetically mediated pain, is the high rate of failure to produce lasting pain relief. Most series report lasting pain relief from sympathectomy alone in only 60% to 70% of patients, but rapidly engaging the sympathectomized patient in a physical restorative program or introducing sympathetic interruption early after the onset of the dysautonomia seems to bring greatly improved results. Results also seem to be better in patients who exhibit a more classical clinical picture and who consistently obtain at least short-term relief from sympathetic anesthetic blocks. Not uncommonly, relieving the sympathetically mediated pain leaves untreated a sizable component of pain transmitted over somatic peripheral nerves or arising from a central deafferentation pain state. These persistent pain states require additional specific therapy.

7

Surgical Therapy

Surgical therapy of the failed back syndrome can be restorative and reconstructive or neuroablative and destructive. Obviously, restorative surgery is inherently more desirable than destructive surgery, but one must keep in mind that ill-advised or ill-performed restorative surgery may yield a destructive result. By definition, all patients with a failed back syndrome have undergone previous back surgery. Nonetheless, to attempt to undertake a restorative operation merely on the assumption that the patient's previous operation was inadequately or improperly performed is to court disaster. The decision whether or not to recommend surgical therapy for a failed back syndrome sufferer is rarely life or death in the sense of survival, except for the patient who contemplates suicide as an alternative to suffering (see page 140). However, the decision about surgery in these patients is quite frequently of life or death magnitude in a more figurative sense. Most of these patients face a normal life expectancy, and the prospect of facing this in constant pain is not a happy one. On the other hand, if the decision is made to undertake further surgery and this surgery produces greater discomfort and disability than the patient suffered before, this patient now faces the prospect of a normal life span in a "living hell" of even greater pain and suffering. Thus, the choice of whether or not to recommend surgery for these patients is a serious responsibility for the surgeon. The prospect of creating greater pain and suffering is intimidating, but the prospect of allowing a patient to continue a life of suffering when surgical intervention might bring relief is also distressing. Surgeons who are not constantly conscious of this awesome responsibility do a disservice to the public they serve. One of the great paradoxes of the practice of medicine entails the twin facts that one cannot practice good medicine without being objective in one's decision making, and yet one cannot make wise decisions unless one is empathetic and sensitive to the patient's emotions and social needs.

Repeat Laminectomy

The most common second operation that sufferers from the failed back syndrome are subjected to is *repeat laminectomy.* Both the published medical literature and my impression after two decades of working with these patients strongly suggest that the rate of successful amelioration of painful or disabling symptoms following second laminectomy is considerably smaller than that following initial laminectomy for low back disease. This is true even if one considers that the term *laminectomy* covers a considerable spectrum of specific operative interventions in the lumbar spine. Statistical data of the results of specific variations of surgical laminectomy as applied to precisely defined variations of the failed back syndrome are difficult to collect because of the complexity and variety of disorders that afflict the postoperative lumbar spine and the imprecision of most published reports. Few published studies address in detail the question of the precise diagnosis and whether surgery was tailored to treat a precise condition. The importance of such precise analysis is evident if one considers this example: resecting an asymptomatic intervertebral disc for the second time in an effort to relieve sciatica will do little good if the patient in reality suffers from adhesive arachnoiditis or lateral recess stenosis. Most conscientious surgeons attempt to tailor repeat operations to specific clinical and anatomic features of the patient's clinical condition, but the flexibility and variability with which this is done varies from surgeon to surgeon, and medical literature gives little hint about the success of these efforts at operative tailoring.

Spinal fusion surgery and surgery aimed principally at neural structures (rhizotomy, lysis of arachnoiditis) are usually not considered to be laminectomies, although these operations are often combined with laminectomy as a single surgical procedure. Technically, *laminectomy* means surgical removal of a lamina. This can be done either unilaterally as a *hemilaminectomy* or bilaterally, including the spinous process, as a *total laminectomy. Laminotomy,* or surgical windowing through a lamina, is a convenient term that is often substituted for the more accurate term *partial hemilaminectomy.* The laminectomy, by itself, may be therapeutic if the lamina is the offending structure, as in spinal stenosis. More often, however, the laminectomy simply offers access to the spinal canal to permit the surgeon to "wreak a cure" on the offending structures contained therein or accessible therethrough.

A number of different therapeutic goals are addressed through the *variations of laminectomy.* Included among these variations are decompression, disc excision, and repair of abnormal structures or conditions.

Decompressive Laminectomy

The principal goal of surgical decompression by laminectomy is the relief of compression of neural structures to bring about an improvement in pain or functional inhibition. Decompression of vessels supplying neural structures is probably also part of surgical decompression for at least some patients.

Spinal stenosis (see pages 29 and 83) is a condition in which the congenitally narrowed spinal canal is further narrowed by degenerative changes. The result is a global or circumferential compression of all of the neural elements contained within the canal at each affected level. Because the thecal sac is compressed circumferentially, adequate decompression necessitates total laminectomy or bilateral medial facetectomy with laminal undercutting. Adequate decompression also necessitates that each level of stenosis be decompressed; this is an important consideration, since lumbar spinal stenosis customarily affects two, three, or occasionally more laminal levels. Computerized tomography (CT) scans nicely document the severity of bony impingement at each level scanned, but myelography is helpful in determining how many levels should be decompressed. Magnetic resonance imaging (MRI) scans also give a linear depiction of spinal encroachment, but they do not distinguish bone as well as CT scans or subarachnoid space as well as myelography. The most important differential diagnosis, especially when a single level appears to be involved, is midline disc protrusion, a differential diagnosis that is usually apparent on CT scans and is usually beautifully demonstrated on MRI scans. Even in patients with multiple levels of spinal stenosis, the acute decompensating event may be midline or lateral herniation of an intervertebral disc. The resulting clinical picture may mimic acute lateral disc rupture or classic spinal stenosis, depending on whether there is compression principally of a single exiting nerve root or the entire thecal sac.

The surgical *technique for decompression of spinal stenosis* is aimed at removal of one or more lumbar laminae without damaging underlying neural tissues and without inducing unnecessary instability of the lumbar spine (Fig. 7.1). Bone removal needs to be carried far enough laterally to decompress all of the neural elements but should include only the medial portion of the facets. Once the laminae and spinous processes have been removed, the facets become even more important in providing posterior stabilization. By definition, spinal stenosis involves tight encroachment of dorsal bony elements against the soft and vulnerable thecal sac and its contained neural elements. Removing the laminae by inserting one jaw of a heavy rongeur beneath the lamina entails a significant risk of producing further damage to the compressed nerve roots. An alternative and preferable technical approach to this form of decompression is also useful in spinal decompression in thoracic and cervical levels for a variety of disorders. This *technique* involves making bilateral channel laminectomies by biting downward onto the dorsal surfaces of the laminae adjacent to the facets on either side with a narrow-nosed rongeur. This process can be facilitated by adding, or substituting, power-driven burrs. The idea of this approach is to cut through the bone from dorsum to ventrum without inserting any instrument between the ventral surface of the bone

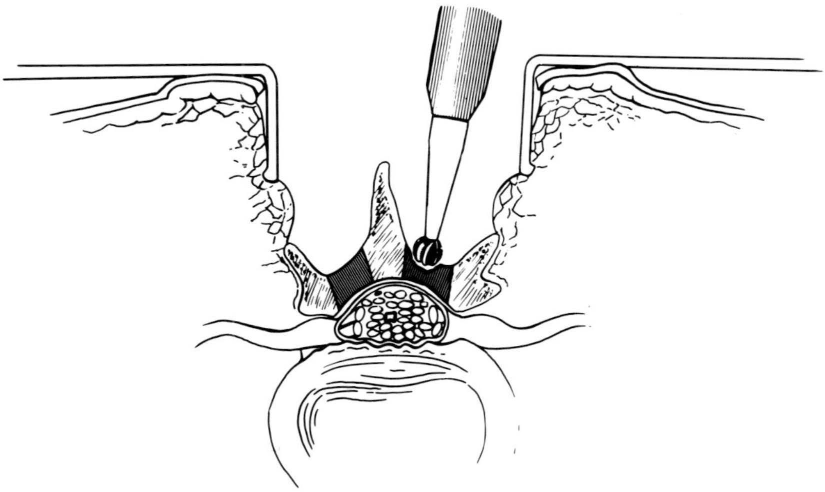

FIGURE 7.1. Surgical decompression of spinal stenosis will usually promptly relieve neurogenic claudication. With neural structures tightly packed within the spinal canal, insertion of instrumentation beneath the lamina must be strictly avoided. Decompression is carried out by cutting "channel" laminectomies into the bone on both sides, permitting removal of the central dorsal arch.

and the compressed thecal sac. Once channels have been cut bilaterally, the ligamentum flavum and interspinous ligaments may be sectioned in the midline to permit removal of laminae and spinous processes *en bloc*.

An alternative to total decompressive laminectomy is *bilateral medial facetectomy with laminal undercutting,* performed at each level of stenosis. Although I have no personal experience with this technique to permit me to evaluate its technical difficulty, safety, and effectiveness, it is logically conceived, and available published results compare favorably with those achieved by total laminectomy. Since spinal stenosis involves segmental compression maximally at the facet joints, with relative sparing between, this technique is designed to decompress the areas of maximal compression while preserving the integrity of the laminal arch and spinous process. Whether this reduces postoperative pain, loss of spinal mobility, instability, disfigurement, or risk of injury to dura and nerve roots more than total laminectomy remains to be demonstrated.

After bony removal is accomplished, a considerable "dead space" is created. This is only partly occupied by the herniating thecal sac, and it is my practice to insert *autogenous fat grafts* along the length of the dural exposure. This not only helps to reduce the dead space but also helps to limit the severity of secondary epidural scarring. I do not customarily leave epidural drains in place but I do leave a layer of thrombin-soaked gelatin foam dorsal to the fat graft as added protection against postoperative bleeding into the space created by the bony removal. *Closing the paraspinal muscles* should be done at the "corners" of the muscles where they were originally attached to the junction point between lamina and spinous process. Failure to approximate muscles at this level will leave a larger dead space than necessary. Also, attempting to place sutures more laterally in the retracted muscle results in the sutures being placed on the ventral surface of the muscle belly so that tightening sutures is either not possible or results in tearing of the muscle (Fig. 7.2). My preference is to use chromic catgut for this aspect of the closure. I often employ a 4-0 widely spaced subcuticular silk suture to prevent widening of the skin incision and then complete the skin closure with skin tapes or a running locked suture of nylon or monofilament stainless-steel wire. Postoperatively, patients should not require external bracing and usually may be allowed out of bed as soon as the effects of anesthesia wear off. Of course, if the *dura has been torn* during the course of the decompression, the dural leak should be tightly repaired, and it is probably wise to maintain the patient on strict bed rest for a minimum of four or five days to limit the hydrostatic cerebrospinal fluid (CSF) pressure against the dural suture line.

Decompression for lateral recess stenosis does

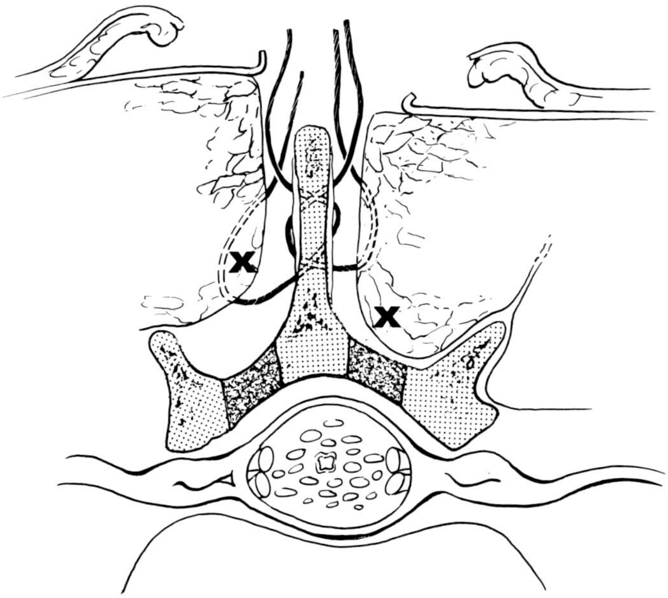

FIGURE 7.2. Deep paraspinal muscles must be closed carefully if they are to perform their optimum function of tamponading the laminotomy defect (heavy shading). The suture on the right is properly placed, entering the muscle superficially to the corner, which was initially attached to the bone at the junction between lamina and spinous process (x). The suture on the left has been placed too far inferolaterally, including the corner. This results in stretching and elevation of the muscle away from underlying laminotomy defect, allowing room for collections of blood, serum, or spinal fluid.

not need to be as extensive as that required for spinal stenosis. Lateral recess stenosis is by definition confined to the lateral recesses of the spinal canal and spares the central theca or spinal sac. Clinically, lateral recess stenosis may mimic lumbar disc rupture, causing predominantly sciatica, though nerve root entrapment signs are commonly lacking. Myelographically, lateral recess stenosis may be difficult to confirm because of the lack of thecal compression. CT scans or MRI scans are usually the most definitive diagnostic studies if they demonstrate bony and soft-tissue narrowing of the lateral corner of the spinal canal at the appropriate spinal level in a patient with sciatica. Surgeons should be especially aware of the possibility of lateral recess stenosis in patients with sciatica and little or no myelographic defect. This condition will not be improved by a small laminotomy and disc excision, and is likely to be compounded if the surgeon attempts a microsurgical disc excision through a tiny laminotomy or dorsal opening limited to resection of the yellow ligament. Patients with congenitally narrow lateral recesses are particularly subject to develop sciatica with even small disc protrusions, and the sciatica may persist despite disc excision if perineural inflammation and scarring develop in association with the disc rupture.

Operatively, lateral recess stenosis should be strongly suspected if one attempts to trace the nerve root caudally into its foramen of exit by passing a small flat dissector beneath the caudal lamina and the instrument does not pass readily into this space. The *operative technique* dictated in this situation is simply removal of enough bone to decompress the involved nerve root, usually a hemilamina resected laterally to the edge of the facet. When decompression is completed, the vertical medial surface of the pedicle should be readily apparent (Fig. 7.3).

Decompression of the neuroforamen, or *foramenotomy,* is similar in several respects to decompression for lateral recess stenosis (Fig. 7.4). In this disorder, the nerve root is compressed as it leaves the spinal canal through the neuroforamen. Whereas the compression in lateral recess stenosis is usually based on a congenitally narrowed canal, the nerve entrapment in foramenal compression is almost always the result of degenerative arthritic spurring, with or without an element of spondylolisthesis or forward slippage of vertebral bodies and facets. As is true with lateral recess stenosis, foramenal entrapment usually produces a picture of sciatica with little or no abnormality on myelography attributable to the foramenal encroachment. Since degenerative changes are rarely limited to the region of the neuroforamen, myelography in these patients is more likely to be abnormal due to the more central extension of the degenerative lipping. Plain radiographs are strongly suggestive of this diagnosis, especially if oblique views are taken to delineate the extent of the degenerative spurring.

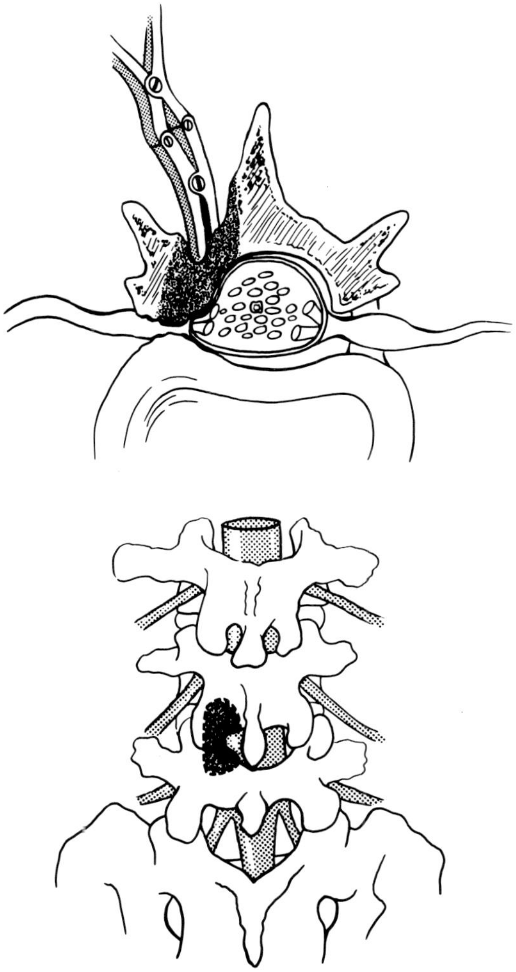

FIGURE 7.3. Surgical decompression of lateral recess stenosis does not necessitate total laminectomy, but does necessitate unroofing the lateral recess by removing laminal bone laterally to the pedicle.

CT scans, with or without three-dimensional reconstructions, and MRI scans should be diagnostic, but accurate diagnosis may be confounded by technical limitations imposed by slice thickness or angle. As is true with lateral recess stenosis, patients may present with a failed back syndrome because of persistent sciatica following simple discectomy that did not include decompression of the foraminal stenosis.

Laminectomy for Disc Excision

Laminectomy for disc excision may be useful to the failed back syndrome sufferer for several reasons. As discussed under improper or inadequate surgery in Chapter 2, some of these unfortunate sufferers will still retain their original disc rupture because the original surgery was performed at an *incorrect level.* If the previous incorrect level was operated upon because of the surgeon's error, repeat diagnostic studies may well confirm persistent abnormality at a level different from that previously operated upon. Unfortunately, it is not always easy to be sure on plain radiographs where the previous level of surgery was performed, especially if no radiopaque markers were left at the time of that surgery. Even with repeat myelography there may be little indication of surgical intervention, especially if that surgery was carefully performed, albeit at a wrong level. The presence of a dorsolateral defect or dural outpouching one interspace level away from a ventrolateral defect suggests that the previous surgery was performed at a wrong level, causing the dor-

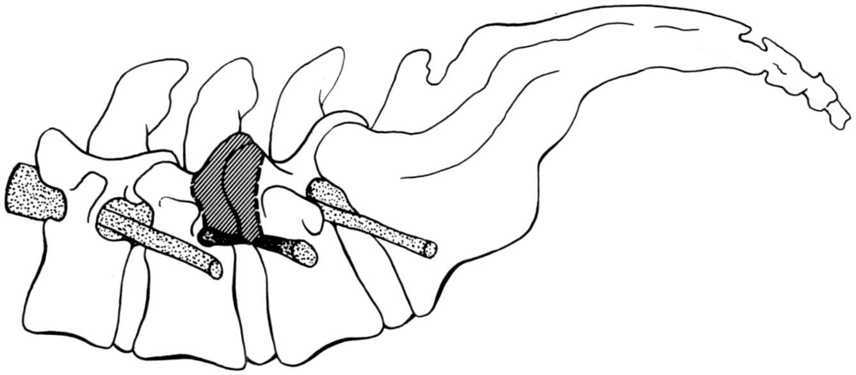

FIGURE 7.4. Foramenotomy may be necessary for decompression of nerve roots compressed laterally within the neuroforamen by overgrowth of degenerative bone spurs. This decompression must include essentially the entire facet region. Care must be taken not to injure the delicate and compressed nerve roots while removing bone that already impinges upon the root. Shading depicts the area of bone to be removed.

solateral abnormality but failing to correct the ventrolateral defect. CT or MRI scans usually image the site of surgical intervention as well as the persistent disc rupture, with the surgical site marked by a bony defect or, more often, by evidence of scar tissue extradurally, within the spinal canal, or in dorsal muscles and fatty tissue planes. Other patients will have undergone discectomy, or at least laminectomy, at an incorrect level because of *insufficient preoperative localizing* information. In some of these patients, a minor abnormality on myelography, CT scan, or MRI scan may have been present at the wrong level and the true disc rupture may have been missed. If this patient was then operated on at the level of imaged abnormality, the correct disc level may have been missed. For the patient who was operated upon solely on the basis of clinical symptoms and signs, an adjacent defect may well have been overlooked. Although surgeons who operate on lumbar discs without the benefit of imaging studies often routinely perform two-level laminectomies, it is possible to overlook an L3-L4 disc rupture if the original suspicion was L4-L5 and the original surgery was carried out at L4-L5 and L5-S1.

So-called *microsurgical discectomy* has recently captured the public interest. To some, this technique is defined as operating through a microscope and through a microscopic exposure. This, by definition, precludes adequate lateral decompression and persistent foramenal compression and accounts for some of the failures seen following this glamorous technique. Although it is quite a feat to be able to operate "through a keyhole," I am always reminded of this folk saying: "One can admire a horse through a keyhole, but one needs to open the barn door to take the horse outside." I have employed magnified vision (either loupes or the operating room microscope) for many years. I do not advocate long skin incisions, but I do advocate adequate bony decompression. Although my skin incision for a simple single-level laminectomy exceeds 4 cm or 5 cm only in the most obese patients, my laminotomy usually measures approximately 20 mm by 25 mm. Exposing a greater area of dura and nerve root permits more gentle nerve root retraction and more adequate exploration and decompression. This plus improved visualization of epidural veins, permitting more precise bipolar coagulation, lessens the risk of postoperative scarring, even though it exposes a greater area of dura and nerve to that risk. Shielding these surfaces from postoperative scarring by placing autogenous fat grafts in the bony defect thus assumes even greater importance. The operating microscope provides excellent illumination and binocular visualization through a small opening, and thus less extensive dissection and less vigorous retraction of paraspinal muscles are required. This plus short incisions, more precise control of epidural bleeding, and more precise visual guidance of nerve root retraction all usually result in reduced postoperative pain and more rapid convalescence. Limited-exposure microsurgery will indeed prove adequate and beneficial to the patient if a "microrupture" of a disc is the sole problem, but application of this technique places the surgeon under the absolute mandate of arriving at a precisely accurate preoperative diagnosis so that he does not overlook and fail to deal adequately with any of the other conditions that may mimic lumbar disc rupture. More limited exposure also increases the risk of inadvertent surgery at the wrong interspace and increases the value of intraoperative radiographic localization, especially for initial laminectomies at L3-L4 and L4-L5.

Laminectomy for disc excision is also useful when performed at the same level if the patient suffers from *retained disc fragments*. Retained disc fragments are more likely to be overlooked following limited microsurgical exposure. They are likely to remain present as a cause of a failed back syndrome in patients who complain of sciatica that persists unabated following their initial surgery or who develop sciatica for the first time immediately following their first operation. Not all of these patients harbor retained disc fragments; some have sustained direct injury to the nerve root, and some have suffered all along from an alternative diagnosis such as lateral recess stenosis or arachnoiditis. Precise diagnosis of a retained disc fragment may be difficult indeed. The history and physical examination are extremely useful tools in this situation. A history of persistent or newly developed sciatica ever since surgery plus physical findings of sciatic neuropathy and sciatic nerve root entrapment suggest a retained disc fragment as at least a strong possibility. Electromyography (EMG) may help to confirm sciatic neuropathy and to differentiate between peripheral neuropathy and nerve root involvement; it is usually incapable of distinguishing the etiology of the nerve root involvement and so cannot diagnose the presence of a retained disc fragment. Myelography may demonstrate an anterolateral defect overlying the vertebral body, rather than the interspace, if a fragment has migrated rostrally or caudally more than laterally. Far lateral retained fragments, of course, may leave no defect on the myelogram. Myelography that demonstrates evidence of previous operative scarring or focal arachnoiditis may be misleading if these changes obscure whatever findings may have been caused by the retained disc fragment. CT and MRI scans can demonstrate the presence of local soft-tissue mass but may not be able to discriminate disc material from scar. The addition of contrast enhancement (see page 67) may detect vascularized scar as distinct from avascular disc material, but this distinction is not always clear or reliable. Nerve root displacement away from the intraspinal soft tissue seen on any of the imaging studies implies an extradural (or at least extraarachnoidal) compressive mass and makes recurrent disc rupture or a retained fragment more likely. In contrast, nerve roots that veer toward or seem to be incorporated in the mass imply arachnoiditis or constrictive scar.

Patients suspected clinically on the basis of history and physical examination of harboring a retained disc fragment become strong candidates for surgical exploration. Despite the difficulty in establishing a firm diagnosis of this condition, surgical excision of a symptomatic mass lesion is the procedure of choice. Because of the diagnostic uncertainty inherent in this situation, the surgeon will be hard-pressed to decide how long to continue nonoperative therapies such as enforced rest, antineuralgic drugs, or extradural or intrathecal steroid injections. Destructive, neuroablative injection therapy is probably not warranted in patients with a clinical history and imaging studies that strongly suggest the possibility of a retained disc fragment until a repeat surgical exploration has been undertaken. At the time of surgical exploration, the surgeon should be acutely aware of the alternative etiologies of persistent or newly developed sciatica. If he fails to confirm the presence of a retained disc fragment, the surgeon must be prepared to search for alternative etiologies and to undertake appropriate surgical correction. This may necessitate lateral recess decompression, foramenotomy, extradural or intradural neurolysis, or even surgical sensory rhizotomy.

Repeat laminectomy at the same level may also be useful for *recurrent disc ruptures*. The question remains unanswered whether the risk of secondary rupture of a disc at the same level is diminished by extensive removal of intervertebral disc material at the time of initial surgery or whether more radical discectomy simply leads to an increased risk of interspace collapse and back pain. No matter what technique is employed, disc material can reform and recurrent ruptures can occur. A brief report confirms such an example:

Case 15

A 45-year-old plant manager injured his back while lifting at work. He developed acute onset of severe right sciatica with some back pain. Symptoms became more severe despite five days of bed rest with anti-inflammatory drugs. Myelography demonstrated a large anterolateral disc rupture at L4-L5 on the right. Physical examination showed evolving mild weakness of dorsiflexion and sensory loss of the shin and dorsomedial foot. Early laminectomy was undertaken. This revealed a large fragment of ruptured disc material at L4-L5, still contained within an attenuated posterior longitudinal ligament but severely distorting the nerve root. The herniated portion of nuclear material was removed and the interspace was thoroughly cleaned with curettes and rongeurs of a total of 9 ml of degenerated disc material. Postoperative recovery was characteristically dramatic. The patient was ambulating on the day following surgery, was discharged five days postoperatively, and was able to return to his managerial duties five weeks following surgery.

Unfortunately, ten months following discectomy the patient slipped on an icy walk and landed firmly on his buttocks. He immediately experienced a recurrence of severe right sciatica. Symptoms were partially controlled with a period of bed rest, antineuralgia drugs, and nonnarcotic anodynes. He attempted to return to work but was prevented from doing so by recurring bouts of sciatica. After three months, myelography was repeated. It demonstrated a large, smoothly contoured anterolateral defect at L4-L5 on the right. A previously placed metal marking clip had migrated to a new position within the interspace but confirmed that this was the same level previously operated upon. At reexploration a large fragment of disc material was found protruding through the opening in the posterior annulus and again impinging upon the nerve root. Following the removal of this fragment, an additional 4 ml of presumably newly formed disc material could be removed with rongeurs and curettes from the intervertebral disc space. Because of this large amount of disc recurrence and in fear of lateral development of severe back pain, a modified interbody bone fusion, or Christoferson procedure, was performed. Postoperatively, sciatica was completely relieved. The patient remained free of significant back pain or sciatica until he was lost from follow-up 18 months later.

The presence of a *recurrent disc rupture* can be clinically suspected if new or recurrent symptoms develop after an asymptomatic interval. As is true of disc rupture in general, there may or may not be a history of trauma or work-related physical stress in association with the development of recurrent symptoms. Myelography is more likely to be abnormal in these patients than in patients with retained disc fragments. The dorsal and lateral epidural scarring left by the previous disc rupture and surgical excision may leave as the pathway of least resistance a dorsomedial migration of the fragment in or against the thecal sac, making myelographic recognition more obvious (Fig. 7.5). Unfortunately, previous scarring or focal arachnoiditis may also obscure the diagnosis of recurrent disc rupture. If the nerve root at the level of previous disc rupture is moderately restricted in motion by epidural scarring, even a small recurrent disc rupture may become acutely symptomatic. CT and MRI scans usually will demonstrate an extradural compressive mass at the site of previous surgery and contrast enhancement usually proves helpful if disc rupture is difficult to discriminate from scar. However, since small disc protrusions may be severely symptomatic in areas of epidural scar, even clear imaging of a small extradural mass may not be able to confirm whether or not this mass is symptomatic.

Therapy of recurrent disc ruptures does not always necessitate repeat laminectomy, since many disc ruptures can be cured by nonoperative therapies, including bed rest, other enforced inactivity, and anti-inflammatory or antineuralgia drugs. Patients who should be strongly considered for repeat laminectomy for possible recurrent disc rupture are those who develop new symptoms of sciatica with back pain after an asymptomatic interval, whose physical examinations confirm nerve root entrapment, and whose imaging studies demonstrate an abnormality (even if this abnormality is not strictly characteristic of a disc rupture) at the appropriate level. Of course, if such a patient is discovered at reoperation not to have a recurrent disc rupture despite persistent sciatica and an imaged abnormality, the neurosurgeon must be prepared to look for and correct other possible causes of this clinical picture. This may entail lateral laminal decompression for lateral recess stenosis or intradural lysis of localized arachnoiditis.

Repeat laminectomy and discectomy at the same operative level on rare occasions may be justified for *discogenic pain*. Patients with back pain, elevated sedimentation rate, and acute inflammatory discitis are not candidates for discectomy because they respond well to immobilization, systemic anti-inflammatory drugs, or intradiscal injections of

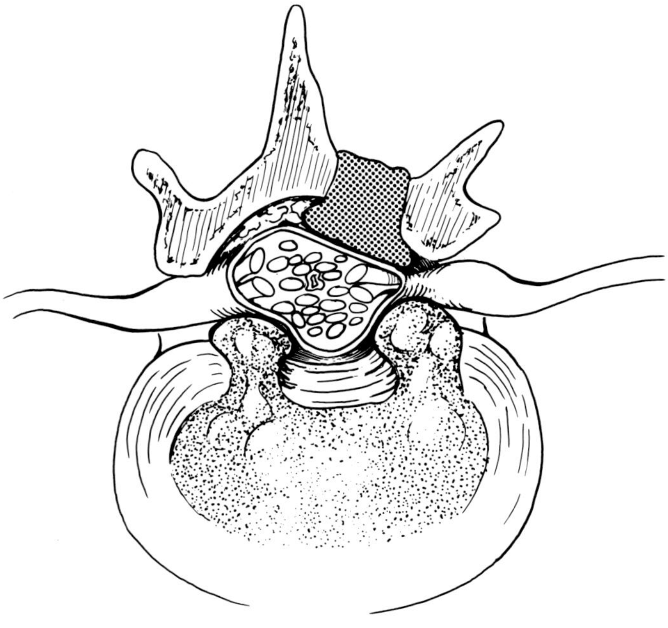

FIGURE 7.5. Postoperative epidural scar may leave a nerve root much more vulnerable to compression by underlying disc protrusion or arthritic spurring. The nerve root on the left has enough room and mobility to escape compression by the small disc protrusion shown on that side. On the right side, a disc protrusion of similar size causes severe compression of a nerve root displaced ventrally and fixed in position by an epidural scar (heavy stippling).

adrenal corticosteroids. Patients with typical discogenic pain suffer predominantly back pain with radiation into buttock or posterior thigh but not below the knee. Characteristically, the back pain is severely aggravated by activity or bending. These patients may show degenerative changes or interspace narrowing on plain radiographs or CT scans. Imaging studies may show the intraspinal areas to be normal or may show changes consistent with scarring or limited arachnoiditis. The diagnosis is confirmed at discography by the production of severe pain on intradiscal injection of contrast material, local anesthetics, or even saline. Local injections of anesthetics intradiscally should significantly reduce the back pain. Intradiscal injections of adrenal corticosteroids should be attempted prior to surgical intervention, because this may occasionally produce long-lasting benefit. As discussed under low back pain in Chapter 3, the diagnosis of discogenic pain remains somewhat controversial, although I am convinced that such an entity actually exists. If nonoperative therapy fails, surgical intervention should be considered. However, I am quite pessimistic about the prospects of simple discectomy alone for this condition, since in my experience this has given disappointing results. As a result, I usually couple disc excision with either interbody, posterior, or posterolateral spinal fusion.

Reparative Laminectomy

Repeat laminectomy may also be done as a reparative procedure. These operations often do not fit the technical definition of laminectomy because they need not involve bone removal. Simply reopening the previous laminectomy defect through soft-tissue removal may suffice for adequate exposure.

Additional bony exposure is usually indicated if *epidural neurolysis* is proposed. This surgery aims to remove extradural scar that is causing pain through restriction or compression of nerve roots or the entire thecal sac. The clinical picture of such epidural scarring usually involves significant sciatica but may also include low back pain. Both the sciatica and the back pain may be aggravated by activity or by stretching or bending. The back pain may be specifically aggravated also by erect posture, coughing, sneezing, or jogging (see pages 18, 28, and 45). These patients usually develop symptoms insidiously months following their initial surgery. A history of a stormy postoperative course with confirmed or suspected wound infection hemorrhage may be elicited. Myelography usually discloses a rough and irregular defect that may be most severe ventrolaterally or dorsolaterally, usually at the previous operative site. EMG may confirm evidence of nerve root involvement but may be unable to differentiate between newly acquired and residual root involvement following an initial disc rupture. CT or MRI scans usually show obliteration of epidural fat; epidural scar is often not symptomatic but, conversely, may cause severe symptoms with no evident mass effect or displacement of theca or nerve roots.

At the time of *surgery for epidural neurolysis* an attempt is made, usually employing magnifying loupes or the operating microscope, to strip away scar tissue from the dura and nerve roots throughout the entire operative area without tearing the attached dura—often a technically challenging exercise. Some bony removal is usually required, since scar tissue usually extends beneath the overhanging residual bone (Fig. 7.6). Once scar tissue has been removed, the surgeon's problem is that of preventing reaccumulation of similar scar. Careful irrigation and meticulous hemostasis in the area will eliminate some potential sources of later exuberant scar formation. Prophylactic antibiotics should be started preoperatively and should be continued for one to three days postoperatively in patients whose epidural scar is or might be related to previously documented wound infection, even though this infection may have occurred more than six months previously. A useful adjunct in attempting to limit recurrent scar formation is the placement of autogenous fat around the nerve root and thecal sac in the entire area of operative exposure (Fig. 7.7). Reexplorations, which I have done in more than a score of patients, at intervals varying from a few months to several years following placement of epidural fat grafts at the time of lumbar laminectomy, have disclosed nearly all of these grafts to be viable. One exception was Case 19 (see page 211). In most patients, fat has remained present in the epidural space, leaving the underlying dura relatively mobile and providing an easy cleavage plane in the epidural space. Placing depository adrenal corticosteroids in this area may or may not be beneficial, but probably should be avoided in patients with previously documented wound infections. Similarly, the role of systemic anti-inflammatory or corticosteroid therapy for a period of one to three weeks following epidural

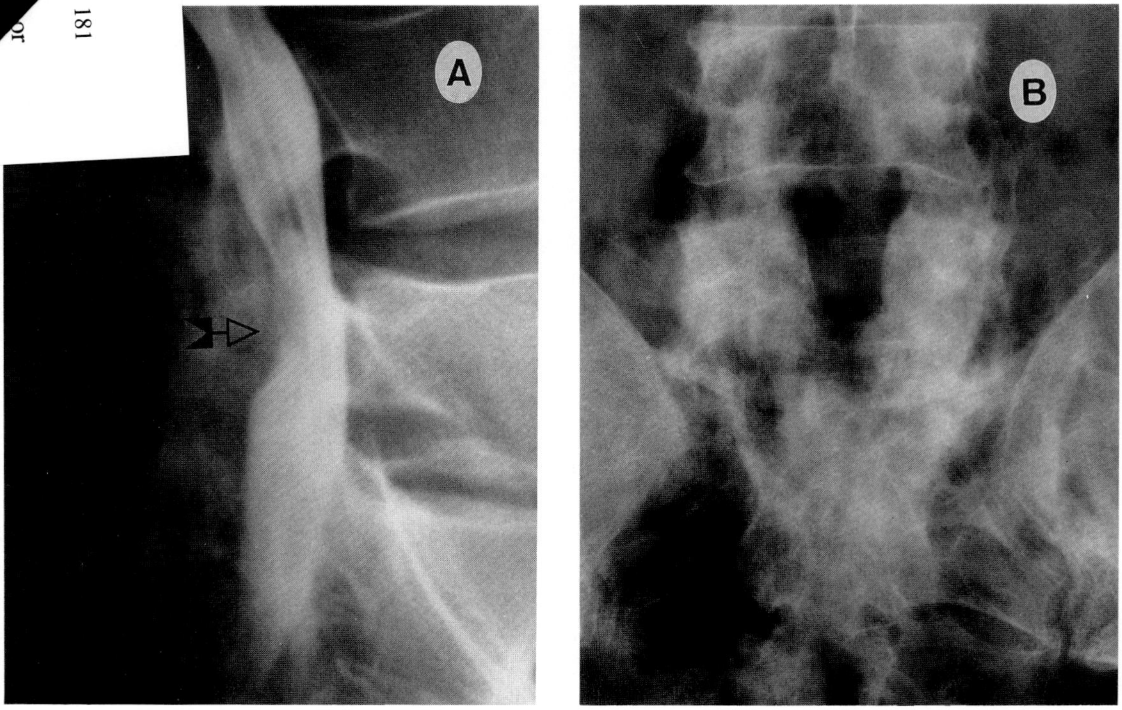

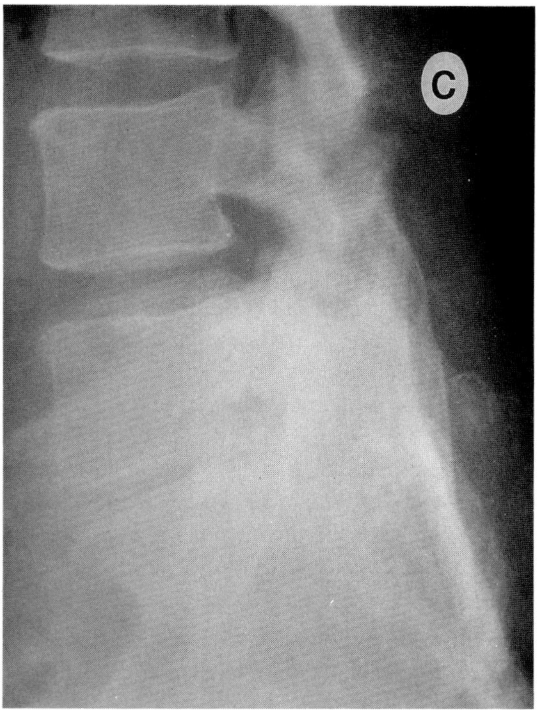

FIGURE 7.6. Severe dorsal epidural scarring caused a pseudostenosis in this patient. Despite several operative interventions, he was left with severe local back pain, aggravated sharply by standing or sitting, in addition to cramping pain in both legs with prolonged walking. **A:** Myelogram demonstrated a dorsal defect (arrow) at the level of previous laminectomy and fusion. **B and C:** Needle insertion into this area revealed soft tissues that were extremely tender. Local anesthetization dramatically relieved his back pain, but steroid injection gave no lasting relief. Surgery disclosed hypertrophic extradural scar tissue sharply confined to this area.

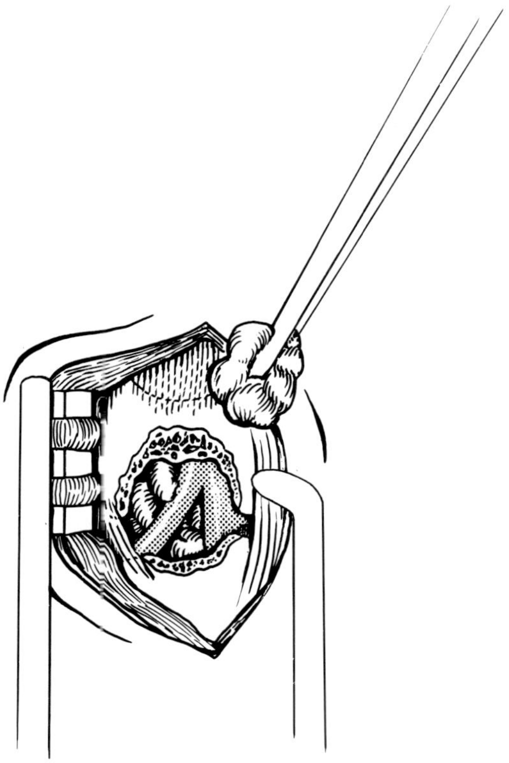

FIGURE 7.7. Pads of autogenous fat placed around the nerve root and exposed lumbar dura at the time of laminectomy seemed to help limit the severity of postoperative perineural scarring and adhesions. This is important at the time of primary disc surgery or other laminectomy, but is even more important at the conclusion of laminectomy for recurrent disc rupture or for lysis of preexisting epidural and perineural adhesions.

neurolysis is of unproven value, although the rationale is an attempt to limit re-formation of adhesions.

Restorative laminectomy is specifically indicated in patients suffering from postoperative *dorsal arachnoidal cysts* (see page 31) or *pseudomeningoceles* (see pages 18–19). These two related conditions are both initiated from dural tears. These tears usually occur at the time of initial surgery but may be the result of subsequent trauma, especially if the dura has been tensed and tethered by extradural scar. Arachnoidal cysts are usually confined within the spinal canal and consist of outpouchings of arachnoid through a defect in the dural sac. They characteristically cause back pain, but may cause intermittent or constant sciatica if nerve roots herniate into the cyst periodically or if they become fixed in a prolapsed position through a narrow neck. Pseudomeningoceles develop when there has been a tear through both dura and arachnoid with spinal fluid leakage. Occasionally, leaking spinal fluid will fail to reach the surface (to cause a CSF fistula) but instead will build up as a fluid pocket in the soft tissues of the back between the paraspinous muscles. Over the passage of weeks this fluid causes the development of a pseudomembranous wall and leads to the development of so-called pseudomeningoceles. These cystic outpouchings remain in communication with the subarachnoid space. Like dorsal arachnoidal cysts, they cause principally lower back pain that is aggravated by activity, erect posture, coughing, or sneezing. Also like arachnoidal cysts, they can cause leg pain to develop if nerve roots herniate into the pseudomeningocele cyst. Myelography will show these cystic lesions if nerve roots do not block their opening, but delayed films or special views with the patient supine may be required. The larger lesions are usually clearly seen on CT or MRI scans, but small cysts, especially arachnoidal cysts, may be missed.

Even though surgical correction of these cystic lesions requires reopening of the previous laminectomy, new bone removal is usually not necessary. *Repair of arachnoidal cysts* requires identification of the dural defect through which the arachnoidal cyst has herniated. Usually, the arachnoid can be pushed back into the subdural space, although occasionally herniated nerve roots may become trapped and require further opening of the defect or surgical lysis of adhesions.[98] When the arachnoidal outpouching—with any nerve roots contained within it—has been replaced, the dural defect can usually be repaired by suturing and reinforcing the suture line with a small patch of muscle or fascia. *Pseudomeningoceles are repaired* by curetting away much of the pseudomembrane then identifying the dural defect. At times, this may have stretched to a rather large opening. Herniating nerve roots are replaced within the thecal sac. Closure of the dural defect may necessitate placement of a dural graft. The material for the graft can usually be obtained from lumbodorsal fascia, or occasionally a particularly well-developed section of the pseudomembrane may be used. Defects are rarely large enough to require removal of fascia lata for dural grafting. I have been reluctant to use artificial dural replacement materials in an already scarred lumbar region for fear of inducing further local scar formation. Once the dural defect has been repaired, autogenous fat is left in the epidural space and paraspinal muscles are tightly reapproximated to the interspinous ligament.

On rare occasions, reopening a lumbar laminectomy for persistent sciatica may disclose, usually unexpectedly, a *neuroma of the extradural nerve root*. I have confirmed this condition only twice, but was able, by excising the neuroma, to relieve the patient of sciatica that had been present constantly ever since the laminectomy. No attempt was made to reanastomose the proximal and distal ends of the cut nerve root, but care was taken to ensure that no spinal fluid was leaking from the proximal stump. No obvious functional regeneration took place, and both patients enjoyed prolonged relief of sciatic pain. The etiology of such neuromata is presumably a direct injury to the nerve root at the time of initial surgery.

Repeat Spinal Fusion

Failed back syndrome sufferers may require repeat lumbar spinal fusion because of painful instability, overgrowth of fusion bone, or resorption of fusion bone. Painful *pseudarthrosis or instability* most commonly develops spontaneously because of improper knitting of the multiple bony fragments used to perform a spinal fusion (see the discussion of fusion problems in Chapter 3). Occasionally, a history of later trauma to the back is elicited as an initiating event in the development of a painful pseudarthrosis. Pseudarthrosis may develop between the bony fragments or between the bony fragments and the subjacent laminae and facets in a posterior or posterolateral fusion, between the bony inserts and the adjacent vertebral body in an intervertebral fusion, or between the fusion bone and adjacent normal bone as a *kissing pseudarthrosis*. Painful pseudarthrosis usually results in back pain greater than leg pain. However, if hypertrophic scar develops beneath the pseudarthrotic line, epidural scarring may become intense. This can produce traction or compression on nerve roots and can lead to sciatica in addition to back pain.

An *overgrowth of fusion bone* may cause difficulty by producing a kissing pseudarthrosis through impingement on adjacent normal bone. Alternatively, an overgrowth of fusion bone may cause difficulties if it produces an *iatrogenic spinal stenosis* with compression of the thecal sac. In actuality, this probably occurs more commonly because of overly vigorous packing of fusion bone. The resulting spinal stenosis typically causes a picture of neurogenic claudication. This is characterized by diffuse aching pain in the back and legs that is specifically aggravated by walking or sustained activity and is associated with little or no evidence of nerve root entrapment on physical examination.

Painful instability of a fusion may also develop as a result of an exactly opposite process, *resorption of fusion bone*. This uncommon process can occur spontaneously with gradual dissolution of previously placed bone material. Postoperative wound infection can be implicated as a causative factor in some cases, but certainly not all. *Osteomyelitis* of the fusion bone can produce localized areas of resorption and presents special problems, since surgical correction of this form of infection usually requires excision of the infected bone and six to eight weeks of appropriate antibiotic therapy prior to considering attempted surgical restoration of the fusion.

Not all pseudarthroses produce pain, and determining when a pseudarthrosis is symptomatic can be difficult and challenging. Historically, the patient with a painful pseudarthrosis usually describes back pain greater than leg pain, although the exceptional patient will describe severe sciatica as well. The back pain may begin immediately following discontinuance of postoperative back bracing, may begin insidiously several months or years after fusion, or may begin precipitously following an injury to the back. The pain is characteristically severely aggravated by activity or bending and is largely relieved by rest. Anti-inflammatory drug therapy may bring permanent relief, or at least is usually transiently beneficial. The physical examination may reveal local back tenderness to percussion or manipulation, but is notable primarily for painful limitation of back bending. Depending on the type of pseudarthrosis, the pain may be more severe with forward, lateral, or backward bending. External bracing of the back characteristically adds greatly to the patient's comfort and, in fact, may be curative (see the discussion of back supports in Chapter 5). Relief of back pain through external bracing is often used as one of the major clinical determinants of the presence of symptomatic pseudarthrosis. Patients who do not obtain relief of back pain through external bracing are generally considered poor candidates for spinal fusion or revision of a previously placed spinal fusion. Care should be taken in this interpretation, however, to ensure that the patient has been adequately braced. Simply placing a patient in a canvas corset is usually insufficient. Firm bracing usually requires a steel or full torso back brace, often an extensive brace like the Taylor or Orthomold hyperextension back brace.

Radiographic diagnosis of a pseudarthrosis can be frustratingly difficult (see page 62). Instability that permits at least 10 degree of angulation on flexion/extension radiographs can usually be detected, but not all painful pseudarthroses result in instability of this degree. Bending radiographs of the lumbar spine cannot diagnose fusion instability unless the patient bends well enough to produce clearly visible motion of nonfused spinal segments. Since these patients are usually being studied because of back pain aggravated by bending, obtaining diagnostically useful bending radiographs usually requires that the patient be adequately premedicated with analgesics and muscle relaxers. The pseudarthrotic line often rambles irregularly across the mass of bone fragments used in the performance of a spinal fusion and may be difficult, if not impossible, to detect on plain radiographs. Laminagrams and CT scans that demonstrate isolated defects in fusion bone likewise do not confirm that the fusion is unstable. Radioisotope scans may be helpful in determining if a pseudarthrosis is present and if it is likely to be symptomatic, but not all symptomatic pseudarthroses produce abnormally increased uptake on isotope scans. Resorption of fusion bone can usually be demonstrated on plain radiographs, as can hypertrophic fusion bone causing kissing pseudarthrosis with adjacent normal bone. An overgrowth of fusion bone causing iatrogenic spinal stenosis can usually be documented most convincingly by myelography or CT scan (see pages 67 and 84).

Confirmation of the symptomatic nature of pseudarthrosis may require *diagnostic needle procedures* (see the discussion of diagnostic injections in Chapter 4). Anesthetization of the point of contact in a kissing pseudarthrosis may be necessary to determine whether this contact is a source of pain. Similarly, anesthetizing the pseudarthrotic line, or the regenerated facet nerves that innervate the pseudarthrotic area, may be necessary to determine whether a presumed pseudarthrosis is symptomatic or even whether such a pseudarthrosis exists.

Once it has been determined that revision of the previous fusion is indicated, the *technique or type of fusion* to be performed must be selected. If a painful pseudarthrosis of the fusion or resorption of the fusion has been documented, the decision must be made whether to simply repair the previous fusion or to expand the fusion by incorporating additional portions of the vertebrae at the segmental level. If an overgrowth of fusion bone is the cause of the patient's failed back syndrome, reduction of the fusion mass may be required.

Revision of Fusion

When a simple pseudarthrotic line through the body of a posterior or posterolateral fusion is confirmed at surgery, with the bulk of the fusion bone remaining intact, *local revision of the fusion* may be all that is necessary. Local revision involves two basic steps. First, the pseudarthrotic line must be fully identified and excised. Excision should include all fibrous tissue interposed between adjacent bone and should include all corticated opposing bone surfaces. Careful exploration should be carried out beneath the pseudarthrotic line in search of secondary epidural adhesions. These should be carefully lysed from dura and nerve roots and autogenous fat should be added in their place to limit re-formation of adhesions. Second, new bone must be added into the pseudarthrotic defect (Fig. 7.8). Quite commonly this new bone can be obtained from the local area without reexposing a separate donor bone site. If an extensive amount of fusion bone remains, there are usually areas where the thickness of the fusion is unnecessarily great or where irregular outcroppings of bone are present on the surface of the fusion. Quite commonly it is possible to remove sufficient bone from these sites to repair the pseudarthrosis without jeopardizing the stability of the remainder of the fusion. When this is not possible, donor bone should be obtained from the posterior iliac crest.

Even if abnormal mobility of a fusion is demonstrated radiographically on flexion/extension films, *documentation of pseudarthrosis* at the time of surgery is not always easy. On rare occasions I have encountered a solid mass of dorsal or posterior fusion bone firmly attached to the sacrum and immovable in relationship to the sacrum. Only after drill-

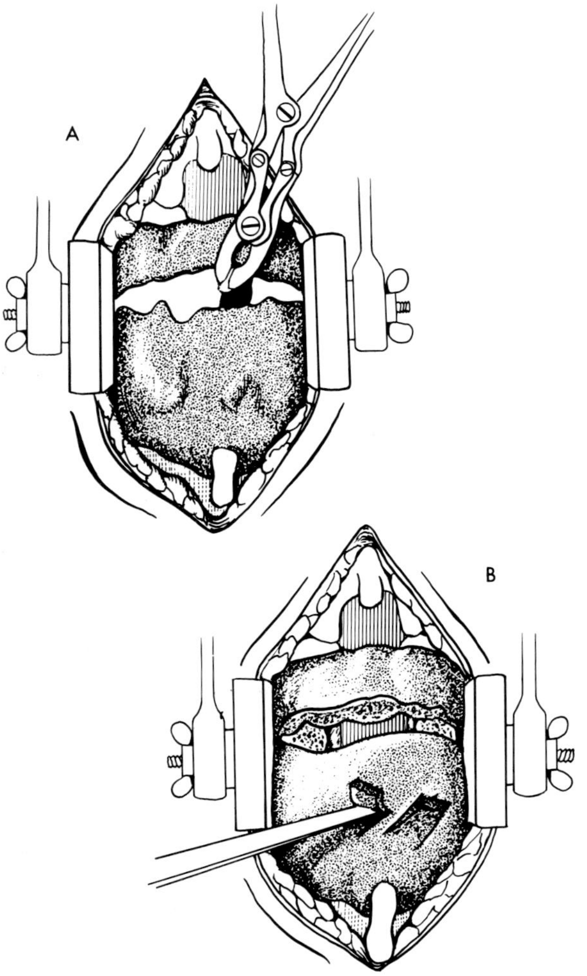

FIGURE 7.8. Two basic steps are involved in the surgical repair of a symptomatic pseudarthrosis of a lumbar fusion. **A:** The first step involves removing soft tissue scar from the pseudarthrotic line and decorticating or "freshening" adjacent bone edges. **B:** The second step involves placing additional fusion bone in the defect. Fusion bone can often be obtained locally from areas where the previously placed fusion bone is unnecessarily thick. Curls or chips of bone can be removed from these areas with an osteotome (as shown here), to be packed in the bony defect.

ing away the fusion bone at the site of suspected instability was I able to document that the fusion bone had failed to attach to the underlying vertebral arch so that the abnormal fusion and pseudarthrosis was between the upper vertebra and the fusion bone. In these instances, the dorsal mass of fusion bone is quite intact, and only conviction and persistence will disclose the true nature of the painful pseudarthrosis. More commonly, the pseudarthrotic line will not be clearly visible at the time of initial surgical exposure. The degree of mobility demonstrable at the operating table may be relatively slight, and the pseudarthrotic line is frequently obscured by overlying soft-tissue scar. In these instances, carefully removing attached scar tissue from the dorsal surface of the fusion bone usually will eventually reveal the cleft or fissure in the bone; as this is more fully revealed, the extent of mobility across the pseudarthrotic line usually becomes more evident.

Extension of Fusion

If extensive resorption of bone is discovered at the time of surgery or if the operating surgeon is uncertain whether the previously placed fusion is sufficient to produce adequate stabilization of the spine, consideration should be given to performing an *extension of the fusion* at the same spinal level. The most common fusion extensions of this type are the addition of a posterolateral or transverse process fusion to a posterior fusion or the addition of a posterolateral fusion to an interbody fusion.

Occasionally, it is deemed advisable to *add an interbody fusion* to an existing posterior or posterolateral fusion. This usually cannot adequately be performed from the posterior approach because this approach necessitates widely spreading the adjacent laminae and posterior rim of the intervertebral disc space. The intervertebral space normally has a greater height anteriorly than posteriorly, and adequate entry into this space requires mechanical opening of the posterior rim of the disc space. Spreading of laminae is also important to permit greater exposure of nerve roots and to allow the surgeon to work around these nerve roots more safely. Interbody fusion by the posterior route can be accomplished through wide fenestration of the posterior fusion and extensive removal of the posterior margins of the intervertebral disc space, but adequate interbody fusion by this technique is usually a technical *tour de force* that results in placement of limited amounts of bone in the interspace. Alternatively, anterior interbody fusion requires a transabdominal or retroperitoneal approach to the anterior portion of the vertebral body. Neurosurgeons and orthopedic surgeons are less familiar with this approach than with the traditional posterior approach. Care must be taken to avoid damage to ureters, retroperitoneal blood vessels, and nerves. Nonetheless, the exposure of the intervertebral disc space is excellent, removal of the disc may be complete or nearly complete, and large amounts of fusion bone can be inserted. This technique may be desirable in situations in which posterior or posterolateral fusions have spontaneously resorbed. That this technique is rarely used as an adjunct to an existing posterior or posterolateral fusion attests to its technical difficulty. Use of this approach would also leave uncorrected the posterior pseudarthrosis, which would imply a conviction on the part of the surgeon that adequate correction of the posterior fusion could not be successfully accomplished or that adequate stabilization of the spine could not be accomplished through posterior fusion alone.

A different type of extension of a preexisting spinal fusion involves *extension of the fusion to a new interspace level.* Extending a fusion to a new level almost always involves including a higher or rostral interspace level and usually entails adding L4-L5 to an L5-sacrum fusion or adding L3-L4 to an L4-sacrum fusion. Extending a fusion in this manner is indicated when it can be proven with reasonable certainty that a patient's pain arises from an interspace adjacent to the upper level of a previously operated upon and previously fused level. In some patients, such an extension may be made necessary because the original surgery was performed at a level caudal to the level of principal symptomatology. Fusion at a more caudal level may have occurred through operative inaccuracy or an inaccurate interpretation of where operative intervention was carried out prior to the fusion. Proving that this is the case once a patient has undergone spinal fusion with or without discectomy may be difficult if not impossible. A history of persistent symptomatology unchanged by previous surgery and subsequent confirmation of a severely symptomatic interspace at the level above a previous fusion are at least suggestive that the initial fusion was not performed at the level of principal symptomatology. On the other hand, many patients will give a history of significant improvement following their initial fusion operation but will later develop new or recurrent symptoms. If a symptomatic painful instability is documented at a rostrally adjacent interspace in these patients, one must question whether this represents (1) further manifestation of the same basic degenerative process that led to the first back problem, (2) a degeneration or "wearing out" of the adjacent interspace secondary to hypermobility at this interspace produced by the adjacent fusion, or (3) some combination of both of these factors.

The *indication for higher extension of a fusion* is intolerably persistent or newly developed pain, usually low back pain, in a patient documented to have painful instability at an interspace rostrally adjacent to a previous, intact spinal fusion. Confirming with reasonable reliability the presence of a painful instability is as difficult in these patients as it is in those patients being considered for primary spinal fusion or addition of a new spinal fusion following previous laminectomy. The techniques by which such a determination is made are essentially the same as those discussed under repeat laminectomy and repeat spinal fusion in this chapter.

The *complications* of extending a fusion are essentially the same as those encountered in revising a previous fusion or performing a new fusion (see the discussion of repeat spinal fusion and primary spinal fusion in this chapter). The technique of extending a fusion is also essentially the same as that already discussed in this chapter. The principal additional technical point is the necessity of carefully decorticating the mass of fusion bone to which the new fusion will be attached prior to placing the new fusion bone.

Reduction of Fusion

Iatrogenic spinal stenosis or *kissing pseudarthrosis* may simply require reduction of the previous fusion rather than re-fusion or re-creation of stability in a previously placed fusion (Fig. 7.9). The *kissing*

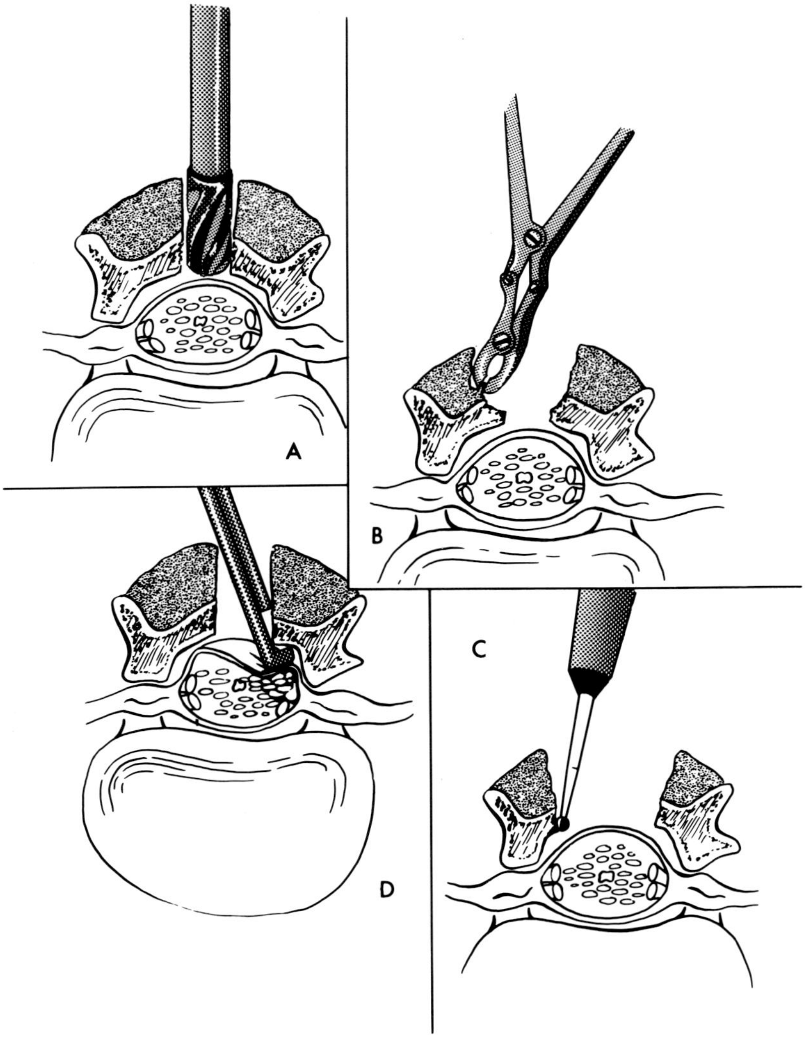

FIGURE 7.9. Revising a spinal fusion through reduction of the fusion mass overlying the spinal theca may be necessary in the treatment of iatrogenic spinal stenosis. In this condition, an overgrowth of fusion bone can lead to compression of the spinal sac causing neurogenic claudication—pain and neurologic loss brought on by walking. **(A)** Once initial fenestration is accomplished with a large burr or drill, **(B)** the opening should be widened by biting away the bone dorsally, and **(C)** by using a small burr. **(D)** Attempting to place the biting foot of a metal instrument beneath the bone can damage already compressed spinal nerve roots.

pseudarthrosis can usually be handled quite simply by rongeuring away fusion bone at the site of contact with adjacent normal bone. Heavy application of bone wax to the cut bone edges probably impairs further exuberant bone growth at this site, and careful closure of soft tissues in the space between the previously juxtaposed bones should further lessen the chance of re-formation of a kissing pseudarthrosis.

Iatrogenic spinal stenosis may be caused by the hypertrophic scar that forms beneath a pseudarthrotic line and an unstable fusion or may be the result of impingement of exuberant fusion bone into the spinal canal. In the latter condition, fenestration of a posterior or posterolateral fusion in the midline with preservation of fusion bone laterally may suffice to decompress the spinal contents while leaving the fusion still intact. Fenestration of the fusion can most easily be performed with the drills used to place burr holes for a craniotomy. A craniotome or Hudson brace with a Devilbiss burr is placed over the center of the fusion at the estimated area of maximum impingement on the underlying theca. It is necessary to drill through the bone and through residual laminae, usually to a depth of 1 cm or 2 cm. Drilling must be terminated as soon as soft tissues of the epidural space are reached. Smaller power drills, such as the Neurotome or Midas Rex instruments, may be used if care is taken not to tear the dura or nerve roots. Epidural fat or scar is then carefully stripped from the undersurface of the bone with angled dissectors such as a small dental dissector. If the compression of the underlying neurostructures is not too extreme, the burr opening can be enlarged rostrally and caudally with Kerrison rongeurs. Great care must be taken in the presence of spinal stenosis not to injure nerve tissue by forcing the footplate of this instrument into a tight spinal canal. In the presence of spinal stenosis, it is usually preferable to use a Leksell or similar rongeur to remove as much bone as possible from the dorsal midline of the fusion. Deeper bone should then be removed with a power-driven drill. The air-driven drills are usually safer to use in this situation than the mechanically driven drills because they stop more rapidly when soft tissues are encountered. Central bone removal should be continued until probing beneath residual midline bone confirms adequate decompression of the underlying thecal sac laterally to the pedicles. Autogenous fat, obtained from the patient's subcutaneous fat layer, is then placed in the epidural space and the residual fusion is carefully tested for stability. If sufficient fusion bone remains to provide adequate stabilization, the central fenestration can usually be left widely patent. If there is any uncertainty about the stability of the residual fusion bone, bone dust and bone chips removed during the fenestration can be loosely repacked into the fenestration dorsal to the epidural fat. Alternatively, the surgeon may elect to extend a posterior fusion laterally to include the transverse process.

Complications of Repeat Fusion

The *complications* of repeat fusion include wound infection or hemorrhage into the operative area. The risk of *wound infection* is particularly great for patients whose previous surgical wounds became infected. *Hemorrhage* into the wound may cause disruption of newly placed fusion bone, may produce severe epidural scar, may compress nervous tissue within the spinal canal, or may simply cause local wound pain. When repeat fusion necessitates fenestration of a previous fusion or revision of a pseudarthrosis through the body of the previous fusion, the possibility exists of dural tears or nerve root injury. *Dural tears* can result in CSF leakage or formation of dorsal arachnoid cysts or pseudomeningoceles. *Instability* is a much less common problem following revision of a fusion than following placement of a primary fusion. Even in the presence of pseudarthrosis, the bulk of the previously placed fusion is usually intact, and revision requires relatively limited alterations in the fusion itself. Extension of a fusion likewise is less likely to become unstable because of the considerable stability provided by the previously placed fusion bone. The addition of an interbody fusion carries a risk of nerve root injury if the posterior approach is used. The anterior approach carries the risk of injury to abdominal contents or retroperitoneal structures.

Primary Spinal Fusion

The *indications for lumbar spinal fusion* are quite controversial and vary widely from surgeon to surgeon for patients with "virgin" low back problems. When a patient develops a failed back syndrome following laminectomy without spinal fusion, those who are more enthusiastic about the benefits of spinal fusion for low back problems are likely to take an "I told you so" attitude and recommend the addition of spinal fusion as a second operative procedure. Even those surgeons who are reluctant to recommend spinal fusion surgery as a primary procedure often temper their initial recommendations with the observation that "we can always do a fusion later if necessary." Most patients with severe spondylolisthesis undergo spinal fusion as their first operation, but occasionally patients exhibit a first-degree spondylolisthesis and present with principally sciatica. These patients may be subjected to discectomy or laminal decompression only, without spinal fusion; if they develop a failed back syndrome, the recommendation for addition of spinal fusion is usually readily forthcoming.

Unfortunately, the attitude that "the patient didn't get well with laminectomy alone so obviously he needs a fusion" is limited and potentially dangerous. Although it is quite valid to consider the addition of spinal fusion in this situation, the *decision to recommend fusion* to a patient should be based on specific indications. Among the most useful of these specific indications is a consideration of the patient's symptoms. The patient most likely to benefit from subsequent spinal fusion seems to be the patient who continues to complain predominantly of pain in his back with relatively little sciatic radiation. Much of the controversy about primary spinal fusion surrounds patients who initially present with this symptom pattern. Many patients who initially present with predominantly back pain undergo spinal fusion, but many others are offered laminectomy alone, some with the option of a later secondary fusion. This course of action is justifiable because many patients in this category will indeed achieve satisfactory improvement following laminectomy alone. These patients are then spared the expense, prolonged recovery, and very real risks of spinal fusion. Other patients, however, develop back pain following laminectomy or obtain relief of severe sciatica only to remain disabled by back pain. Patients who respond best to secondary spinal fusion seem to be patients with low back pain of the "mechanical" type. These patients characteristically complain of back pain that is aggravated by weight bearing, bending, lifting, or other activities that stress the back. Characteristically, they obtain at least partial relief from recumbency. Since many patients obtain dramatic relief of back pain through the use of anti-inflammatory drugs, it is probably wise to include the obverse as an indication for surgery (i.e., a failure to respond to a useful degree to anti-inflammatory drug therapy).

An extremely useful adjunct to a symptomatic determination of the advisability of secondary spinal fusion is a *clinical trial of back bracing*. Patients who obtain good to excellent relief from back pain through the use of a steel or full torso back brace, yet fail to obtain progressive improvement or lasting symptomatic control through use of the brace alone, are likely to be good candidates for spinal fusion. Patients whose back pain is controlled with a canvas corset or lumbosacral belt are less suitable candidates for the major undertaking of spinal fusion surgery for two reasons. First, the inconvenience of wearing a lumbar corset probably is not sufficiently great to justify the major undertaking and risk that spinal fusion entails. Second, lumbar corsets and belts actually provide relatively little stabilization to the lumbar spine and suggest the strong possibility that these patients may improve through enforced activity therapy, anti-inflammatory drug therapy, or merely with the passage of time.

Laboratory confirmation of the necessity of primary fusion is of limited usefulness. *Radiographic or CT* demonstration of degenerative spurring, interspace narrowing, or spondylolisthesis should all be carefully considered. Degenerative changes that are present at multiple levels in the lumbar spine raise serious question about the advisability of spinal fusion, but do not absolutely preclude fusion if a more focal process can be convincingly demonstrated in addition to the diffuse degenerative disease. If only diffuse degenerative disease is present, the addition of spinal fusion at one or two interspace levels is not likely to stop all of the patient's back pain. Furthermore, fusion may well lead to an acceleration of the development of degenerative changes at the adjacent interspace, which now must become hypermobile to compensate for the loss of mobility in the fusion area. Severe *focal degenerative changes* on the margins of the interspace or in the facet joints, in contrast, suggest that spinal fusion may be helpful in a patient who seems symptomatically to be a suitable candidate for spinal fusion. Interspace narrowing alone is a very weak indicator of the need for spinal fusion, since interspace narrowing may occur as a normal variant and frequently occurs in asymptomatic patients following discectomy. On the other hand, interspace narrowing suggests that the facet joints may be forced into misalignment, thus acting as a source of back pain. As mentioned earlier, demonstration of severe *spondylolisthesis* usually leads to primary spinal fusion so that postlaminectomy failed back syndrome patients are unlikely to exhibit more than first-degree spondylolisthesis. Although this feature, like interspace narrowing, suggests the possibility of a localized source of back pain, first-degree spondylolisthesis occurs in many asymptomatic persons. It is certainly possible that a patient with a first-degree spondylolisthesis is disabled not by his spondylolisthesis but by back pain arising from some other etiologic process.

Two *needle procedures* may help in deciding when spinal fusion is necessary. Diagnostic *discography* may be helpful, especially if done under local anesthesia. Discography that proves to be abnormal at a spinal level other than the one originally operated upon does not necessarily suggest the need for spinal fusion, although some surgeons consider spinal fusion advisable in patients who have undergone two-level disc excision solely due to the increased risk of instability that this creates. Discography will always be abnormal when performed at a previously operated level. This level will accept greater than *normal* amounts of contrast material, and radiographs will demonstrate extensive central filling if not posterior extravasation. One type of abnormality on discography, however, does suggest the possible usefulness of spinal fusion. Injection into a previously operated but well-healed interspace should produce little or no pain despite the abnormal radiographic picture—at least in those instances in which posterior free extravasation does not occur. Under these circumstances, if contrast injection into a previously operated intervertebral disc produces severe back pain similar to the patient's customary pain, this suggests that the intervertebral disc may be the source of the patient's pain. As discussed earlier, many of these patients obtain sufficient relief through the use of anti-inflammatory drugs or intradiscal steroid injection (see pages 128 and 151). Intradiscal injection of anesthetics that causes a prompt improvement in the patient's preexisting pain likewise suggests that this interspace is the source of the patient's pain. Patients with painfully abnormal, previously operated intervertebral discs who fail to respond to anti-inflammatory drug therapy, intradiscal steroid injection, and other vigorous nonoperative therapies should be considered potential candidates to benefit from primary spinal fusion.

A second needle procedure that may be helpful in determining the need for primary spinal fusion is *facet nerve anesthetization*. Although the demonstration of facet abnormalities on plain radiographs does not reliably implicate these structures as the source of the patient's pain, temporary alleviation of the patient's pain through selective anesthetization of the facet nerves strongly implicates the facets. Because of the short length of the facet nerves, lasting denervation of the facet joint is not a feasible goal. However, single or repeated anesthetizations of the facet nerves may be coupled with facet neurectomy, intrafacet steroid injections, anti-inflammatory drug therapy, enforced activity or inactivity, or other nonsurgical therapies to achieve lasting relief in some of these patients. Patients who obtain gratifying but short-lived relief following facet nerve anesthetization on several occasions but who remain disabled principally by back pain should be considered potential candidates to benefit from primary spinal fusion.

Once a decision has been made that a primary spinal fusion seems indicated for a given patient, a decision must be made about the *type of fusion to be performed*. Three basic fusion techniques are available: posterior or posterolateral fusion, interbody fusion through the posterior approach, or interbody fusion through the retroperitoneal or transabdominal approach. Posterior or posterolateral fusions and interbody transabdominal or retroperitoneal fusions are most commonly performed by orthopedic surgeons, usually with a neurosurgeon. Interbody fusion through the posterior approach is probably performed more commonly by neurosurgeons than orthopedic surgeons.

Posterior and Posterolateral Fusion

The standard type of lumbar spinal fusion for many years was the *posterior or posterolateral fusion* (Fig. 7.10). These procedures provide stabilization of the intervertebral disc space indirectly through destruction and fusion of the facet joints and through fusion stabilization of the dorsal spinal arch.

The principal *advantage of these procedures* is that they may be performed largely through the same operative exposure made to remove the intervertebral disc or to perform other operations on the lumbar thecal sac and nerve roots. Another major advantage is that a larger bony surface is available for fusion: The posterolateral fusion entails application of fusion bone to transverse processes, facets, laminae, and at least the base of the spinous processes. This wide fusion base provides excellent triangular stabilization of the posterior arches and usually provides adequate secondary stabilization of the intervertebral disc space.

The extensive area of bone to be fused, however, also provides part of the *disadvantage of these procedures*. They both require much more extensive posterior soft-tissue dissection and bony exposure than does interbody fusion by way of the posterior approach. Likewise, the larger bed of fusion bone that is required increases the risk of improper fusion of the multiple bone fragments used in these procedures, with a higher incidence of pseudarthrosis.

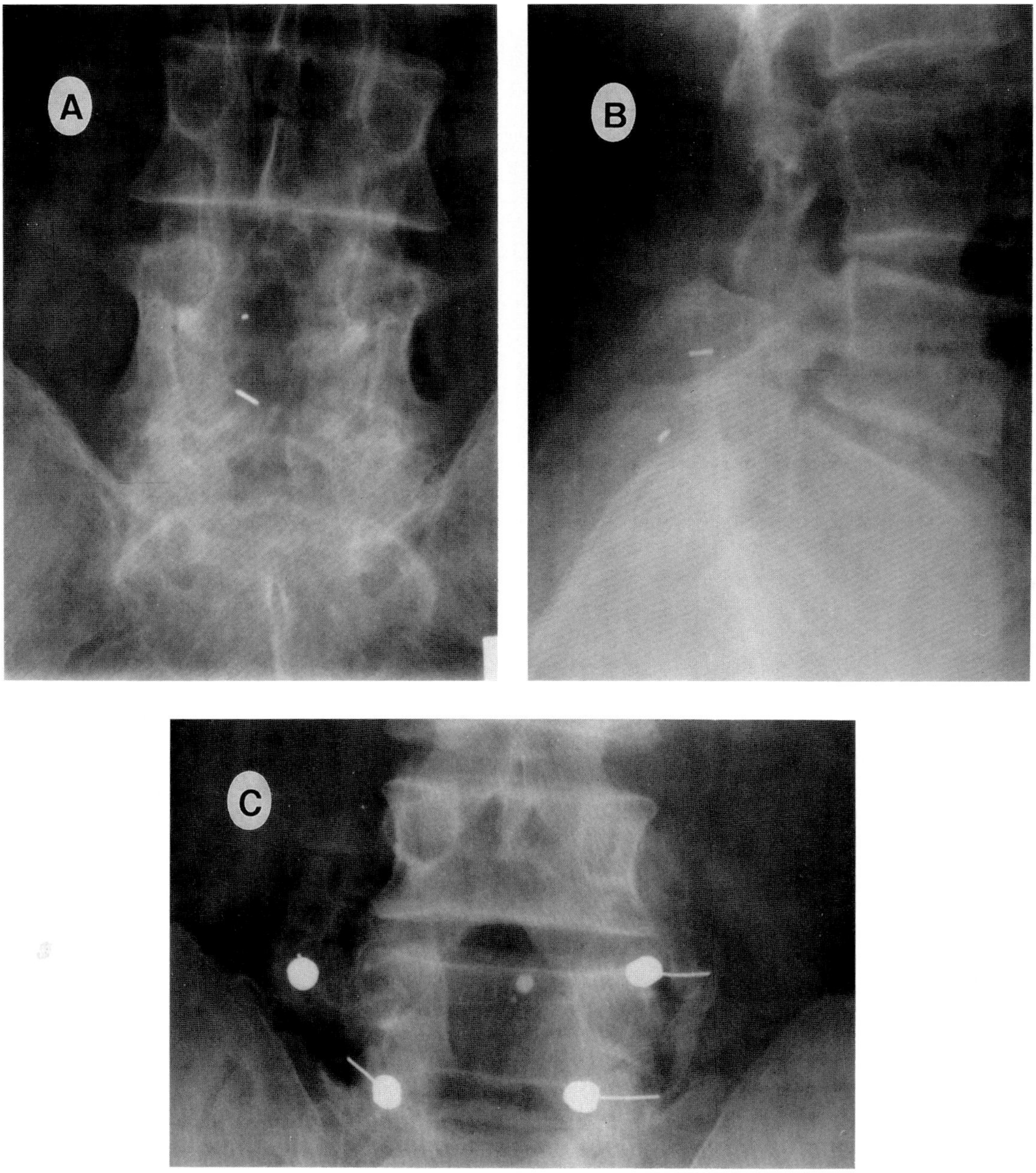

FIGURE 7.10. Posterior and posterolateral spinal fusions grow together as solid masses of bone from the initial confusion of bone chips placed over the decorticated spinal segments. **A and B:** Radiographs demonstrate a standard posterior fusion, with bony fusion of laminae and the base of the amputated spinous processes of L4 to upper sacrum. **C:** Radiograph demonstrates a posterolateral fusion of L4 to upper sacrum, with additional masses of fusion bone incorporating the transverse processes bilaterally.

In fact, the instance of pseudarthrosis has been estimated to be as high as 20% for each interspace level fused. As is frequently stated, the presence of a pseudarthrosis alone does not necessarily imply a failed back syndrome, since patients with pseudarthroses may remain asymptomatic.

The *technique of posterior fusion* and of *posterolateral fusion* is similar (Fig. 7.11). A midline incision is made from at least the spinous process rostral to the proposed upper limit of the fusion and extending caudally to overlie the midportion of the sacrum. Some surgeons prefer to continue the midline incision in a lateral sweep out onto the posterior iliac crest to provide access to this region for *donor bone*. More commonly, however, a secondary incision is made paralleling and slightly lateral to the medial one third of the posterior iliac crest to provide access to donor bone. At the midline incision, soft tissues are divided in the midline and the lumbar dorsal fascia is separated bilaterally from the tips of the spinous processes of the vertebrae that are to be fused, over the next most rostral vertebra, and over the upper half of the sacrum. Muscular attachments are stripped subperiosteally from spinous processes, laminae, and facets. If a posterolateral fusion is planned, the bony exposure must be wider than that needed for a posterior fusion and must be continued lateral and ventral to the facets to reach and expose the transverse processes. This additional exposure provides greater bony stability but increases the risk of injuring nerve roots that lie just ventral to the transverse processes. The exposed area of bone to be fused is then decorticated or denuded of its outer layer of cortical bone by using rongeurs, curets, or osteotomes. Some surgeons prefer to remove the cortical bone entirely, saving the bone to add later to the mass of fusion bone. Others simply "shingle" or elevate strips of cortical bone without completely removing them. This provides access for osteoblasts to the underlying cancellous bone for fixation of the fusion. The *facet joints* are usually destroyed with greater or less vigor with osteotomes and curets, although rarely is more than the caudal half excised. Some surgeons attempt to add further to the facet fusion by drilling holes through the center of the facet for the placement of metal screws or bone dowels, but this is commonly done only in special situations. If the spinous processes remain intact following a previous laminectomy or one done at the same session as the secondary spinal fusion, the surgeon may elect to leave them intact and undecorticated, or he may simply remove and morselize them—being content to use the base of the amputated spinous process as the apical fixation point for the posterior or posterolateral fusion. Donor bone is usually obtained by exposing the medial one third of the posterior iliac crest and clearing its posterior face sub-

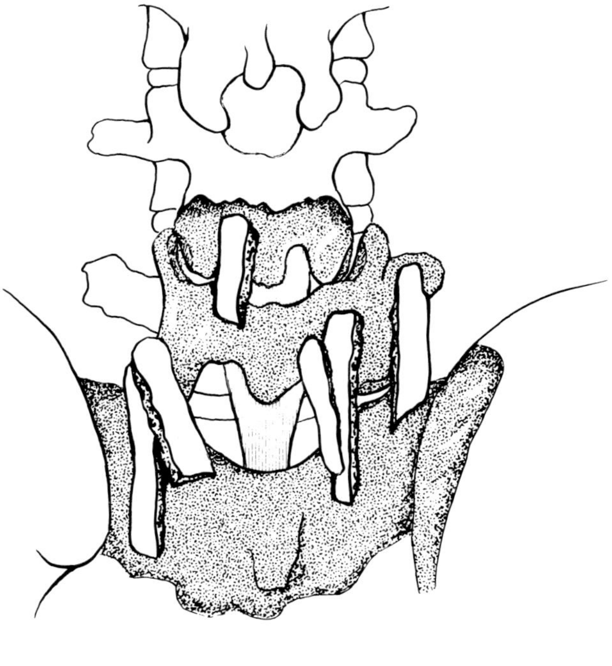

FIGURE 7.11. Posterior and posterolateral spinal fusions have been the most common forms of lumbosacral spinal fusion currently done in the United States. Posterior spinal fusion involves decorticating laminae, removing spinous processes, surgically destroying facet joints, and placing multiple bony chips in contact with the exposed cancellous bone (left side). Posterolateral spinal fusion includes the additional maneuver of decorticating transverse processes and placing additional bone chips further laterally (right side). This provides a broader-based fusion, which is inherently structurally more stable, but also entails more extensive and time-consuming surgery.

periosteally of muscle attachments. The posterior or caudal cortical surface is removed as single or multiple large bony plates. The interior cancellous bone is then removed with curved osteotomes or large curets as multiple fingerlike pieces of bone. The cortical bone may be either morselized or fashioned into a rough H to be wedged in place between the spinous processes of the two adjacent vertebrae that are to be fused. The remaining decorticated bony surfaces of the upper sacrum and posterior arches of the target vertebrae are then packed firmly with cancellous and morselized cortical bone. These are held in place by tight closure of overlying soft tissue, muscle, and fascia. Bleeding from decorticated bony surfaces may be controlled with anticoagulant powders or gels. *Bone wax* should not be used because it has been demonstrated to interfere with optimum bone fusion. Persistent bloody oozing from the bony surfaces may necessitate placement of a wound drain, even though this clearly increases the potential risk of infection. Prophylactic antibiotics should not be required if careful intraoperative asepsis and postoperative wound care are maintained. If the surgeon elects to use prophylactic antibiotics, these should be started immediately prior to surgery and usually need not be continued for more than 48 or 72 hours postoperatively. Postoperative fever (as high as 101 or 102 degrees) and mild leukocytosis are expected and are sometimes termed *bone fever.* These indications of local inflammatory response to extensive bony injury must be followed carefully lest they merge without detection into evidence of wound sepsis.

Lumbar posterior or posterolateral spinal fusions are almost always anchored to the sacrum and therefore include fusion of L5 and S1. Only on rare occasions is a so-called *floating fusion* performed. This term refers to a lumbar fusion that does not incorporate the sacrum, usually a fusion at L3-L4. The practice of anchoring the fusion to the sacrum is based on appreciation of the vulnerability of the lumbosacral disc space, as well as the statistical fact that more than nine out of every ten lumbar disc ruptures occur at either L4-L5 or L5-S1. If L4 were fused to L5 but not to the sacrum, the added stress and strain on the lumbosacral disc would be great. Most likely, this would rapidly cause excessive wearing of the disc, with rupture or painful degeneration. On those rare occasions when a floating fusion is performed at L3-L4 or higher, some orthopedic surgeons like to couple this with the use of small compression rods in hopes of providing better immediate stabilization and better long-term fusion. A patient in whom this technique was employed is presented in Case 5 on page 102.

The principal *complications of posterior or posterolateral fusion* include the specific risks of injury to nervous tissues in addition to the nonspecific risks of wound infection and blood loss. With extensive bony exposure, *blood loss* can at times be severe, although this need not be essential to the procedure. Working together, Dr. Joseph Abate, a talented orthopedic surgeon also interested in diseases of the lower back, and I frequently were able to perform laminectomy and posterior spinal fusion without replacement blood transfusions. The risk of *neural injury* may take several forms. The risk of lateral paraspinal nerve root injury during exposure, decortication, and fusion of transverse processes in a posterolateral fusion was referred to earlier. Neural structures, either proximal extradural nerve roots or the thecal sac itself, may be injured during decortication of laminae or the upper sacrum. Sacral decortication with osteotomes must be done particularly carefully, since some areas of the dorsal arch of this bone are at times quite thin. As discussed on page 25, injury to neural structures can also occur from excessively vigorous packing of fusion bone over areas of previous laminectomy. The resulting bony encroachment on the spinal canal can result in an iatrogenic form of spinal stenosis. *Bleeding* can also lead to neurologic complications if this occurs following wound closure. The development of a hematoma at the fusion site may lead not only to disruption of the fusion but also to compression of underlying neural structures. Even if compression does not occur, extravasation of blood into the epidural space can lead to *excessive scarring* with secondary irritation or compression of nerve roots and thecal sac. Postoperative *paralytic ileus* is so common following lumbar spine fusion that it is more properly considered an expected concomitant rather than a complication. The ileus rarely lasts more than a few days and usually does not necessitate gastric or intestinal intubation, although patients should be maintained NPO (nothing by mouth) until active bowel sounds return. Both the lumbar pain and the narcotics used to control the pain aggravate paralytic ileus. The enforced bed rest tends to prolong ileus and promote constipation, so preoperative cleaning enemas are desirable.

Interbody Fusion—Posterior Approach

The second type of spinal fusion is interbody fusion through a posterior approach. For more than half a decade this has been, and remains, my preference and exclusive recommendation for new one- or two-level lumbar fusions. This technique is not as popular as posterior or posterolateral fusion, but it has many staunch advocates.

The major *advantage of posterior lumbar interbody fusion* (PLIF) is that it provides immediate bony stabilization, rapid relief of pain and early patient mobilization. Most of my patients leave the hospital seven to ten days following one- or two-level posterior interbody fusion—some as early as four days postoperatively—and many do not require narcotics at the time of discharge. Posterior interbody fusion can be performed through the same posterior midline incision used for laminectomy. It entails less extensive bony disruption than posterior or posterolateral fusion, and I have rarely needed to transfuse patients to replace blood loss. A full interbody fusion requires exposure of the posterior iliac crest to obtain donor bone if the facets are to be fused as well, but bone bank bone performs well for the interbody bone plugs, since larger bone grafts are devitalized and must be replaced entirely by creeping bone substitution. A modified interbody fusion, as advocated by Christoferson, can be performed with bone obtained locally at the laminectomy site (Fig. 7.12) but is now rarely performed.[7] Interbody fusion entails placing bone in the intervertebral disc space, so extensive posterior decortication is not required. My modification of interbody fusion entails the addition of destruction of the paired facets at the level of the fusion, packing these spaces with bone, and wiring the spinous processes together to clamp the interbody bone in place and to limit mobility at the facet fusion sites (Figs. 7.13 and 7.14).

There are two major *disadvantages of posterior interbody fusion*. Although, theoretically, directly fusing the interspace seems the most logical way of stabilizing a diseased disc space, in reality it may be more *difficult to obtain adequate stabilization* by fusion of the interbody space alone than by posterior or posterolateral fusion. The reason is that the bone surface available for fusion is limited in area. The intervertebral disc usually cannot be removed entirely from the posterior approach, so resection is usually limited to the nuclear portion, with preservation of the annular portion. As a result, the area available for fusion is usually less than 10 square cm. Much of the pull of back muscles against the intervertebral disc is transmitted through a levering effect from the dorsal arch so that a fusion between the vertebral bodies is subjected to even greater stresses than a posterior or posterolateral fusion. The addition of bilateral facet fusion and wiring, as in my modification of the interbody technique, provides effective four-point stabilization of the disc space and includes direct posterior stabilization of the facet joints. The second major disadvantage of this procedure is that it involves *approaching the interspace through the epidural space*. The nerve root must be displaced to permit wide access to the interspace and greater care must be taken to avoid nerve root injury. If interbody bone plugs do slip, as has now happened to two of my patients during violent vomiting in the first few days postfusion, the posteriorly migrating plug can severely compress the nerve root. A potential third disadvantage of the procedure is that it *customarily does not involve destruction or fusion of the facet joints,* although this is included in my modification of the technique. Since much of the back pain experienced by failed disc syndrome sufferers may originate from the facet joints, not fusing the facets could limit the effectiveness of interbody fusion alone in providing pain relief. Because the posterior approach involves working in close juxtaposition to nerves and in a confined space, and since this bears some similarity to anterior cervical spine fusions, this procedure is generally more popular among neurosurgeons than orthopedic surgeons. As mentioned earlier, posterior interbody fusions are usually not feasible as an extension of or an addition to a previously placed posterior or posterolateral fusion.

The *technique of posterior interbody fusion* begins with unilateral or bilateral laminotomy or partial hemilaminectomy. Although I usually pack the disc space bilaterally from a unilateral laminotomy, many surgeons advocate bilateral laminotomy, nerve root retraction, and interspace packing. After exposure of the lateral epidural gutter and resection of ruptured disc material, if any is present, the nerve root is retracted carefully 10 mm to 15 mm medially. Generally, at least half of the superior and inferior hemilaminae must be resected to gain adequate rostrocaudal exposure. The posterior longitudinal ligament is divided across the midline. It is usually necessary to curet or rongeur away a

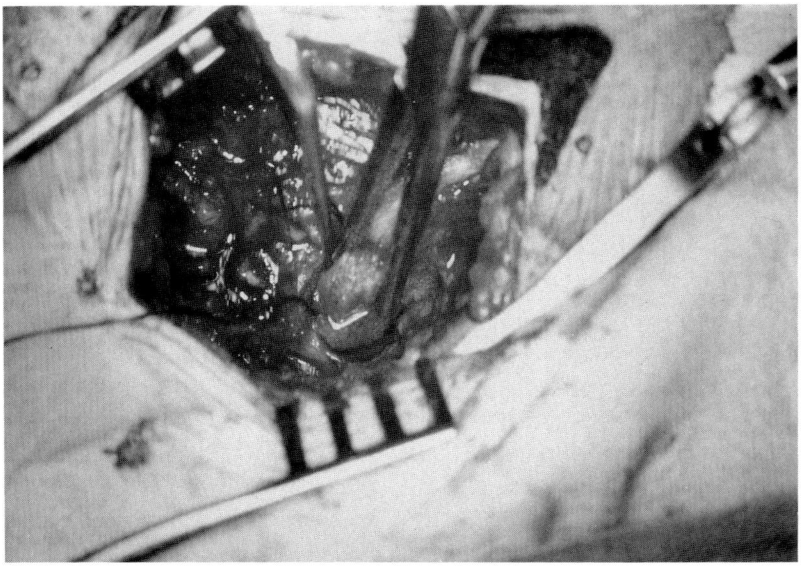

FIGURE 7.12. This operative photograph shows a bone plug or dowel fashioned from the spinous process being maneuvered into position for seating within the interspace as part of a Christofersen procedure. Care must be taken to protect the nerve root by medial displacement during this maneuver.

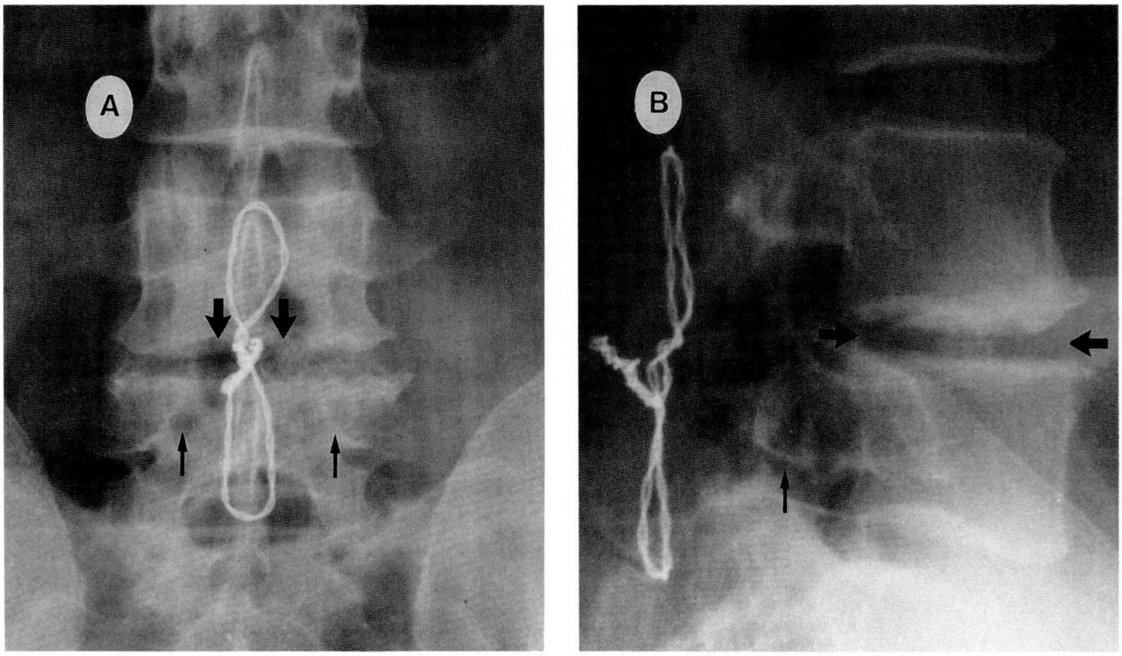

FIGURE 7.13. Postoperative AP (**A**) and lateral (**B**) radiographs following interbody-facet fusion and wiring document interbody blocks of bone (heavy arrows), partial facet fusions (small arrows), and a dorsal figure eight loop of heavy wire holding the areas of fusion in apposition.

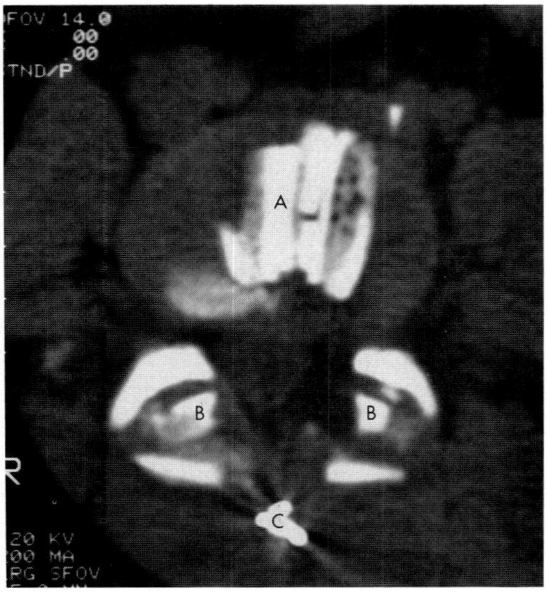

FIGURE 7.14. Interbody-facet fusion and wiring includes: **(A)** blocks of bone-bank bone in the disc space, **(B)** small pieces of autogenous bone in the partially resected facet joints, and **(C)** heavy gauge stainless steel wire around and approximating the adjacent spinous processes.

portion of the posterior rim of the vertebral body until the measured height of this entry into the disc space is similar to the measured height of the anterior portion of the exposed disc space. The interspace must be meticulously cleared of nucleus pulposus and cartilaginous end plates in the entire area of proposed fusion. This can be done with large curets or small osteotomes. Once this has been completed, the height and depth of the interspace are carefully measured. This can be done by placing osteotomes or periosteal elevators of various widths in the interspace until a width is encountered that barely or snugly fits into the interspace. I use bone bank bone for the interbody bone plugs, shaping them with an oscillating saw and rongeurs. If autogenous *donor bone* is to be used, it is usually obtained from the posterior medial iliac crest through a separate skin incision. The crest is exposed on both its dorsal and ventral surfaces and full-thickness segments of bone are removed with a wide osteotome. The width of each plug should be equal to or a few millimeters greater than the measured height of the interspace. The length of bone removed should be no greater than the measured depth of the disc space exposure. Once donor autogenous bone dowels are available, they are shaped slightly to facilitate their entry into and snug fit within the interspaces; then they are hammered, with the aid of bone sets, into the interspace. Care must be taken to protect the medially displaced nerve root. The first dowel to be inserted for a full fusion should be displaced medial to or across the midline using a levering motion and a long narrow bone set or periosteal elevator. If a unilateral laminectomy has been performed, it is important to displace this bone dowel as far across the midline as possible before placing a second or third dowel. It is important that bone dowels not be longer than the available opening in the interspace so that protruding bone is not left in the canal to compress nerve roots. At this point in the procedure I also perform a *fusion of the facet joints* at the level of interbody fusion. This is accomplished by removing the caudal two thirds of the superior facet on each side by making a bone incision dorsolaterally over the facet joint. The cartilaginous surface of the inferior facet is shaved off with curved osteotomes and narrow-nosed rongeurs. Small chips or sticks of donor bone from the patient's iliac crest are then packed into the joint spaces on each side. It is usually possible to expose enough of the iliac crest to obtain this limited amount of donor bone by dissecting laterally through subcutaneous tissues from the single midline incision. I then stabilize the interbody and facet portions of the fusion by pulling the spinous processes together by tightly twisting an 18-gauge *stainless-steel wire* wrapped around the base of each spinous process. Autogenous fat is usually placed over the exposed posterior surface of the bone plug, which should be recessed several millimeters below the posterior longitudinal ligament, and soft tissues are closed with catgut or silk as they would be following a laminectomy.

The major *complications of posterior interbody fusion* that are specific to this procedure involve immediate or late neurologic damage. *Blood loss* is usually less extensive with this procedure than with posterior or posterolateral fusion. The major immediate *risk to nerve roots* comes during the forceful insertion of bone dowels past the retracted nerve root. If a spicule or fragment of bone should catch the nerve root, immediate laceration may occur. Even if this does not occur, the forceful retraction that is necessary may lead to nerve root injury. This can result in either transient, painful neuropathy or more lasting intraneural scarring with chronic painful neuropathy. The risk of delayed nerve injury also includes the risk of posterior displacement of the interbody bone plugs. I customarily keep patients in a rigid back brace for two to three months following a full posterior interbody fusion. This is done to permit adequate union of the bone before permitting the patient to resume flexion and extension. The risk of persistent, painful *pseudarthrosis* is related to the relatively smaller area of bone available if fusion is limited to the interbody area only, as discussed above. The addition of bilateral facet fusion and wiring, which I advocate, seems to improve stability. If pain arises from abnormal facets, even slight mobility of the interspace may still allow generous movement of the facets, an amount of movement that may well be sufficient to generate severe pain on movement or weight bearing. By fusing the facet joints directly, the likelihood of painful fusion pseudarthrosis through persistent *facet pain* is likely to be lessened.

Interbody Fusion—Anterior Approach

The third alternative approach to lumbar spinal fusion is *interbody fusion through an anterior approach*. The anterior approach is usually retroperitoneal, but some surgeons prefer a transabdominal approach. Many neurosurgeons and orthopedic surgeons are familiar with the retroperitoneal approach to the lumbar spine for surgical correction of bone tumors, fractures, or other disease primarily affecting the vertebral bodies. This procedure is generally considered the most extensive of the three forms of fusion and is the least frequently performed. Its most common use seems to be as an extension of or addition to a posterior fusion in patients who persist with mechanical back pain or who repeatedly develop pseudarthroses of their posterior or posterolateral fusions. As discussed under repeat spinal fusion in this chapter, the decision about extension of or addition to a preexisting fusion is one that should be made carefully. It is not sufficient to assume that persistent mechanical back pain is arising from the interspace for which posterior or posterolateral fusion was attempted, since other structures in the back may give rise to a similar type of pain.

The chief *advantages of interbody fusion through the anterior approach* are that it provides greater surface area for stabilization than interbody fusion through the posterior approach and that it can be performed successfully despite a previous posterior or posterolateral fusion. The retroperitoneal approach allows wide exposure of almost the entire intervertebral disc space. By this approach, the entire disc may be removed, including annulus as well as nucleus pulposus. This provides a significantly larger bone surface for fusion and placement of thicker bone grafts.

The chief *disadvantages of this procedure* are its extensive nature and the limited access that it provides to structures dorsal to the intervertebral space. The retroperitoneal approach entails some risk of injury to ureters or abdominal structures and significantly increases the likelihood of postoperative ileus. The anterior approach to the disc space severely limits the surgeon's access to many of the other structures or disorders that may affect the lumbar spine and its contained neural structures. Although additional disc material can be resected through an anterior approach, this approach cannot realistically encompass the same type of extradural exploration that can be accomplished through laminectomy at the time of posterior or posterolateral fusion. Consequently this procedure has, as its almost exclusive goal, the production of a stabilizing spinal fusion, so the surgeon must ascertain preoperatively with as much exactitude as possible whether this is likely to produce adequate pain relief.

The *technique of interbody fusion through an anterior approach* necessitates simultaneous exposure of both the anterior intervertebral disc and a source of fusion donor bone, unless bone bank bone is to be used (Fig. 7.15). The retroperitoneal approach is probably preferable to a transabdominal approach and entails a skin incision in the midaxillary line over the lateral abdominal wall. Abdominal muscles are divided, but the peritoneum is left intact. The peritoneum usually strips easily, anteriorly along a plane of retroperitoneal fat. The spinal column is encountered as a prominent midline bony mass. At its base the ureter and exiting nerve roots are encountered. Over its lateral surface retroperitoneal veins, major arteries, and intercostal vessels extending posteriorly to the neuroforamina are encountered. These structures must be identified, a procedure that usually requires intraoperative radiographic confirmation of actual vertebral level. The intervertebral disc is resected by sharply incising the longitudinal ligament and annulus at the point of attachment of the annulus to the superior and in-

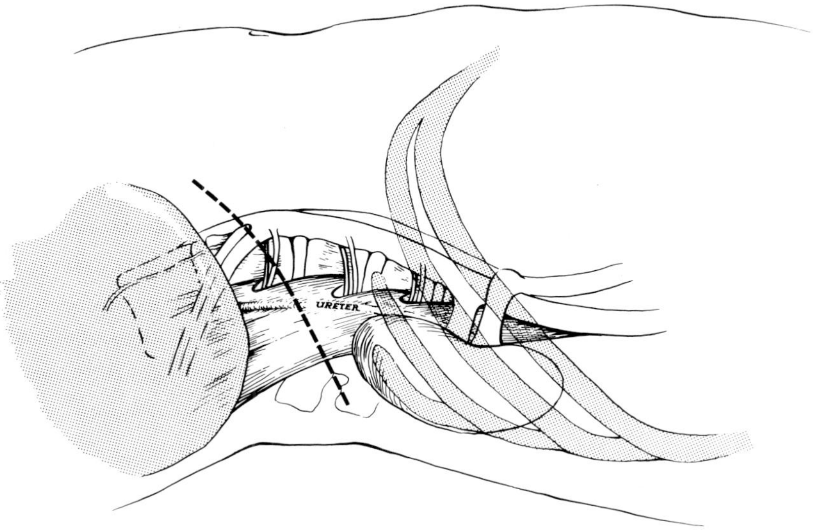

FIGURE 7.15. Interbody fusion, by way of an anterior approach, affords wide exposure of the vertebrae and interspaces and permits total removal of nuclear and annular portions of the disc. This provides a greater bone surface for fusion. Care must be taken during surgery to avoid damage to ureters and important retroperitoneal blood vessels.

ferior margins of the adjacent vertebral bodies. Usually the anterior longitudinal ligament is left intact on the contralateral side of the disc space, both as an aid to stabilization of the fusion and as protection against damage to vessels and ureter on the opposite side. Similarly, an effort is made to retain the posterior longitudinal ligament intact, with or without a portion of the posterior annulus, to protect the spinal canal. If recurrent disc protrusion is suspected, some exploration of the anterior epidural space can be accomplished through the bed of the interspace, although this may necessitate the use of small mirrors. Bone bank bone usually works well, since the large size of the bone blocks results in fusion by "creeping substitution" as osteoclasts and osteoblasts infiltrate the block of nonviable bone (bank bone or autogenous) and slowly replace it with new bone. If autogenous bone is to be used, donor bone is usually obtained from the anterior iliac crest by exposing this bone through the lower end of the flank incision. Full-thickness bone dowels or plugs are removed in similar fashion as described for interbody fusion through the posterior approach. Since a larger bone area is available for fusion, larger bone dowels must be obtained. After these have been driven into place in the interspace, the surgeon should check carefully to ensure that they do not extend posteriorly into the spinal canal. As is true with the other interbody fusion technique, the wedge shape of the intervertebral disc space offers a considerable element of stability and protection for the spinal canal. When the cartilaginous plates are removed it is usually possible to leave intact lips of cortical bone protruding from the superior and inferior vertebral bodies along their posterior margins, thus further protecting the spinal canal from unintentional impaction or displacement of bone into the canal. Some surgeons prefer to improve the immediate stability of the interbody fusion by clamping the vertebral bodies tightly together mechanically. This can be accomplished by applying one or more small metal plates to the side of the vertebral bodies or by inserting stainless-steel screws into the sides of each vertebral body and connecting these tightly together with heavy-gauge stainless-steel wire. With or without internal mechanical stabilization, patients are usually placed in a plaster or fiberglass body jacket for a period of four to six months.

The potential *complications of interbody fusion through an anterior approach* have been alluded to already. Care must be taken to prevent injury to or disruption of the *ureter* and *major retroperitoneal arteries and veins*. Intercostal arteries are relatively vulnerable. Damage to these vessels is usually well-tolerated but can lead to *infarction of the conus medullaris*, although this is rare. Neural structures may be damaged by driving bone plugs backward into the spinal canal or by fracturing the posterior wall of the vertebral body when bone plugs or dowels are driven into place. *Nerve roots* may also be injured paraspinally as they lie in the retroperitoneal space and muscle. Injury to abdominal contents is rarely a problem, but nearly all patients experience at least transient *ileus*. If surgeons are aware of this likelihood, they can prevent serious complications or patient distress by maintaining their patients on intravenous fluids until active bowel sounds return and by inserting a nasogastric or intestinal tube if gastric or intestinal dilatation becomes symptomatic.

Lysis of Arachnoiditis

Lysis of lumbar adhesive arachnoiditis is a procedure that I have generally reserved for patients with widespread back and leg pain, significant neurologic deficits, and myelographically or radiographically documented complete transverse obliteration of the lumbar thecal sac. Patients with such severe transverse lumbar adhesive arachnoiditis at times develop progressive neurologic deficits or progressively increasing pain. Some of these patients respond to intrathecal steroids or noninvasive therapy, but those who continue to progress clearly become candidates for microsurgical lysis of their arachnoiditis.[36,99] The following two cases illustrate some of the variability of this disease:

Case 16

At age 34, this stove assembler underwent three separate lumbar laminectomies for back and left leg pain. He ultimately improved enough to return to work despite some residual discomfort.

In 1970, 19 years following his back surgery, he developed urinary retention, and prostatitis was diagnosed. Recurring bouts of retention led to transurethral resection one year later. There was no evident cutaneous sensory loss in the saddle area. In 1973, after repeated heavy lifting at work but with no specific trauma, he rapidly developed severe pain in his back and both legs, greatest in the right leg—contralateral to his previous pain. Over several weeks, bilateral leg numbness appeared and he became totally unable to void. Symptoms progressed despite hospital therapy with bed rest. Myelography showed hypertrophic bony changes and complete transverse obstruction at the level of L4-L5. Cystometrography documented an atonic, neurogenic bladder.

Laminectomy was performed at L4 and L5. Dense transverse adhesive arachnoiditis was encountered with a large ossified plaque. The plaque was partially removed and partial nerve root lysis was performed. No dural graft was placed. Pain relief was dramatic and numbness rapidly cleared. Although he became able to void with the aid of bethanechol (Urecholine), he continued to have some voiding difficulty. Six weeks postoperatively, he was able to return to his heavy manual work in the stove company. He remained employed there despite brief hospitalization in 1974 and in the spring of 1978 for urinary retention. He was hospitalized briefly in December 1978 for a flare-up of low back pain that responded to nonoperative therapy.

Case 17

This 66-year-old diabetic homemaker, mother, and laundry worker came under my care in November 1966 with an acute episode of intolerably severe left sciatica. She gave a history of 10 or 15 years of intermittent low back and left hip pain, attributed to diffuse arthritis. Her present symptoms began spontaneously three weeks before and failed to remit despite hospital bed rest therapy. Under observation she developed a mild left footdrop. Myelogram showed an extremely large left lateral defect at L4-L5. At operation a large free fragment of disc material was recovered, but dense epidural adhesions around the nerve root and disc fragment were noted. In the course of dissection, a small tear was opened in the dura and arachnoid, but this was promptly sutured.

Postoperatively, she was rapidly relieved of left leg pain. Weakness and numbness cleared over the next few weeks. Unfortunately, she developed a persistent superficial skin infection that was treated with local applications, but healed only after excision of a sinus tract, including a sequestered silk suture from the lumbodorsal fascia.

Approximately six weeks following surgery she complained of increasing discomfort in her low back and right or contralateral leg. This was associated with increasing difficulty initiating urination and a sensation of numbness in her saddle area and right medial thigh. Examination revealed mild weakness of dorsiflexion and plantar flexion of right ankle, persistent mild weakness of dorsiflexion of left ankle (although this was considerably improved over her preoperative status), and hypalgesia over the perineum, medial right thigh, and anterior and lateral aspect of both feet and calves. Straight leg raising to 40 degrees on the right and 50 degrees on the left caused ipsilateral severe leg pain. Urinary difficulties rapidly progressed to complete urinary retention requiring insertion of a Foley catheter.

She was afebrile when she was hospitalized two months following her initial surgery. Her white count was normal and her wound was well-healed. Myelogram disclosed a complete subarachnoid obstruction with ragged border at L4-L5, consistent with adhesive arachnoiditis. Spinal fluid was normal chemically and microscopically. Intrathecal methylprednisolone (Depo-Medrol) brought considerable improvement in pain and sensory loss. Bladder control gradually improved with the aid of bethanechol (Urecholine).

In less than a month, symptomatic improvement faded and complete urinary retention again developed. In February 1967, laminectomy was performed at L3 through L5. There was no evidence of infection, although she was given perioperative prophylactic antibiotics. Intradural exploration revealed a band of dense whitish arachnoidal adhesions transversely across the entire thecal sac at L4-L5. The area of dense adhesions measured less than 1 cm in rostrocaudal thickness. Adhesions were freed by blunt and sharp dissection and 80 mg (1 ml) of methylprednisolone acetate was instilled prior to meticulous dural closure. Postoperatively, severe pain rapidly subsided, but she continued to require nonnarcotic and occasionally opiate analgesics for the subsequent year. Sensory loss rapidly cleared over a few weeks, but unpleasant dysesthesia and hyperesthesia appeared over the lateral aspect of the right foot. This was controlled with antineuralgia drugs and had completely disappeared eight months following lysis of arachnoid adhesions. Bladder control returned to normal, although she continued to complain of chronic constipation. When examined one month after surgery both ankle reflexes and right knee reflex were unobtainable. There was a mild weakness of dorsiflexion and plantar flexion of right ankle and patchy impairment of pinprick perception distally over both lower extremities but not in the perineal region. Straight leg raising was now possible to 70 degrees bilaterally with stiffness rather than pain.

It is less clear whether patients with transverse or obliterative adhesive arachnoiditis should be *considered for such surgery* if they exhibit a relatively static clinical picture of severe, diffuse back and leg pain with relatively limited neurologic deficits and if they fail to respond to other therapy. Uncertain also is the role of lysis of arachnoiditis for patients who present with predominantly sciatica and whose myelogram or CT/myelogram discloses a limited defect at one or two adjacent nerve root pouches. In these patients it is often difficult to determine preoperatively whether the defect represents recurrent disc rupture or focal arachnoiditis. Certainly if exploration for possible disc rupture is planned, intradural lysis of arachnoidal adhesions should be considered if exploration fails to disclose a significant disc fragment or mass of extradural scar tissue. Occasionally, patients are encountered who continue to complain of sciatica following an exploratory laminectomy that failed to encounter ruptured disc material. If these patients' focally abnormal myelograms remain relatively unchanged preoperatively and postoperatively, the likelihood is great that their symptoms are due to localized arachnoiditis. It is unclear whether these patients are better served by attempting to perform microsurgical lysis of this localized arachnoiditis or whether one should consider sensory rhizotomy. Certainly the patient's philosophy and wishes must be weighed heavily in reaching this decision, since the uncertainty of microsurgical lysis must be weighed against the uncertainty and induced sensory loss of rhizotomy.

In 1979, I presented what was then the *second largest reported series of patients subjected to surgical lysis of lumbar adhesive arachnoiditis* (see the discussion of adhesive arachnoiditis in Chapter 3).[38] Most of these seventeen patients developed symptoms within one or two years following initial laminectomy or continued with severe symptoms despite laminectomy, but three developed symptoms after back trauma or hypertrophic spinal stenosis developed eight, nineteen, and twenty-one years following laminectomy. One patient clearly developed spontaneous arachnoiditis, and several others were suspected of having developed spontaneous arachnoiditis that was initially misdiagnosed as lumbar disc disease. Of course, I have encountered many other patients with asymptomatic or symptomatic arachnoiditis who were not subjected to lysis of their arachnoiditis, such as the patient presented in Case 13 on page 163. All of the patients included in this series were operated on because of severe back and bilateral leg pain. Fourteen patients also suffered progressive neurologic involvement. Five were confirmed to have multisegmental arachnoiditis and twelve were found to have single-level annular or subtotal adhesions at the site of previous discopathy. At surgery an attempt was made to lyse the arachnoidal adhesions intradurally, using an operating room microscope or magnifying loupes. Individual nerve roots were separated by blunt or sharp dissection. At the conclusion of surgery, all but two patients were treated

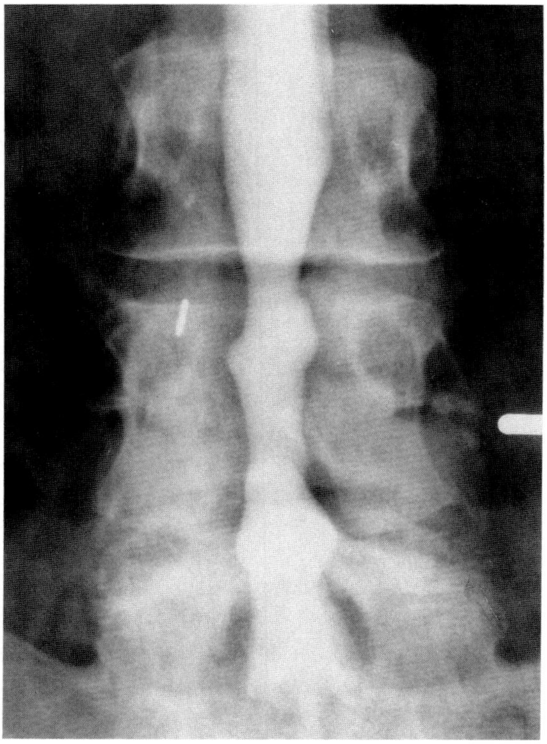

FIGURE 7.16. Persistence of arachnoiditis following microsurgical lysis. This myelogram was obtained when this woman developed increasing low back and sciatic pain 15 months following microsurgical lysis of arachnoiditis and two-level sensory rhizotomy (without placement of metal clips on distal nerve ends). Preoperatively, she demonstrated total transverse obliteration. Despite recurrence of pain there was no neurologic worsening. Note the ragged appearance of the thecal sac caused by the bilateral arachnoidal scarring.

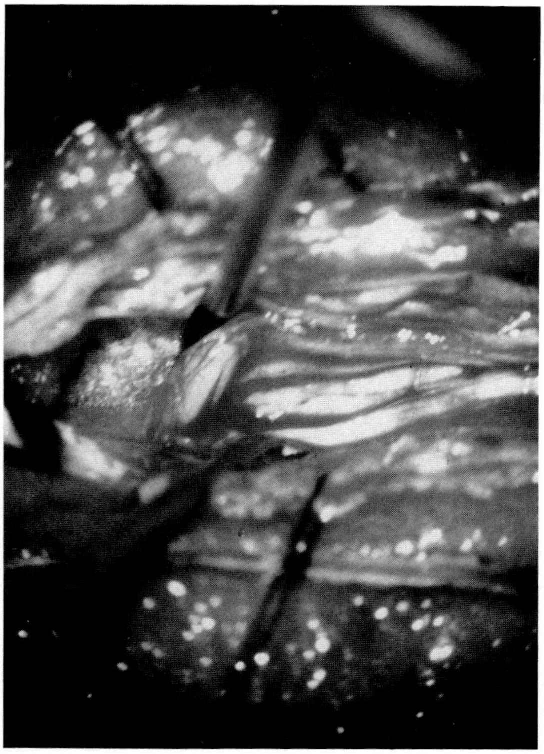

FIGURE 7.17. Microsurgical lysis of arachnoiditis is documented in this photograph taken through the operating room microscope. Dense arachnoidal adhesions make identification of nerve roots difficult and require sharp dissection for separation of the nerve roots. Intrathecal and systemic steroids are often used in an effort to retard reformation of these adhesions.

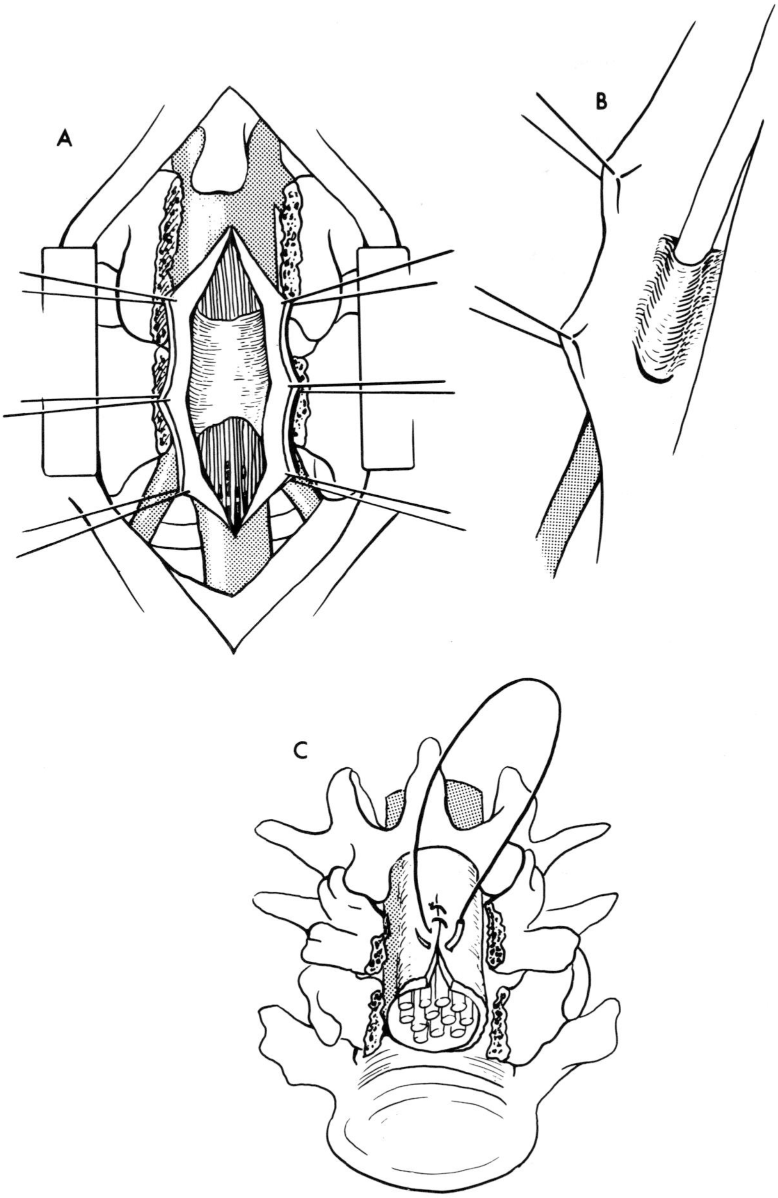

FIGURE 7.13. **A:** Surgical lysis of adhesive arachnoiditis requires total laminectomy at two or more levels for arachnoiditis of the transverse type. **B:** Hemilaminectomy may suffice for localized, monoradicular arachnoiditis. **C:** In either situation, adherent epidural scar should be left attached to the dura to facilitate water-tight closure.

with intrathecal, systemic, or combination corticosteroids. During the first year after surgery, 76% of these patients experienced improvement in pain (35%, good to excellent) and 71% experienced improvement in neurologic status. Follow-up for greater than one year revealed that only 50% still enjoyed pain relief and 45% experienced neurologic improvement. Four out of five patients followed for more than five years maintained good pain relief. The only two patients to suffer pain relapses more than twelve months following surgical lysis did so after trauma or pregnancy.

The *diagnosis of arachnoiditis* can be made either by myelographic or CT/myelographic demonstration of a complete or near complete spinal block or by plain radiographs that demonstrate loculated and immobile iophendylate (Pantopaque) in the lumbar region in patients whose spinal fluid could not be obtained during attempted lumbar puncture in this area (Fig. 7.16). MRI scans may be able to show extensive arachnoiditis, but usually are not able to provide detailed information.

The *technique of surgical lysis of lumbar adhesive arachnoiditis* requires use of magnified vision (Fig. 7.17). An operating room microscope is preferable. High-powered magnifying loupes can be used, but they deprive the surgical assistant of a magnified view. Decompression may at times be gratifyingly successful even without complete lysis of adhesions (as in Case 17, above), but the ideal goal of this operation is complete lysis of adhesions throughout the involved region. This necessitates a total laminectomy covering the area of involvement (Fig. 7.18). If the documented upper level of obstruction extends more than one segmental level above the site of previous operation, the disease is likely to extend throughout the entire lumbar region. On the other hand, if the upper level of obstruction is near the site of previous disc surgery, the obstruction is likely to be confined to the one or two levels that were previously operated upon and presumed to have been the site of previous disc disease. As discussed earlier, this implies that (1) surgery caused the arachnoiditis, (2) disc disease caused the arachnoiditis, or (3) arachnoiditis was present initially but was misdiagnosed as lumbar disc disease. In any event, in this group of patients it is usually necessary to perform laminectomy at only two or three levels. Unless they are obviously involved in arachnoiditis, it is usually not necessary to expose the lowest lumbar and upper sacral segments, unless intradural exploration confirms that the arachnoiditis is more extensive than normally encountered. The exposed dura is incised in the midline. At times, there may be a cleavage plane between the dura and the underlying thickened arachnoid, but this plane may be difficult to identify. It is not necessary to dissect arachnoid from the dura; in fact, doing so can weaken the dura and increase the risk of CSF leakage postoperatively. Great care must be taken not to injure nerve roots. Depending upon the severity of the arachnoiditis at a given level, nerve roots may be completely encased in dense white arachnoidal scar that is similar in color to nerve roots (Type III), may be "plastered" to the dura circumferentially by arachnoidal thickening with a patent central opening (Type II), or may be surrounded by arachnoidal adhesions only near their point of exit through the theca (Type I). In some patients the arachnoidal adhesions are relatively delicate and nerve roots can be dissected free with fine blunt dissectors. In most patients at least some areas will be encountered where the arachnoidal scarring is sufficiently tough and dense that attempted blunt dissection risks serious injury to the nerve root, which may be more delicate than the scar tissue. In these instances, a small scalpel blade is used and scar tissue is carved away from nerve roots millimeter by millimeter while the surgeon constantly strives to differentiate white nerve roots from white scar tissue. This differentiation is aided by observing the fine blood vessels in the nerve roots and by observing and palpating their round configuration. A surgical laser can be used but risks cutting nerve roots or dura if it penetrates too deeply through unexpectedly thin or soft adhesions. Areas of *ossification,* or new bone formation, within the arachnoidal scar can occasionally be dissected free and removed. At times it is necessary to cut through thin plaques of ossification with heavy scissors or even with bone-cutting instruments. Care must be taken not to sever nerve roots contained within the areas of ossification when the bone is cut or when it fractures unexpectedly. Dense arachnoidal ossification that completely incorporates nerves usually cannot be safely resected. Prior to dural closure it has been my practice to instill 1 ml (80 mg) of methylprednisolone acetate (Depo-Medrol) intrathecally in hopes of limiting the formation of recurrent arachnoidal adhesions. This can be most easily accomplished by closing the dura almost completely with interrupted and running sutures of 4-0 or 5-0 neuralon, then injecting the corticosteroid with a blunt lumbar puncture (LP) needle just prior to tying the last suture. Dural closure must be watertight. Special care is necessary if thickened arachnoid has been dissected away from the dura, leaving this membrane attenuated. The dural suture line is reinforced with a thin strip of half thickness gelatin foam to promote scarring and early waterproof sealing. Autogenous fat is then left in the bony defect.

The primary *complication of microsurgical lysis of arachnoiditis* is *nerve root injury.* Nerve roots may be severed at the time of initial opening if the dural incision carries too deep and interrupts nerve roots adherent to the undersurface of the dura. Nerve roots also may be cut, torn, or contused at the time of their dissection from dense arachnoiditis or during attempted dissection of ossified arachnoid. The late onset of *hyperpathia* can be a discouraging sequel following otherwise successful lysis of adhesive arachnoiditis. Patients who experience sensory loss preoperatively may experience sufficient improvement in nerve root functioning that sensory stimuli are for the first time able to pass through the damaged area. Unfortunately, if these stimuli are transmitted in a "garbled" or distorted way, the result may be the perception of a painful stimulus. This distorted sensory perception, or *hyperpathia,* may result in either spontaneous pain or painful distortion of otherwise nonnoxious cutaneous stimuli. A third potential and serious complication is that of *CSF leakage.* This is particularly likely to occur if one attempts to strip thickened arachnoid away from dura at the site of dural incision. This may leave behind a thinned, attenuated dura that may easily tear during suturing. Even if tears do not occur, the puncture holes made by the sutures may stretch slightly, and large volumes of CSF may persistently leak from a tiny pinhole that develops at the site of suture penetration through a thinned area. The likelihood of persistent leakage may be augmented by the instilled corticosteroid because of some impairment of wound healing. The risk of CSF leakage can be limited by not dissecting thickened arachnoid away from the dura at the incision site, by meticulous dural closure, by reinforcing the dural suture line with gelatin foam, and by leaving patients at complete bed rest for a minimum of four or five days postoperatively. If CSF leakage does occur through a pinhole opening at a suture puncture site through an attenuated dura, attempting to place additional dural sutures may simply add further perforations. In this instance, repairing the CSF leak will usually require oversewing a patch or graft of autogenous fat or muscle. I do not advocate primarily closing dura with a graft or patch because, in my experience, it is usually not necessary to expand the dura to decompress nerve roots involved in arachnoiditis, and the risk of CSF leakage seems to be significantly greater when primary dural grafting is performed

Excision of Local Tender Areas

Whereas repeat laminectomy, fusion revision, and primary fusion are the three most frequently executed operations performed on failed back syndrome sufferers, *excision of local tender areas* is undoubtedly the least common (Fig. 7.19). Needle therapy of various types on focally tender sites was discussed under corticosteroid and anesthetic injections of local tender areas and prolotherapy in Chapter 6. In that discussion it was pointed out that needle therapy often provides optimum therapy for many of these conditions. Indeed, local needle therapy with adrenal corticosteroids or prolotherapy often works better than all of the noninvasive therapies and usually works sufficiently well to preclude surgical intervention. Unfortunately, needle therapy often brings the patient relief lasting for only two to three months, rather than effecting a permanent cure. A series of needle injections, coupled with back-strengthening exercises to toughen the area, may gradually bring permanent relief or may continue to bring prolonged intervals of relief. Most patients who obtain excellent relief lasting several months following each needle procedure are content to receive repeated needle therapy rather than contemplate further surgical intervention. A few patients tire of the necessity of repeated needle therapy and request direct surgery. If these patients have consistently suffered with a single focally painful site and have consistently achieved short-term relief from anesthetization or other needle therapy, it is not unreasonable to consider *en bloc* resection of these foci. I have on very few occasions resected two such types of focally tender and painful foci: fusion bone donor sites and trigger points. Scar tissue that forms along the posterior iliac crest at the site of resection of fusion donor bone may contain single or multiple painful neuromata. Trigger points usually prove to be nearly normal histologically, showing principally the scarring that has resulted from previous needle therapy but rarely, if ever, showing neuroma formation. Extremely thin patients who develop focal trigger points over extremely prominent posterior iliac spinous processes seem to be particularly distressed by them, presumably largely because of their lack of local padding. It is these patients who seem most often to request local surgical resection. Surgical resection of focally tender and painful sites can be extremely gratifying, as illustrated by Case 13 on page 163. Unfortunately, not all cases respond so well, as the following report illustrates:

Case 18

This 57-year-old woman was referred from another state after having undergone three laminectomies, spinal fusions, and revisions of spinal fusions over the preceding nine years. In the four years since her last operation she remained disabled for work, although

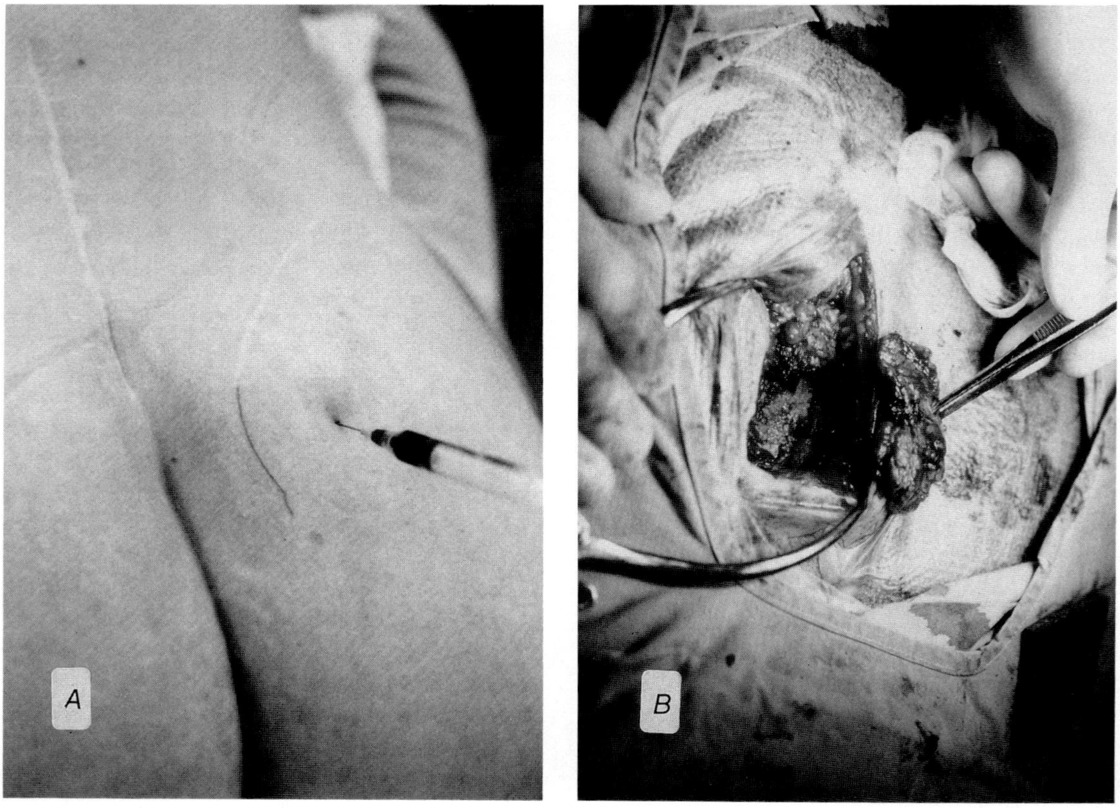

FIGURE 7.19. Excision of painful local tender areas is indicated on rare occasions. **A:** Injection of the center of the tender area with blue dye prior to anesthetizing the patient. In this case, the tender area was the donor site for fusion bone in a woman who had received good temporary relief after each of a long series of steroid and prolotherapy injections at this site. **B:** An en bloc resection of the blue-stained material, including the periosteum. Microscopically, this tissue contained several small neuromas.

she was able to do occasional shopping or other chores. She continued to take dihydrocodeinone compound (Percodan) several times a day and meperidine (Demerol) several times a week chiefly because of pain localized over the right sacrum. When examined in office consultation she had exquisite and sharply focal tenderness at the site of her maximum pain, approximately overlying the right sacroiliac joint. At that same office visit the area of maximum tenderness was locally infiltrated with 6 ml of 1% lidocaine (Xylocaine), 4 ml of 0.5% bupivacaine (Marcaine), and 1 ml (40 mg) of methylprednisolone acetate (Depo-Medrol). She reported dramatic and almost total relief of pain for the first time in years. Immediately following anesthetization of this trigger point she could bend forward to touch mid shins, previously having been able to bend forward only to touch her knees. Follow-up reports from the patient and from her referring physician in her home state documented that she obtained approximately one month of excellent pain relief following this injection. Her referring physician attempted to repeat the injection but achieved only partial pain relief.

The patient requested local resection of her trigger point and, largely because of the distance involved, I agreed to undertake this surgery. Prior to induction of general anesthesia, the area of maximum local tenderness was identified by palpation and by needle insertion. Indigo carmine dye (0.5 ml) was injected into the center of the painful area. Surgical exploration and subsequent histologic examination revealed no obvious abnormality of the resected block of tissue other than the deep blue staining from the injected dye. Immediately postoperatively she complained of severe local pain but by six days after surgery she had weaned herself from narcotics and reported good improvement in spontaneous pain and pain on attempted bending. Initial reports following her return home were quite optimistic. Unfortunately, within three months following trigger point resection she reported that her original pain had returned in full severity.

The surgical *technique for resection of focally tender and painful sites* is essentially that which was briefly described in Case 18. The target area should be identified prior to induction of general or spinal anesthesia both by palpation and by needle insertion. Ideally, local anesthetization should be carried out as further confirmation. With the area identified in this fashion, blue dye, usually indigo carmine, can be injected as an aid to subsequent local *en bloc* resection. Since trigger points commonly involve periosteum at the site of muscle attachments, this periosteum should be included in the resection. For thin patients with prominent posterior iliac spines, the spinous processes may be flattened with osteotomes and curettes. Muscle reattachment is probably facilitated by not using bone wax generously but by controlling bone bleeding with gelatin foam or other absorbable anticoagulant materials.

The *complications of such resections* are essentially those of wound infections and local hemorrhage. The *major limitation of these resections* is that they may fail to relieve pain and may cause additional local pain and tenderness because of the periosteal disruption that is involved.

Dorsal Column Stimulator Implantation

Dorsal column stimulation (DCS) provides pain relief through *competitive sensory stimulation* of the dorsal fibers of the spinal cord, which transmit tactile and postural information.[100-103] DCS implantation offers carefully selected patients with failed back syndromes the possibility of pain relief without destruction of nervous tissue and with relatively limited risk. The outcome of DCS implantation is generally better in patients who have obtained at least partial pain relief from *transcutaneous stimulation (TNS)* and seems especially applicable to those patients with widespread back and bilateral leg pain in whom the scope of TNS is not sufficiently wide to relieve the entire painful area. Patients with symptomatic adhesive arachnoiditis or patients who remain severely symptomatic despite extensive surgery and stable fusions are most commonly selected for this technique.

DCS electrodes can be *inserted percutaneously or by open surgical laminotomy* and can be attached to temporary external connections for testing prior to permanent implantation. The simpler technique of *percutaneous electrode placement with temporary externalization* permits preliminary testing of the adequacy of pain relief before committing the patient to more extensive surgery for implantation of a costly internalized device. Unfortunately, two major problems restrict the usefulness of this technique. Despite all precautions, the temporary percutaneous device carries a distinct risk of sepsis. Equally important is that the easily placed percutaneous electrodes do not maintain their position well relative to the spinal cord and tend to shift as the patient resumes a more active life-style, thus losing their effectiveness.

The alternative surgical technique, which I prefer, is to proceed directly with *permanent implantation* once the patient has been determined to be a reasonable candidate, based in large part on the patient's prior response to TNS. Patients who obtain no pain relief whatsoever from TNS have a much reduced chance of obtaining benefit from an implanted system. The epidural stimulating electrode is implanted through a short low thoracic skin incision. One very satisfactory electrode system consists of four small contact plates in a ribbon of Silastic rubber. This can be inserted obliquely in the epidural space across the dorsum of the spinal cord in the low thoracic region from a laminotomy on one side to a laminotomy at a higher level on the opposite side. The combination of four contacts allows a variety of stimulation patterns. The wires from the electrode are tunnelled subcutaneously around the chest to a subcutaneously created pocket over the lower anterior rib cage. Alternatively, the wires may be tunnelled over the shoulder or around the upper thorax above the breast to a pocket in the pectoral area. Either a receiver/transducer or a self-powered stimulating unit is then attached to the electrode wires and implanted in the subcutaneous pocket. Many surgeons prefer to use local anesthesia with light neuroleptanalgesia for DCS implantation rather than general anesthesia. Having the patient awake during the procedure allows intraoperative stimulation for confirmation of electrode placement but requires a cooperative patient and may increase the risk of wound infection by increasing the complexity and duration of the operation.

The *implanted systems themselves vary widely.* The simpler systems involve a single fixed output to one channel, so one pair of electrodes must be preselected through external testing, through manipulation of the electrodes under local anesthesia, or through reliance on anatomical probability. Other systems provide for multiple channels or selection of different channels after implantation. The unit that is implanted may be either a radio receiver/transducer or a battery-powered self-contained unit. The receiver/transducer units are powered by externally applied antennae, and stimulus parameters are easily set by the patient using the power transmitter, which operates through the antenna. Although this can be more inconvenient than the completely implanted battery-powered systems, the need for surgical intervention to change batteries is obviated. Under normal usage, batteries generally last several years. Stimulus parameters and power output can be changed on the battery-powered implanted systems through a transcutaneous control device. If the patient is to control the stimulus parameters, this entails purchase of an extra and expensive unit; alternatively, all settings can be made by the surgeon or his designee. The battery-powered units can be turned on and off with a simple magnet held in proximity to the device.

Complications from DCS implantation include sepsis, spinal cord compression, device failure, or pain or discomfort. As mentioned earlier, infection is a major consideration in percutaneously tested systems, but any chronically implanted device has the potential for early or later infection, usually necessitating removal of the device, particularly when there is a deep infection. Occasionally the electrode has elicited a fibrous reaction, possibly related to the tearing of small epidural vessels, which has caused later spinal cord compression. This rare complication requires removal of the electrodes and decompression of the epidural mass. *Device failure* is most commonly encountered when simple electrodes shift their position. Even well-placed and permanently secured electrodes will give varying results depending on patient posture. As the patient bends forward or backward, the spinal cord moves within the subarachnoid space, moving either closer to or further from the epidural stimulating electrode. Although this is rarely a major problem, it can be annoying to some patients, especially those who have to change positions frequently. A progressive failure to produce pain relief does not necessarily imply device failure, especially if the patient continues to obtain sensory input. On the other hand, a progressive fading of sensory awareness of stimulator input can be due to epidural fibrosis, interruption of implanted wires, corrosion of contacts, or failure of the implanted receiver or battery-powered generator. Relatively inexpensive devices are available for percutaneous measurements of the output of the implanted device, but confirmation and correction of the problem often require surgical intervention. A number of patients request removal of the device because of discomfort or pain, especially if the original pain for which the device was implanted has not been adequately controlled. Patients commonly experience pain either at the site of electrode penetration into the spine or from the subcutaneous bulk of the implanted receiver or generator. Subcutaneous implantation of the receiver or generator over the upper chest or lower rib cage is preferable to subcutaneous implantation over the abdomen, where the device can be painfully compressed by the rib cage on trunk flexion. At any location, compression by constricting clothing, especially belts or brassieres, can provoke discomfort, and this consideration should also influence device placement.

Implantation of Epidural or Subdural Catheters and Pumps

The technique of temporary placement of epidural or subarachnoid catheters for intraspinal injection of morphine or other agents was discussed in Chapter 6.[104] *Permanent implantation of such catheters with implanted pump systems* permits long-term therapy with morphine or other agents in those patients who obtain useful results from temporary infusions. Currently both the Medtronic Corporation and the Infusaid Corporation manufacture fully implantable pump systems. Each version has a reservoir that can be refilled by percutaneous needling, allowing one to two weeks of administration. The catheter is placed epidurally or intrathecally in the lumbar spinal canal through a side-hold Touhey spinal puncture needle after making a small skin incision. Some surgeons prefer direct surgical exposure of the dura through a small bony opening if the catheter is to be placed intrathecally, since this permits placement of a purse-string suture at the dural penetration site. The catheter is tunnelled subcutaneously around the trunk to be attached to the pump, which is inserted into a subcutaneous pocket over the lower rib cage anteriorly. Subarachnoid catheter placement permits the administration of smaller narcotic doses than those required for epidural administration but carries a risk of CSF leakage. Preservative-free morphine, now fairly readily available, has been the most widely used agent for pain relief, though a variety of other agents have been studied. Baclofen (Lioresal) seems to have a useful role in long-term relief of spasticity and may have a useful role in centrally mediated deafferentation pain.[105]

As with temporary catheters, *sepsis remains the major risk* of epidural or subarachnoid catheter and pump system placement. *Careful sterile technique* must be followed in percutaneous refilling of pump reservoirs as well as at the time of surgical implantation. Drug concentrations and doses must be carefully selected, and the dose to be administered must be carefully formulated. Overdosage can cause respiratory arrest, and chemical or bacterial contamination can cause spinal injury or infection. Initial test doses must be given with the patient under close supervision to avoid the risk of oversedation or respiratory depression. Drug formulation and reservoir refilling must be carried out by professional personnel or by carefully trained family members. This requirement for reservoir refilling, generally at intervals of one to three weeks, is one of the major limitations of the use of implantable pump systems, since the process is relatively labor intensive. This can pose a particular problem for patients who live at a distance from the implanting facility or who do not have available competent family members. Fully implantable pump systems are generally expensive, and earlier pump versions resulted in numerous reports of *pump failure or unreliability.* Apparently this failure rate of the devices accounted for some of the early pessimism regarding habituation to long-term administration of epidural morphine, though this remains a significant potential limitation. Before reliable mechanical pumps were readily available, manually activated systems were more commonly implanted, consisting of a subcutaneous and refillable reservoir with a manual pump (often a valve system used for hydrocephalic shunting). These devices were subject to considerable patient error and the possibility of overdosage through accidental overcompression of the reservoir.

Sensory Rhizotomy and Neurectomy

Of the neuroablative procedures for pain relief, the most commonly performed for patients with failed back syndromes are those that involve sectioning of nerve roots. *Sensory rhizotomy,* or *sectioning of the dorsal sensory roots of lumbar or sacral nerves,* holds a traditional, albeit somewhat controversial, role in the management of pain problems. *Facet neurectomy,* or *surgical interruption of nerves supplying the facet joints,* is a more recent addition to the neurosurgeon's armamentarium and is even more controversial than surgical sensory rhizotomy. Percutaneous needle approaches to interruption of these facet nerves have been more favorably received than open surgical section, as discussed under facet nerve injections in Chapter 6.

Surgical Sensory Rhizotomy

Although *surgical sensory rhizotomy* in the lumbar area has been used by neurosurgeons for many decades, the operation remains controversial because of differing reports about its effectiveness in relieving pain.[106,107] Published results vary, with successful outcomes ranging from a low of 25% to a high of 80%. The indications for surgical sensory rhizotomy obviously vary from surgeon to surgeon. At least theoretically, surgical sensory rhizotomy should be reserved for *patients with unilateral sciatica.* The more localized the patient's pain, the greater the expectation that sensory rhizotomy will bring relief. That actual or observed results are so frequently disappointing attests to the complexity of pain and the need for great caution and careful diagnostic studies in attempting to select patients for this destructive type of pain-relieving surgery. I have generally reserved this form of surgery for patients whose pain seems to be transmitted into the nervous system exclusively, or almost entirely, by one or two lumbar nerve roots and in whom nonoperative therapy or reparative or restorative surgical therapy has failed to produce satisfactory pain relief. The clinical impression of pain transmission by one or two lumbar nerve roots is usually based on the history and physical examination, radiographic studies, and diagnostic needle procedures. The history should be consistent with unilateral sciatica with relatively little back pain. Patients with bilateral sciatica or significant back pain rarely obtain relief from either unilateral or bilateral sensory rhizotomy. Sciatica that is associated with symptoms and physical findings suggesting nerve root entrapment should be carefully evaluated to exclude treatable conditions, such as recurrent disc rupture or epidural scar, before subjecting the patient to destructive surgery. Sciatica that is consistent with neuralgic origin (i.e., pain that is more or less constant and burning or tingling in character) should be treated first with antineuralgia therapy before advocating rhizotomy. The physical examination will suggest one or two levels of nerve root involvement if motor, sensory, and reflex findings are confined to one or two segmental levels. Patients who exhibit no motor, sensory, or reflex abnormalities should be carefully screened for significant psychologic problems or low pain thresholds before this form of surgery is considered, though the surgeon must keep in mind that it is possible to have significant nerve pain in the absence of severe nerve damage.

The most useful radiographic study in decision making about lumbar sensory rhizotomy is *myelography.* Patients whose myelograms reveal extensive or multiple nerve root involvement, such as transverse arachnoiditis, must be viewed with great caution as potential candidates for this therapy. If multiple nerve roots are involved, it is highly unlikely that sectioning one or two sensory nerve roots will satisfactorily relieve the patient's pain, so long as pain input continues from other sensory nerves. A myelographic, CT, or MRI abnormality at a single level that is consistent with disc rupture should also signal the need for caution in contemplating surgical sensory rhizotomy, since this patient may suffer from a potentially surgically correctable process such as recurrent disc rupture or focal arachnoiditis. If such an abnormality persists, despite secondary exploratory laminectomy, the likelihood of etiologically significant focal arachnoiditis becomes great. As discussed on page 201, the surgical decision between attempted lysis of arachnoiditis versus surgical sensory rhizotomy then becomes an extremely difficult one to make—a decision that must involve the patient's full comprehension and active participation.

I have insisted on careful *diagnostic nerve blocks* in all patients considered for surgical sensory rhizotomy, even though I share with many of my neurosurgical colleagues a strong impression of the fallibility of these studies as predictors of satisfactory surgical outcome. *Intrathecal anesthetics* (see page 108) rarely interrupt sensory transmission exclusively in one or two nerve roots. Even if the neurologic examination at the time of diagnostic intrathecal block demonstrates objective sensory loss almost exclusively in the expected territory of one or two nerve roots, there is usually at least some sensory interruption in adjacent nerve roots as well. Likewise, *epidural, periradicular nerve root blocks* (see page 105) may cause some "spillover" sensory loss in adjacent nerve roots, but carefully performed epidural root blocks seem to provide the most reliable correlation with surgical outcome. This type of block may be difficult if not impossible to perform in the presence of spinal fusion, and severe epidural scarring may preclude the attainment of high-grade sensory loss in the desired one or two nerve roots. *Paraspinal nerve root blocks* performed lateral to the neural foramina usually produce quite specifically radicular sensory loss, more or less limited to the nerve root or roots that have been injected. Unfortunately, the value of the greater precision that this form of diagnostic nerve block provides may be partly negated by the fact that the block may be performed lateral (or distal) to the site of the pain. As a result, a failure to relieve pain by paraspinal nerve block, despite achievement of excellent monoradicular or biradicular sensory loss, may be observed in patients who nonetheless achieve excellent pain relief following surgical intradural sensory rhizotomy. Of course, even excellent pain relief produced by temporary anesthetic blocks may not correctly predict long-term pain relief, as discussed on page 108 and later in this chapter.

The question of *how many sensory roots to section* is quite troublesome. In my experience, relatively few of the patients considered as candidates for surgical sensory rhizotomy can be assumed to suffer sciatic pain that is transmitted exclusively through a single sensory nerve root on the basis of history, physical examination, myelography, and diagnostic needle procedures. Those patients in whom all of these four categories are in agreement as suggesting monoradicular pain should be offered single-level surgical sensory rhizotomy. Perhaps some of the patients who fail to obtain adequate relief from single-level rhizotomy would obtain relief from a second-level rhizotomy, but my experience with second-level rhizotomy is quite small and largely disappointing, and the medical literature is of little help on this particular question.

Although I consider myself conservative in the number of surgical sensory rhizotomies that I perform, I most commonly section two sensory nerves once I undertake rhizotomy. This tactic is based on my observation that the majority of patients to whom I offer this operation have symptoms that suggest the possibility of involvement of more than one sensory nerve root. Furthermore, I have observed over the years that sectioning two adjacent sensory nerves produces surprisingly limited peripheral sensory loss and rarely causes significant disability for the patient. The complications that I have observed following this operation do not seem to be particularly more severe following sectioning of two nerve roots than following sectioning of a single nerve root.

Is surgical sectioning of three sensory roots ever justified? Perhaps so, but only in those patients who have obtained good to excellent temporary or short-lived pain relief from needle procedures that seem to have interrupted three adjacent lumbar nerve roots, yet who have failed to obtain adequate pain relief from interruption of two adjacent nerve roots. There are several reasons for caution in recommending three-level sensory rhizotomy. First, pain that is transmitted into the central nervous system (CNS) over this widespread area is even more likely to be refractory to focal interruption at the nerve root level, both because it is highly likely that even more nerve roots are involved and because the complex organization of the sensory portion of the nervous system makes it more likely that pain of this widespread origin will continue to find access into the CNS or will persist as central deafferentation pain. Second, the price paid by the patient is likely to be significantly greater following three-level sensory rhizotomy than following two-level rhizotomy. Although these patients still exhibit surprisingly limited areas of cutaneous hypalgesia and frequently never develop any lasting areas of analgesia or total loss of pain perception, they are nonetheless much more likely to experience difficulty with trophic skin ulcers and ankle instability due to impaired proprioception.

The chief advantage of surgical sensory rhizotomy is the prospect of *lasting pain relief.* Patients who have failed to obtain satisfactory relief from noninvasive therapy, including antineuralgia drugs, and who have obtained good to excellent relief, but not permanent relief, from needle procedures often find the prospect of surgical interruption of sensory nerve roots an attractive possible means of obtaining lasting relief. The following case report documents a successful recovery from a failed back syndrome, with therapy that included surgical sensory rhizotomy (Fig. 7.20):

Case 19

This 37-year-old sales representative underwent L5-S1 left discectomy in 1966 with excellent results until he reinjured his back while lifting in December 1979. He developed severe low back and left leg pain and numbness in his left foot and calf. He improved somewhat with chiropractic treatments, then hospitalization for pelvic traction. Five weeks later, symptoms rapidly increased while he was driving. He was referred to the University of Massachusetts Medical Center, where examination showed that straight leg raising to 10 degrees on the left caused severe radiating leg pain. There was hypalgesia of lateral left calf and ankle and absent left ankle reflex. Myelogram disclosed a large left lateral defect at L5-S1. He was treated with rest, systemic dexamethasone (Decadron), diazepam (Valium), and methocarbamol (Robaxin) for muscle relaxation, but with only slight benefit. At surgery in February 1980, encapsulated free fragments of disc material were discovered adherent to the left S1 nerve root. Initial recovery was dramatically rapid, and excellent improvement continued for the next month.

Severe pain soon recurred in his left leg and lower back. Examination was almost identical to his initial examination except that the bowstring test was now positive. He was afebrile with normal white count, but sedimentation rate was elevated to 54. He was treated with oral methylprednisolone (Medrol) without benefit. The L5-S1 disc space was aspirated and barbotaged with saline, but cultures were negative. Barbotage was painful, and intradiscal methylprednisolone acetate (Depo-Medrol) injection brought a marked reduction in his back pain over a period of several days, but severe sciatica persisted. Hydantoin (Dilantin) and thiamine as a neuralgia regimen and TNS both gave only partial relief. At repeat operation in March 1980, the previously placed epidural fat pad had been replaced by dense scar tissue. Intradural exploration showed a few fine adhesions only. Cultures of the wound and disc space were again negative. Methylprednisolone acetate was left intradurally and in the disc space. Postoperatively, relief was again dramatic. Unfortunately, two weeks later, after he had discontinued Dilantin and after depository steroids had worn off, sciatica gradually recurred and again became severe. He was treated with carbamazepine (Tegretol) and enteric-coated salicylates, with some improvement in sciatica.

Within a month of his intradiscal steroid injection, low back pain again recurred and became severe, despite substitution of sulindac (Clinoril) for salicylates. Repeat intradiscal injection of methylprednisolone in April 1980 again improved back pain significantly, although sciatica remained quite troublesome. Hydantoin was added to the neuralgia regimen without signif-

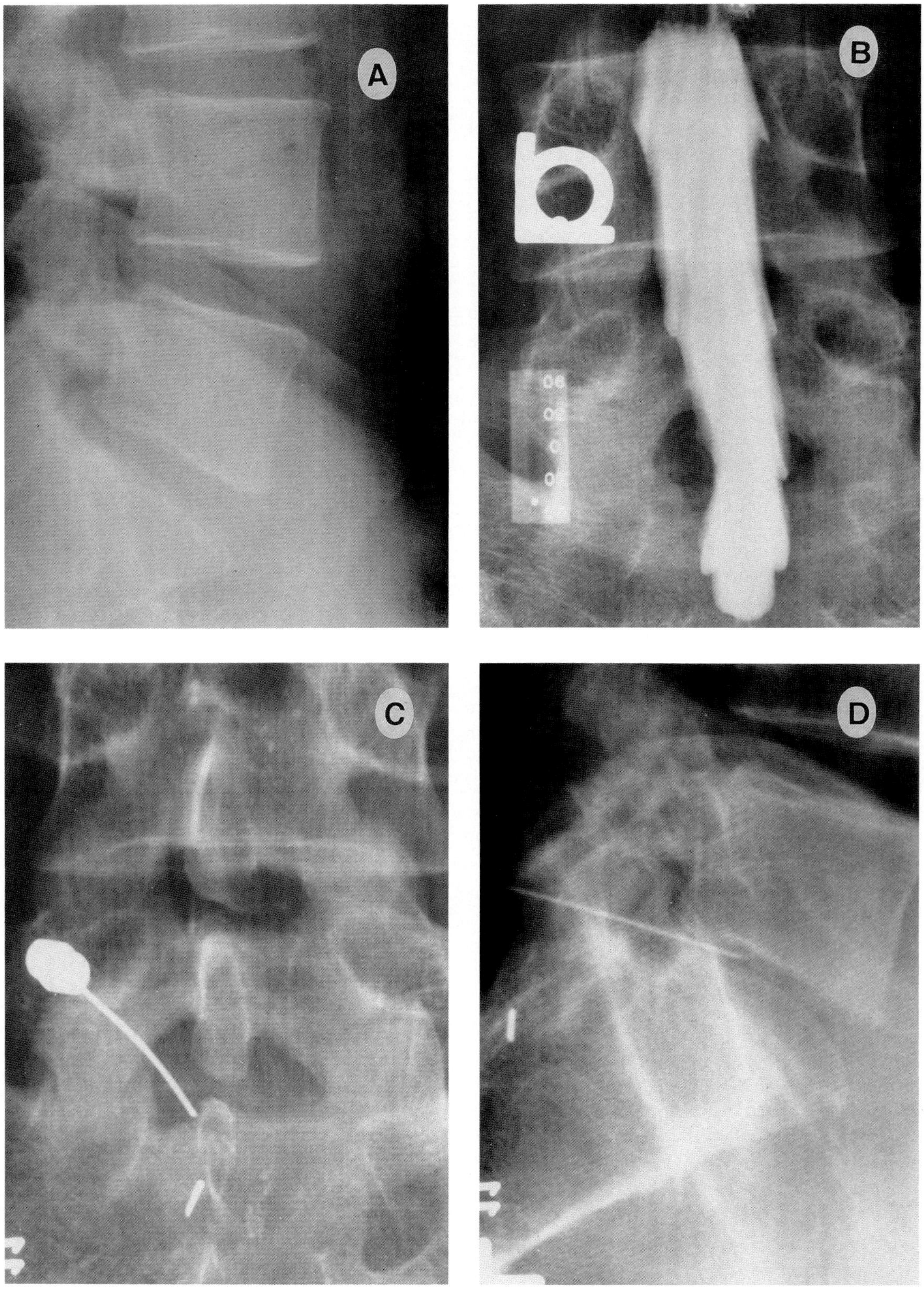
A
B
C
D

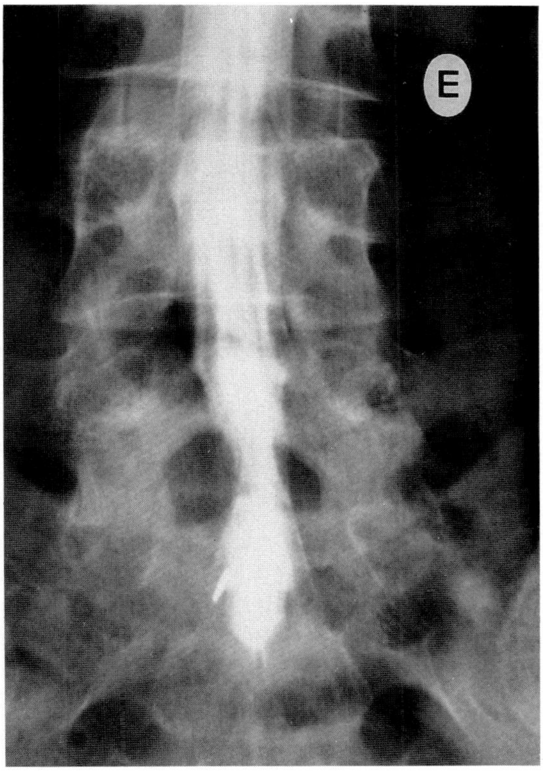

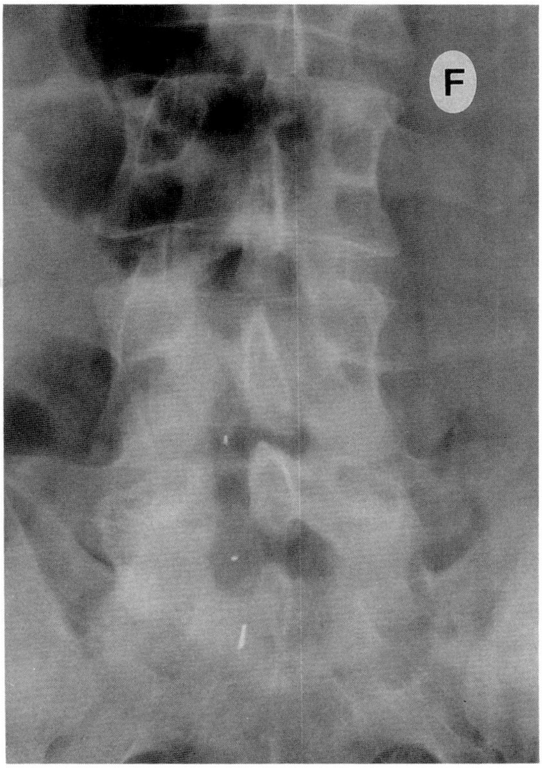

FIGURE 7.20. These radiographs document the successful restoration of the patient discussed as Case 19. **A:** Plain radiographs in January 1980 were normal with little evidence of his previous disc surgery. **B:** A myelogram done on his first University of Massachusetts hospitalization showed a large left anterolateral defect at L5-S1. **C and D:** After he developed severe, delayed, postoperative low back pain, L5-S1 disc aspiration and barbotage (by way of posterior approach) was culture negative, and intradiscal anesthetic and steroids gave dramatic improvement. **E:** Sciatica became progressively more severe and repeat myelogram in March 1980 again showed a large defect at L5-S1 on the left. Surgery disclosed severe epidural scarring and filmy arachnoiditis intrathecally. **F:** Ultimately surgical sensory rhizotomy was required, and gave excellent and lasting relief of sciatica. Surgical defect and metal clips on the distal cut ends of the L5 and S1 nerve roots can be seen. Additional intradiscal steroid injections were required for control of low back pain before the inflammatory discitis gradually "burned out" and became asymptomatic. **G:** This radiograph in September 1981 shows sclerosis and collapse of the L5-S1 interspace at a time when the patient had been asymptomatic and actively working for nearly a year.

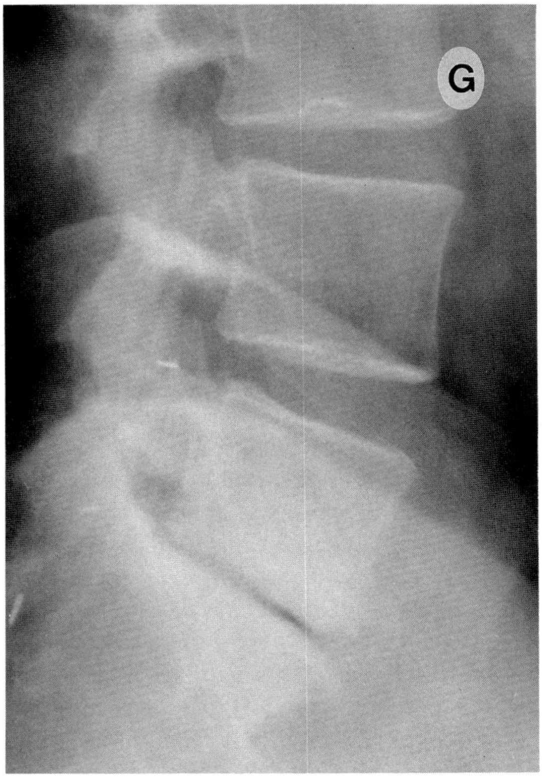

icant improvement in sciatica. In June 1980, he was again hospitalized with intractable sciatica. Repeat myelogram showed a small defect at L5-S1 on the left. Two attempts at intrathecal phenol sensory rhizotomy were unable to produce lasting sensory loss or pain relief, even though initially the dosage was pushed to the point of transient weakness of plantar flexion. At reoperation, dense epidural fibrosis was again discovered. Histologically, this tissue contained multiple foreign granulomas. L5 and S1 nerve roots were densely bound in localized arachnoiditis intradurally. Surgical sensory rhizotomies were performed at both roots, and histologic examination showed perineural scarring. Methylprednisolone was again placed intradiscally. Postoperatively, leg pain was almost completely gone and back pain remained dramatically improved for approximately six weeks.

In July 1980, low back pain recurred again and became progressively more severe. On an outpatient basis he was given his fifth injection of intradiscal methylprednisolone, again with excellent improvement in lower back pain. One month later he required aspirin only for pain relief, and occasionally used his corset during periods of activity.

He was able to return to work in September 1980, even though this involved extensive driving. One year later he had resumed sports activities, remained fully employed, and required only occasional nonnarcotic anodynes. Follow-up radiographs of his back showed apparent spontaneous fusion of the L5-S1 interspace.

Patients must be cautioned that the most careful clinical assessment does not guarantee pain relief. Furthermore, the ability to produce excellent temporary relief by nerve root anesthetization does not guarantee that this relief can be made permanent, because of the *dynamic nature of the nervous system*. With interruption of one pathway, the central pain neurons that have been deprived of input gradually lower their threshold and become even more sensitive to pain input from alternative pathways. As a result, some patients who obtain excellent pain relief following surgical sensory rhizotomy will become late failures because of delayed recurrence of pain. These patients can at least be offered the possibility of ameliorating this late failure through the use of systemic antineuralgia medications or periradicular, epidural steroid injection.

The chief disadvantage of surgical sensory rhizotomy is that it commonly *fails to provide the desired pain relief*. The failure to relieve pain may result from a surgical complication or improper patient selection or simply may reflect the surgeon's limited ability to interrupt the complex anatomy of pain transmission. When failure occurs as a surgical complication, it is likely to be secondary to either sectioning of sensory fibers at the wrong nerve root or failure to section all of the sensory fibers of the proper nerve root. Careful preoperative diagnostic needle procedures and careful intraoperative nerve root identification anatomically and electrically should minimize the risk of improper nerve root identification. Careful inspection of the nerve root under magnified vision in a search for multiple sensory fiber bundles and careful electrical stimulation of each nerve root bundle should help to minimize the risk of incomplete sectioning of sensory rootlets.

As discussed earlier, *cutaneous sensory loss* is an inherent part of the procedure, but for most patients this is of little consequence. For one thing, the overlapping distribution of peripheral nerves is so great that patients almost never exhibit analgesia or complete loss of pain perception, much less anesthesia or complete loss of all sensation, even following three-level sensory rhizotomy. Following monoradicular sensory rhizotomy, even hypalgesia may be difficult to document. Furthermore, most patients who are candidates for this procedure already exhibit some degree of peripheral sensory loss, and most patients are not greatly troubled by the small amount of sensory loss they develop postsurgically—if they develop any detectable additional loss at all. Even if cutaneous sensory loss is limited, many patients note the effect of *proprioceptive interruption* from the ankle, especially following two-level and three-level rhizotomy. This is usually quickly compensated for following two-level and even three-level sensory rhizotomy, but may remain as a persistently limiting ankle instability, especially in walking on rough ground or at night.

The *technique of surgical sensory rhizotomy* varies from surgeon to surgeon (Fig. 7.21). Most commonly, the sensory rootlets are divided intradurally, but a few neurosurgeons prefer an *extradural sectioning* of the sensory rootlets. Extradural sensory rhizotomy requires less bone removal and offers the prospect of more accurate identification of the involved nerve root, since the nerve root is exposed at the site of previous discectomy and through essentially the same laminotomy or partial hemilaminectomy used for the original operative procedure. In the proximal part of the extradural nerve root, sensory fibers are still completely segregated from the motor fibers and lie in the dorsal half of the nerve

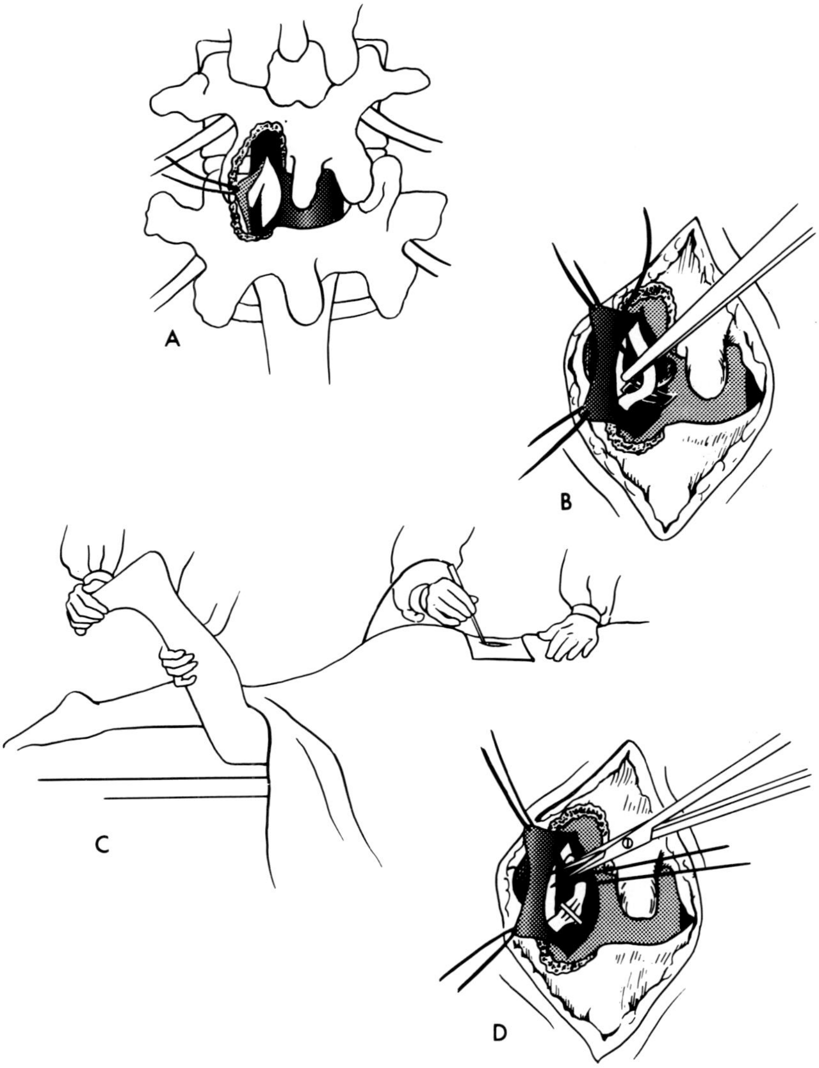

FIGURE 7.21. Surgical sensory rhizotomy may be quite beneficial in carefully selected patients with intractable sciatica. **A:** Surgery begins with laminectomy and dural incision to expose the target nerve root both intradurally and extradurally. **B:** Individual rootlets of the target nerve root are separated and the one or two dorsal rootlets, presumed to be sensory rootlets, are elevated on a fine suture passed beneath the rootlets with a blunt-end-to tiny needle. **C:** Each individual rootlet is then electrically stimulated while a circulator or assistant tests for distal motor movement. **D:** Having confirmed that the proper nerve root has been exposed and that sensory rootlets have been separated from motor rootlets, the rootlets are sectioned with a surgical laser or with microscissors.

root. In an anatomically normal extradural nerve root, the plane of separation between the motor and sensory components can usually be identified relatively easily although this may be difficult in the presence of significant local scarring. Once the separation between sensory and motor fibers is identified by inspection or palpation of the extradural nerve root, the dorsal half of the nerve root is sectioned until the plane of cleavage between the two components is fully visualized. Care must be taken to avoid spinal fluid leakage through sectioning too proximally or close to the thecal sac. Of course, if intradural scarring is also present, as I have commonly found to be the case, one must be concerned whether sectioning peripheral to the site of involvement will prove adequate for pain relief. Certainly, the sectioned nerve root will degenerate in its entirety proximal to the point of incision, but not inspecting the nerve root intradurally may leave undisclosed a significant involvement of adjacent nerve roots, which should be treated by either neurolysis or rhizotomy.

The performance of *intradural sensory rhizotomy* requires more bone removal than simple discectomy, because the nerve root must be identified intradurally rostral to the point of extradural injury or entrapment. Some surgeons prefer to remove the entire lamina of one or even two spinal levels above the point of presumed maximum nerve root involvement, usually the level of previous disc surgery. My preference is to remove only a single hemilamina for each level of rhizotomy that is planned. High-powered loupes will suffice, but the operating room microscope makes it possible for the assistant to see as well as the surgeon. Once the dura has been exposed through laminectomy or removal of overlying fusion bone (see page 187), meticulous extradural hemostasis should be obtained using bipolar coagulation of epidural veins. Epidural packing with thrombin-soaked cottonoids should be kept to a minimum, because this will distort the thecal space. The dura is incised rostrocaudally beginning at the rostral or previously unexposed end, where thecal anatomy is more likely to be normal and not distorted by scar tissue. If possible, I try to leave the arachnoid unruptured until dural opening is completed. This provides some extra protection to nerve roots and allows one to place dural tenting sutures as an aid to continued epidural hemostasis prior to collapsing the thecal sac through evacuation of spinal fluid. To minimize excessive CSF loss and postoperative headache, intradural rhizotomy should be done with the patient in a prone jackknife position with head and thorax lower than lumbar spine.

After the arachnoid is opened, the surgeon must *identify the proper nerve root*. The nerve roots normally enter dural pouches intradurally several millimeters rostral to the extradural point at which they become definable as separate nerve roots. I do not attempt extensive extradural nerve root dissection, but I find it helpful to attempt to identify the nerve root extradurally as an aid to intradural localization of the proper root. This is especially important when localized arachnoidal scarring is present, causing obliteration of intradural root pouches and at times obscuring nerve roots in opaque scar. Additional confirmation can be obtained through *electrical stimulation* of motor roots. For this to be done effectively, the patient must be capable of motor response. The anesthesiologist should be careful not to administer curare or other potent muscle-relaxing medications. Electrical stimulation is done by separating the target nerve root into motor and sensory components. Usually the dorsal and ventral halves of the nerve are readily apparent, but not uncommonly three or four bundles of rootlets are identified. In this instance it is safest to isolate each bundle for individual electrical stimulation. I have found it useful to separate these fibers by passing beneath them the blunt end of a fine needle with wedged-on 5-0 dural closure neuralon. These sutures should not be secured with clamps, but safely can be secured to retractors with small dabs of bone wax. Each segment of the nerve root should be separated by inserting 3×4 mm *microcottonoids* between the individual bundles. A fine electrical stimulator probe attached to a variable power stimulator is then applied to each individual nerve bundle while a circulating nurse or assistant holds the patient's foot in a neutral position beneath the drapes. It is usually wise to begin with stimulation of presumed motor nerve roots to guarantee that the patient is not paralyzed and that the stimulator is working properly. Stimulating motor root bundles should produce obvious motor responses in the foot or leg, but stimulation of the secondary rootlets should produce no motor movement unless a very high level of electrical current is employed, causing spillover into motor bundles. Observing the type of motor response that is elicited can give further confirmation of localization. Ankle plantar flexion, ankle dorsomedial dorsiflexion, and knee extension with some ankle dorsiflexion identify S1, L5, and L4 nerve roots respectively.

Once the sensory bundles have been identified, the surgeon must decide whether or not to apply *metal clip ligatures*. Occasionally, small arterioles enter in conjunction with sensory root fibers, so application of tiny metal clips distal or lateral to the point of planned sectioning may limit the risk of delayed intradural bleeding. Immediately after sectioning, a tiny arteriole may go into tight spasm. If it fails to form a firm clot, bleeding may resume several hours or days later when the vasospasm relaxes. Large metal clips or multiple clips should be avoided, because these clips usually induce significant local scar reaction. Many surgeons advise against applying clips to the proximal end of cut nerve roots for fear that this may provoke continued irritation and pain. Sensory nerve rootlets are sectioned with a surgical laser after placing a cottonoid below the area to be cut to protect the ventral nerve roots and dura. A microscissors can be used if a laser is not available, but a scissor cut does not produce the hemostasis available by using the laser. Dural closure must be performed meticulously with interrupted and running sutures of 4-0 or 5-0 silk or neuralon. The subarachnoid space should be carefully irrigated to remove all blood, since this also can aggravate local scarring. Autogenous fat is placed in the epidural space. I customarily leave gelatin foam along the suture line and in the dorsal bony defect.

Several specific *complications may follow surgical sensory rhizotomy.* These include problems that result directly from surgery and are in addition to the inherent sequelae discussed earlier as disadvantages of this procedure. Lower extremity *weakness* or *autonomic impairment* may result if motor roots are sectioned along with sensory roots. This is more likely to occur if electrical stimulation is not performed. Bowel and bladder weakness or incontinence may also result if motor fibers of the intended nerve and of adjacent more caudal nerves that pass the point of nerve root sectioning are inadvertently damaged. This can occur during dissection of arachnoidal scarring through stretching, compression, or surgical sectioning of motor or autonomic fibers. Patients will not uncommonly complain of *severe pain postoperatively* for several days (although many experience immediate and dramatic pain relief), but persistently increased pain that begins immediately postoperatively must be considered a surgical complication. This may result from damage to sensory fibers and adjacent nerve roots or from incomplete sectioning of sensory fibers in the target nerve root. This may apparently also result from denervating only a portion of the afferent pain impulses. The residual impulses that reach the spinal cord may then be distored due to an imbalance of afferent input. Severe hyperpathia and neuralgic pain may become a persistent problem if partially *deafferented, central pain-activated neurons* progressively lower their threshold and begin to fire more or less continuously as a result of collateral stimulation from adjacent afferent inputs.

With more extensive sensory rhizotomies, the possibility of *trophic ulceration* increases. Patients must be extremely careful to avoid blistering, pressure sores or trauma to partially denervated skin areas. Once skin lesions develop they are characteristically slow to heal in these areas. At times, skin ulcers may spontaneously progress despite meticulous skin care and even despite aggressive local therapy with antibiotic ointments and avoidance of weight bearing. A severe example of this complication is illustrated by the following case.

Case 20

This 37-year-old nurse came under my care in 1972 for low back and left leg pain following an automobile accident three years previously. Her initial symptoms began insidiously in 1953 and led to laminectomy and discectomy at L5-S1 three years later, after myelogram showed a complete transverse block at this level. Back pain recurred within six months, and the following year she underwent L5-S1 posterior spinal fusion with excellent relief for the next 12 years.

Following her automobile accident in 1969, back and left leg pain became progressively more severe. Myelogram showed a similar transverse obstruction at L5-S1 and a partial anterolateral defect at L4-L5 on the left. Little fusion bone could be visualized. At the time of surgery in June 1972, most of the fusion bone had reabsorbed with gross instability and persistent pseudarthrosis between the fusion bone and the lamina of L5. A small disc bulge was resected at L4-L5 and epidural neurolysis was performed at L5-S1. The posterior fusion was extended to incorporate L4 through the sacrum. Back and leg pain was only partially improved and again gradually increased. During this interval she developed progressive cervical radiculopathy with triceps weakness, atrophy, and reflex loss. Anterior cervical discectomy and fusion gave lasting relief of this problem.

In the spring of 1973, flexion/extension back radiographs suggested pseudarthrosis. Repeat myelogram had changed little from her myelogram one year before. Surgery in April 1973 documented partial resorption of fusion bone with instability. Epidural neurolysis was performed, and she was re-fused using local and sacral bone. Following surgery, severe back and left leg pain persisted and again gradually increased in severity. She failed to respond to anti-inflammatory drugs, antineuralgia drugs, or TNS. Intrathecal and epidural steroids gave only temporary relief. In November 1973, fusion was extended to a posterolateral fusion of L4 to sacrum and surgical sensory rhizotomies were performed at S1 and S2 nerve roots. Again, she failed to obtain permanent relief, although she obtained transient improvement following each of a series of intrathecal steroid injections. She continued to complain of pain primarily in the dorsomedial aspect of her foot, at the margin of her area of sensory loss. L5 extradural nerve block seemed to give excellent relief of this residual pain.

In April 1974, an additional sensory rhizotomy of the L5 root was performed, with resection of additional bundles from the remaining S1 nerve root. Unfortunately, severe burning leg and buttock pain persisted. After consultation with another neurosurgeon, right anterolateral thoracic cordotomy was performed in October 1974. This produced good analgesia of the entire left lower extremity and trunk but only about 20% pain reduction. Six months later she required psychiatric hospitalization for severe depression with suicidal ideation. She responded well enough to return to work several months later with the aid of psychotropic drugs, despite persistent leg and buttock pain.

In the summer of 1975, she noted ulcers on the lower aspect of her right toe and foot that were slow to heal. The toe ulcer proved particularly intractable. A lumbar sympathectomy performed by a vascular surgeon improved the warmth of her foot but failed to improve healing of the ulcer and caused an increase in leg pain. Osteomyelitis developed in the toe and amputation of the toe was required in January 1976. Unfortunately, the stump of her amputation failed to heal properly and osteomyelitis in the foot and ankle were diagnosed. A below-the-knee amputation was performed in March 1977, and surgical revision of stump infection was required the following month. She was eventually able to return to work with a prosthesis, but continued to complain of burning pain in her left buttock and lower extremity. The pain was said to be aggravated by activity but not relieved by rest. Various antineuralgia drugs failed to bring relief, and symptoms persisted until she was lost to follow-up in the fall of 1978.

Facet Neurectomy

The *indications for facet neurectomy* were discussed under facet nerve injections in Chapter 6, which dealt with percutaneous needle procedures for facet neurectomy using sclerosing chemicals or

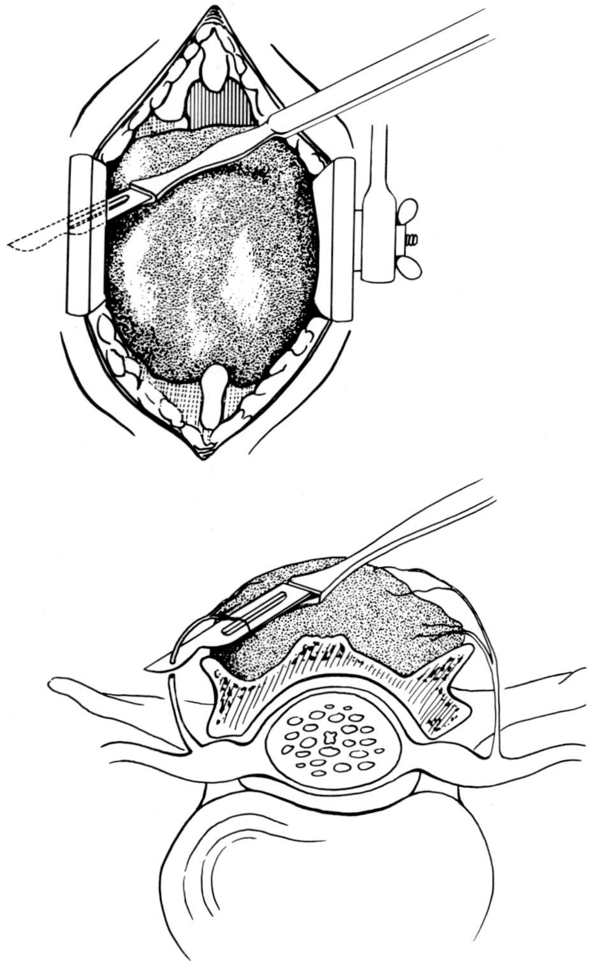

FIGURE 7.22. Facet rhizotomy is probably rarely justified as a separate operation, but may be a useful contribution at the time of primary lumbar spinal fusion or revision of a painful pseudarthrosis. The same recurrent facet nerves that innervate the facet ultimately innervate the mass of fusion bone. These can be cut by a sweeping, oblique incision lateral to the fusion mass. Muscular arteries will usually also be severed, but great care must be taken not to sever nerve roots that lie ventral to the transverse processes.

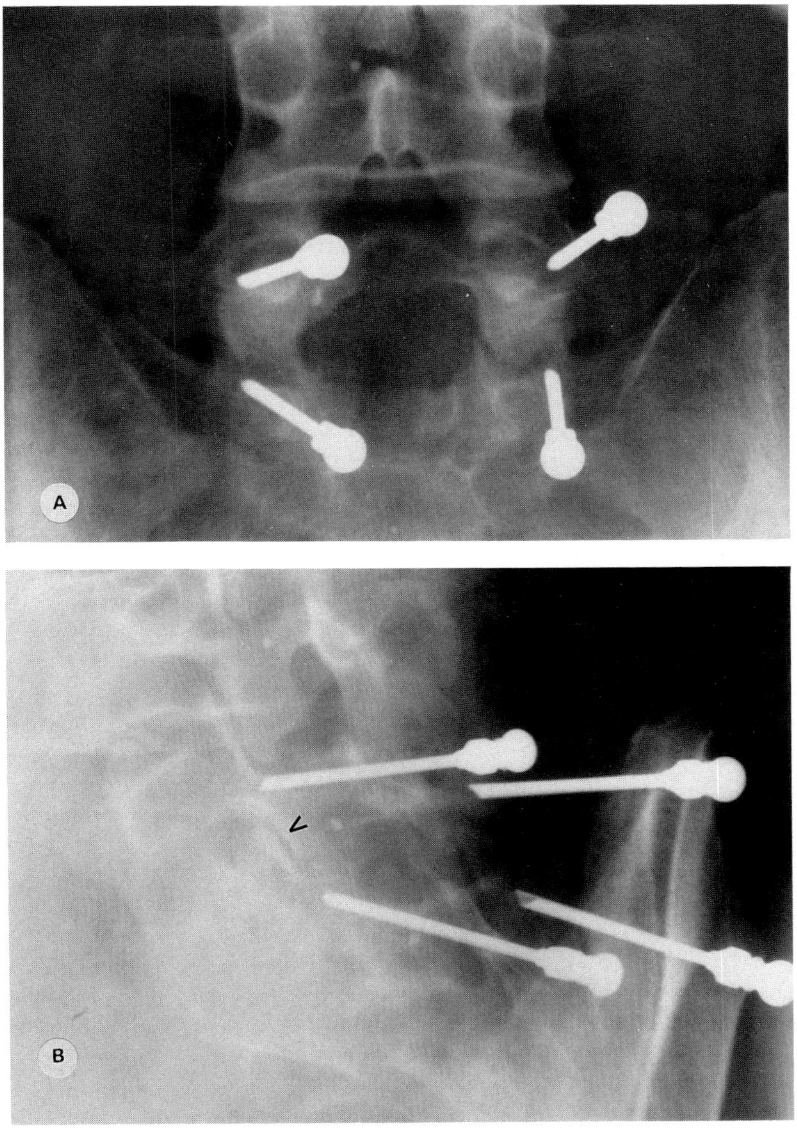

FIGURE 7.23. Facet neurectomy can be accomplished by a percutaneous radiofrequency (RF) needle procedure. These PA (**A**) and oblique (**B**) lumbar spine radiographs, from the patient discussed as Case 7, demonstrate four large diameter guide needles placed at the same four locations where diagnostic anesthetization had given excellent relief of back and posterior thigh pain. The large bore guide needles are used to direct the more delicate RF lesioning electrode to its proper target. Note that lesions are made rostral and caudal to the sclerotic facets (v) to interrupt superior and inferior recurrent facet nerves.

radio-frequency (RF) heat lesioning. Patients who might be considered for open surgical facet neurectomy should be chosen on the basis of similar indications. In my opinion, however, the open surgical procedure should rarely be necessary, since percutaneous approaches seem to be equally effective, yet much simpler and with smaller risk. No matter how these nerves are interrupted, whether percutaneously or by open surgery, their short length makes it almost certain that they will regenerate within a few months. I therefore find it difficult to justify a major open operative procedure for such a short-lived result, especially when a simpler and safer percutaneous alternative is essentially equally effective. In fact, I have performed only one open surgical facet neurectomy as a separate procedure.

This was done in a patient who had obtained excellent pain relief for several months following each of several percutaneous procedures and who specifically requested open surgical intervention. Following this procedure she did obtain good relief of back pain, which lasted nearly four months. But she was not able to enjoy the first month because of postoperative incisional pain.

Facet neurectomy performed as an *adjunct to laminectomy or fusion* is a more attractive procedure than facet neurectomy performed as a separate operative procedure (Fig. 7.22). This procedure is designed to denervate partially the facet and fusion bone for at least the first few months following surgery. The goal is to reduce the amount of postoperative pain to permit an earlier return to more vigorous activity and a more rapid withdrawal from dangerous narcotics. This technique may be particularly useful for patients operated on for painful pseudarthrosis who present with a background of chronic back pain and whose fusion stability is generally reasonably good enough to permit vigorous activity with the aid of external bracing in the first few months following repeat fusion.

The *technique of surgical facet neurectomy,* as I recommend it, differs quite drastically from the early technique described by Rees (Fig. 7.23). His procedure consisted of making bilateral paraspinal skin incisions through which a scalpel blade was swept through the muscles longitudinally, paralleling the lateral borders of the facets. The anatomy of this region raises serious questions whether this technique does in fact reliably interrupt most or even any facet nerves. It seems more logical to approach the nerves medially to laterally. This is done following a midline incision and exposure of laminae and facets or fusion bone laterally. Muscular attachments are separated subperiosteally laterally to the lateral margins of the facets. The facet nerves curve backward from the paraspinal nerve roots as a conjoint branch, which then divides into superior and inferior articular branches. Incising laterally between the two facets and angling slightly ventrally toward the parent nerve root seems more likely to interrupt the common facet nerve more proximally and more reliably than could be done by a vertical incision at the level of the facets. This incision will usually interrupt muscular arteries that must be controlled with electrocoagulation. The surgeon must be careful not to injure the paraspinal nerve root either at the time of his incision or during electrocoagulation of nearby arteries.

The most worrisome *complication of surgical facet neurectomy* is the risk of inadvertent interruption or electrocautery *damage to nearby paraspinal nerve roots.* The additional muscle interruption adds to the immediate postoperative *back pain. Bleeding* from severed muscle arteries can at times be quite troublesome, and adding this additional volume of blood loss to that lost during laminectomy, fusion, or repeat fusion may be sufficient to require blood transfusion.

Cordotomy and Myelotomy

Pain-relieving destructive procedures on the spinal cord are rarely indicated for the failed back syndrome. Two fundamentally different surgical procedures are available. The first is *cordotomy,* an anterolateral incision into the spinal cord designed to interrupt the pain-transmitting lateral spinothalamic tract. This operation is also termed *lateral spinothalamic tractotomy.* Anterolateral cordotomy may be done either as an open surgical procedure in the thoracic region or as a percutaneous RF heat lesioning procedure in the cervical area. The second operative approach is termed *myelotomy* and refers to a midline incision into the spinal cord. It is designed to interrupt decussating spinothalamic fibers. The former procedure interrupts contralateral pain and temperature perception; the latter procedure interrupts pain and temperature perception bilaterally but generally over a much smaller segmental area. Both of these procedures are rarely indicated for nonmalignant disease, but both may at times bring dramatic pain relief in some desperate failed back syndrome cases. An illustrative case report follows:

Case 21

This 38-year-old homemaker had been under active psychiatric care for many years for severe chronic depression of the manic-depressive type. In 1978, she spontaneously developed right sciatica that became progressively more severe despite bed rest therapy and analgesics. Physical examination disclosed limited straight leg raising and "stocking and glove" sensory loss of almost the entire right leg, but no convincing weakness or reflex loss. Myelography showed no obvious abnormality. She was told that no specific therapy was available and that she should learn to live with it. After approximately a year she elected an alternative course and nearly succumbed to a self-administered medication overdose.

Two months later she was referred to me. Her history and physical examination were unchanged, and repeat myelography again showed only minimal nerve root blunting. Discography was severely abnormal at L4-L5. This disc level easily accepted 2.5 ml of 76% diatrizoate meglumide and sodium (Renografin 76). Injection reproduced severe sciatica and back pain and radiographs confirmed posterolateral extravasation.

Injections at L3-L4 and L5-S1 were remarkably different from this, causing little discomfort despite the patient's overt apprehension. In 1979, I performed an L4-L5 laminectomy exposing and excising a small but definite lateral bulging of the intervertebral disc. Immediately postoperatively she was dramatically relieved of pain. She began ambulating actively 24 hours postoperatively and discontinued all narcotics within 72 hours.

Unfortunately, within three months sciatic and buttock pain and tenderness gradually reappeared. Over the next nine months the symptoms became progressively more severe despite treatment with anti-inflammatory drugs, antineuralgia drugs, and a series of local trigger point steroid injections. She undertook a home exercise program with the same enthusiasm that she had exhibited in the early postoperative period, but found that this only aggravated her pain. Repeat myelography again showed only minimal irregularity of the thecal sac. Intradiscal methylprednisolone acetate (Depo-Medrol) instillation at L4-L5 brought no relief. A series of epidural nerve root anesthetizations and steroid injections brought temporary good relief with L5 root anesthetization and excellent relief with anesthetization of both L5 and S1 roots. After considerable discussion with the patient and her husband, and with the concurrence of her psychiatrist, surgical sensory rhizotomy of L5 and S1 was performed in 1980. This relieved her of the lower extremity sciatica, but left her with persistent pain and tenderness in her right buttock. This pain seemed to be aggravated by activity but only partially improved by rest.

Over the next eight months the pain gradually became more severe and she became more overtly depressed, despite continued psychotherapy and the addition of several psychotropic drugs by her psychiatrist "One-legged" diagnostic spinal anesthetization gave apparently dramatic relief, but only with anesthetization of most of the lumbar and sacral segments. Graded diagnostic spinal block provided some pain relief following even the most dilute solutions, suggesting a nonorganic basis for her pain. However, perseverance with this study to the point of analgesia without anesthesia seemed for the first time to provide total relief of pain. Two attempts at intrathecal sensory rhizotomy, using 1 ml and 1.5 ml of 5% phenol in glycerol, respectively, provided pain relief lasting only hours to a few days. At this point the patient had resumed Percodan for pain relief but complained bitterly that the limited amounts of this narcotic that were prescribed for her were almost totally ineffective in relieving her severe pain. In June 1981, she again attempted suicide through medication overdose. Faced with this desperate situation, she and her husband were offered the alternatives of cingulotomy or thoracic anterolateral cordotomy. After considerable discussion it was elected to proceed with cordotomy, fortifying this decision with tryptophane therapy. Surgical thoracic cordotomy was performed in June 1981. Although she complained of some interscapular incisional pain she was immediately dramatically relieved of all buttock and leg pain and rapidly and enthusiastically returned to a full activity schedule. Despite the incisional pain, she discontinued narcotics entirely after ten days. Five months later, severe depression continued to be intermittently disabling. She was bothered by an unpleasant "coldness" of her right foot and leg, but had discontinued tryptophane due to its cost and took codeine for pain several times each week. Over the subsequent three months, pain appeared in the left leg, but the right leg remained pain free.

Thoracic Anterolateral Cordotomy

Anterolateral cordotomy, or *spinothalamic tractotomy,* is designed to interrupt at least a major portion of the spinothalamic tract fibers that carry precise information of pain perception from one hindquarter of the body. The majority of spinothalamic fibers decussate obliquely over a level of several spinal segments to ascend toward the thalamus in the anterolateral quadrant of the spinal cord. Interrupting this bundle of fibers still leaves intact those undecussated fibers that ascend ipsilaterally, as well as a variable number of polysynaptic fibers that carry less precise or *protopathic pain* information. Nonetheless, complete sectioning of the spinothalamic fiber tract usually eliminates the ability to perceive superficial pain and to discriminate hot and cold over the contralateral lower extremity and lower trunk. Fibers that arise most caudally in the body (i.e., from sacral and lumbar segments) lie most laterally and most posteriorly in the fiber bundle. This topographic arrangement of fibers permits the neurosurgeon to perform selective lesioning during the performance of a percutaneous cervical cordotomy, sparing thoracic and upper lumbar sensation. However, the lumbar and sacral fibers lie adjacent to the corticospinal fibers, which transmit voluntary motor control ipsilaterally, and the autonomic control fibers, which are most important in controlling bladder and bowel function. The autonomic control is usually bilateral, so sectioning fibers unilaterally usually does not result in incontinence. In contrast, corticospinal motor fibers transmit precise information and are not bilaterally represented. Damage to these fibers causes weakness in the "good leg," or the leg opposite the painful extremity.

The *technique of anterolateral cordotomy* is adequately described in neurosurgical texts and is well-known to most neurosurgeons (Fig. 7.24). Because this procedure is universally employed for pain relief and is not specifically employed only for treatment of the failed back syndrome, a detailed description will not be given. Open surgical thoracic cordotomy is performed through a midline thoracic incision at approximately T4 to T6. A hemilaminectomy is performed at one level contralateral to the side of the patient's pain. The dentate ligament is identified running the length of the lateral aspect of the spinal cord and is used as a guide to the separation between dorsally situated corticospinal motor fibers and ventrally situated spinothalamic pain fibers. The latter fibers are divided with tiny knives, aided by the use of small hooks. Some surgeons prefer to do this surgery under a combination of local and "wake-up" anesthesia. In this technique

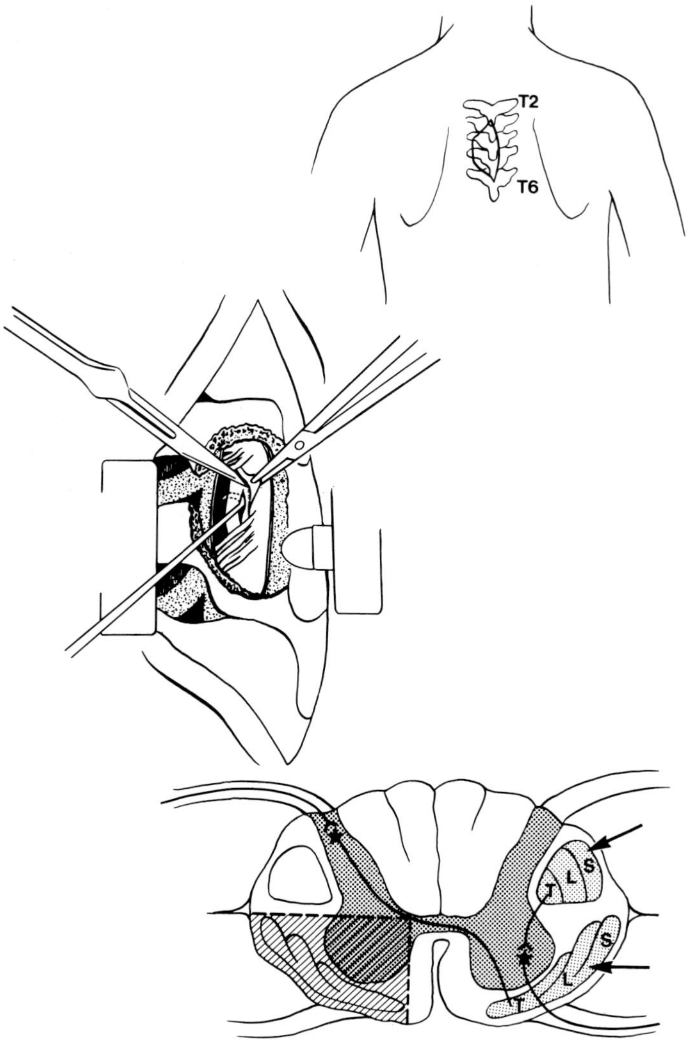

FIGURE 7.24. Thoracic anterolateral cordotomy is designed to interrupt the pain transmitting fibers of the spinothalamic tract (STT). This tract must be incised contralateral to the patient's pain, since incoming pain fibers cross the spinal cord shortly after they enter. Anatomical layering takes place within this tract so that relieving lumbar and sacral pain requires incision of the most dorsolaterally situated fibers (T-thoracic, L-lumbar, S-sacral). These fibers lie close to the voluntary motor fibers of the corticospinal tract (CST). Anatomically, this tract can be spared by confining the incision into the cord ventral to the dentate ligament (shown here, held by the tips of a fine hemostat), since this structure normally arises between the CST and the STT.

the patient is awakened following the spinal cord incision and tested on the operating table for sensory loss. If the ability to perceive a pinprick is not eliminated throughout the entire planned area of the lower extremity, buttock, and trunk, additional fibers can be sectioned. This technique is probably most important in patients who suffer sacral pain, where it is necessary to incise those spinothalamic fibers that lie closest to the corticospinal motor fibers. In general, however, this anesthesia technique is difficult to carry out effectively, and sensory testing is often severely compromised by having to deal with a patient who is confused and in pain.

Cervical Anterolateral Cordotomy

Percutaneous cervical anterolateral cordotomy enjoyed considerable popularity in the past, but presently is much less frequently used, both because of a general waning in enthusiasm for spinothalamic tractotomy and because of an increasing awareness of the significant potential for major complications inherent in this procedure.

Percutaneous cervical cordotomy's *advantage* over open surgical cordotomy is that it requires only a needle puncture rather than a painful and extensive operative incision. The procedure is usually performed in the radiology department with x-ray guidance of a stereotactically placed RF heat lesioning needle electrode. The procedure can easily be done under local anesthesia, which permits precise monitoring of induced analgesia.

The procedure does have several *disadvantages*. When one monitors the results of heat lesioning of the spinal cord or brain by neurologic examination, one must be conscious of the fact that *physiologic interruption* does not necessarily imply anatomic disruption. Patients may demonstrate physiologic disruption for several hours and then show prompt recovery. The result is that an apparently ideal level of analgesia documented at the time of an RF spinothalamic tractotomy may rapidly shrink to an undesirably small size over the next hours or days, as fiber bundles that were merely physiologically interrupted and not destroyed resume functioning. A second disadvantage of the procedure is that it must be done in the high cervical region to avoid damage to adjacent anterior horn neurons that control motor functions in the arm and hand. At high cervical levels, bilateral cord lesioning carries a severe risk of *apnea* or impaired respiratory drive. This impairment of respiratory drive is often referred to as *Ondine's curse*, in honor of the mythical character who was doomed to die if he fell asleep. These patients must be watched very carefully during sleep, since the reduced respiratory drive inherent in the sleep process may allow them to slip into sleep apnea.

The technique of percutaneous cervical cordotomy is adequately described in neurosurgical texts and need not be described here in detail. As was mentioned earlier, the procedure is usually performed in the radiology department with the patient supine on the x-ray table (Fig. 7.25). The RF needle electrode is introduced percutaneously in the lateral cervical spine below the ear or mastoid process and is directed through the C1-C2 neuroforamen. Once the subarachnoid space is reached, the dentate ligament is visualized by injection of air or positive contrast medium for use as an anatomical landmark. RF lesioning of the spinothalamic fibers in the anterolateral quadrant of the spinal cord is usually preceded by electrical stimulation to confirm placement in the pain pathways and sparing of the corticospinal motor pathways. Sensory and motor testing is carried out with the needle tip temperature elevated to the vicinity of 40 to 50 degrees centigrade, a temperature range that induces physiologic blockade without tissue destruction. If proper localization is confirmed, thermal lesioning is then carried out.

The most frequent *complications of percutaneous cervical cordotomy* involve *unintentional damage* to other areas of the spinal cord. This may result from bleeding triggered by the introduction of the needle electrode, from thermocoagulation of sulcal arteries (which supply in part voluntary motor, respiratory, and autonomic fibers), or through unwanted enlargement of the heat lesion. Careful sensory and motor examination during the performance of heat lesioning should prevent the latter complication. The possibility of severe respiratory embarrassment or apnea has been discussed as one of the disadvantages of this technique, almost precluding its applicability as a bilateral procedure in patients with nonmalignant disease.

Median Myelotomy

A procedure designed for bilateral interruption of lumbar and sacral spinothalamic pain-transmitting fibers is *median myelotomy.* This procedure is much less commonly performed for pain relief than is

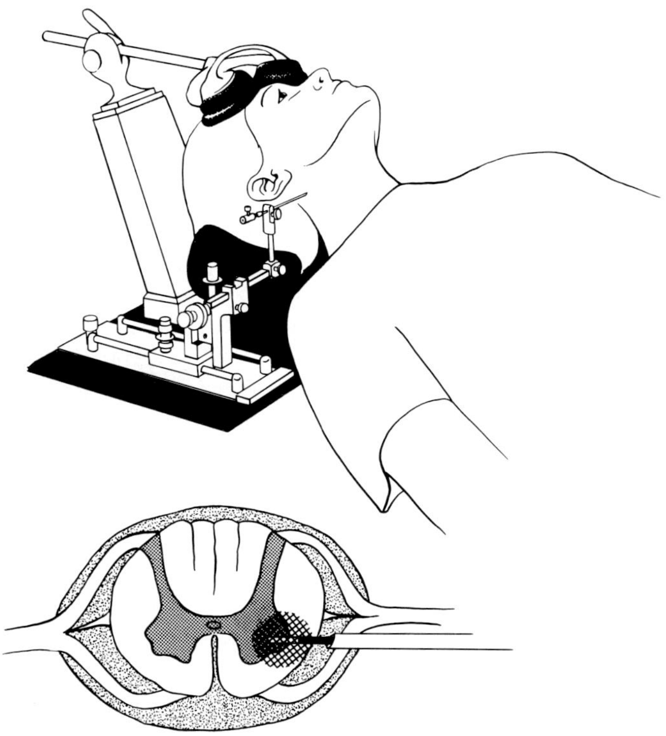

FIGURE 7.25. Cervical anterolateral cordotomy can be performed by a percutaneous needle technique. Using radiographic control, a radiofrequency (RF) electrothermal lesioning and stimulating needle is passed through the large lateral neuroforamen at C1-C2 and is manipulated into the anterolateral quadrant of the spinal cord. Electrical stimulation confirms proper placement before RF lesioning is carried out.

anterolateral cordotomy even in general neurosurgery, and it is rarely performed for the failed back syndrome. It is designed to interrupt pain and temperature fibers arising bilaterally in sacral and lower lumbar regions. Since pain fibers constitute the bulk of spinal fibers that decussate in the midline, a vertical incision lengthwise through the conus medularis and lower lumbar spinal cord will interrupt pain fibers that arise bilaterally. Once the afferent pain fibers synapse in the spinal cord, the secondary fibers ascend obliquely as they decussate so that it is necessary to incise the spinal cord several segmental levels above the point of entry of the peripheral pain fibers. Thus, to denervate upper sacral or lower lumbar levels, the spinal cord must be incised rostrally to the point of entry of middle or upper lumbar nerve root fibers.

The *indications for median myelotomy* must be carefully drawn because of the extensive nature and significant risks of this procedure. Ideally, the procedure should be suitable for the patient suffering from bilateral lower lumbar and sacral pain. Unfortunately, midline pain is difficult to eradicate and some reassurance should be sought about the possible effectiveness of such an extensive operative procedure. Differential diagnostic spinal anesthesia or bilateral lumbar and sacral nerve root blocks that produce good to excellent pain relief are suggestive of a good result, although they are certainly not absolutely predictive. No patient should be subjected to this form of destructive surgery until he has proven to be unresponsive to an extensive trial of nonoperative or needle therapy. Intrathecal steroid injections, microsurgical lysis of arachnoiditis, and intrathecal phenol rhizotomy should be considered as potential alternative therapies.

The major *advantage* of this procedure is that it provides bilateral interruption of pain fibers. Among its *disadvantages* are that it necessitates rather extensive lower thoracic laminectomy and it entails a significant risk of motor weakness or autonomic impairment.

The *technique of median myelotomy* begins with surgical exposure of the conus medularis and lower thoracic spinal cord through thoracic laminectomies at T10, T11, and T12 (Fig. 7.26). The conus medularis, or lower end of the spinal cord, is identified within the cauda equina congregation of lumbar, sacral, and coccygeal nerve roots. When the surgery is performed for failed back syndrome patients, it is usually possible to spare perineal pain and temperature sensations, so that incision into the

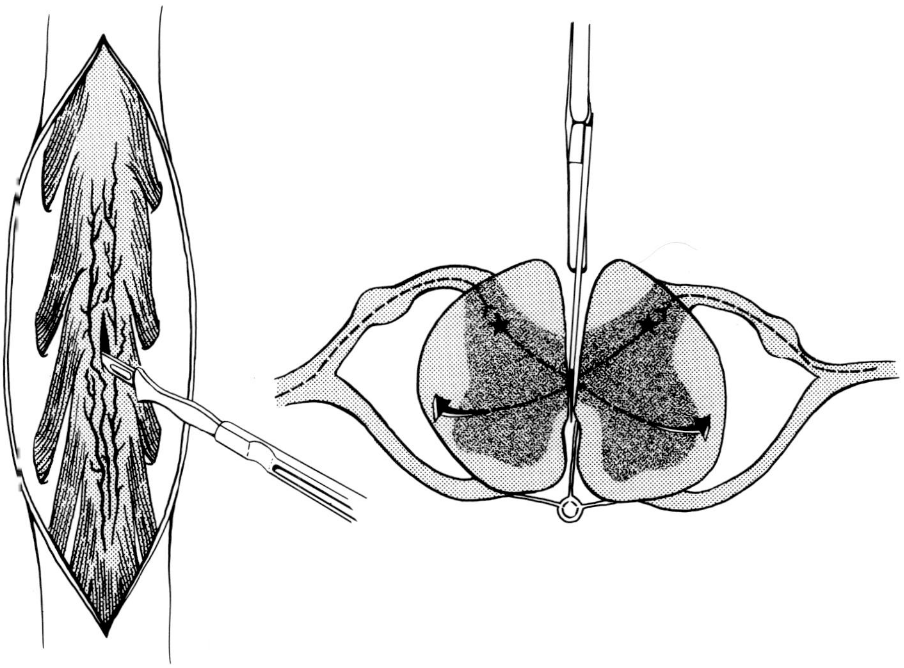

FIGURE 7.26. Lumbosacral median myelotomy is not commonly employed but may be useful for selected patients with bilateral, intractably severe sciatica and sacrococcygeal pain. Extensive surgical exposure of the conus medullaris is required. Microincision of the decussating, midline pain-transmitting spinothalamic tract (STT) fibers of the lower end of the spinal cord will require interruption of some of the cord's superficial vasculature.

spinal cord can begin 2 cm or 3 cm rostral to the lower tip of the conus medularis. From that point, the midline incision through the cord is extended rostrally an additional 5 cm to 7 cm. During cord dissection, care should be taken to avoid damaging the ventral or anterior spinal artery as much as possible. Interrupting this artery at one level usually does not result in major cord injury, but the blood supply in the spinal cord is variable and infarction can result capriciously.

Primary among the *complications of median myelotomy* is the risk of unintended *spinal cord injury* and neurologic deficit. As my friend and teacher, Dr. John Drew, liked to remark, "Operating on the spinal cord isn't like operating on the brain. The spinal cord is delicate!" Spinal cord injury can result from interruption of fine blood vessels, seemingly gentle retraction, or even dehydration of the cord during surgical exposure. The neurologic deficits that can result as a complication of median myelotomy include the production of a *cauda equina syndrome*. In its most severe form, this can produce complete sensory loss and paralysis of the distal lower extremities and saddle region, in addition to loss of bladder and bowel control. Such complications occur infrequently following median myelotomy but must be weighed carefully in the balance of decision making. Median myelotomy may also produce incomplete interruption of pain fiber transmission and leave the patient with *painful dysesthesia* or constant *hyperpathia*—a painful hypersensitivity to peripheral stimuli that is usually coupled with spontaneous burning pain. The risks of *spinal fluid leakage* and postoperative *hematoma* with cord compression are present, as they are with all forms of spinal cord surgery.

Brain-Stem Lesions and Stimulation

A variety of procedures have been described that involve *surgery on brain-stem structures*.[108-112] None of these procedures enjoy widespread application, and many are still considered innovative in nature. The principal anatomical targets have been the *thalamus*, *hypothalamus*, and *mesencephalon*.

All of these procedures have in common the stereotactic placement of lesioning electrodes or chronically implanted electrodes to permit chronic or repetitive electrical or chemical stimulation of specific brain regions. Four general types of operations may be recognized: (1) lesions in the anterior or dorsomedial thalamus to *reduce suffering or anxiety* associated with pain; (2) lesions in the center median or interlaminar thalamus to interrupt the *protopathic* (more primitive and diffusely perceived) component of pain perception or in the dorsolateral tegmental region of the mesencephalon to produce analgesia, or a loss of the conscious awareness of pain, over the opposite side of the trunk and limbs; (3) electrical or chemical *stimulation of the "reward" system* in the lateral hypothalamus to induce a feeling of well-being and to reduce the apparent significance of pain; and (4) electrical stimulation of the periaqueductal region of the thalamus and mesencephalon to interrupt pain transmission or to *modify the intrinsic polypeptide-opiate receptor system* of the brain.

Few patients with a failed back syndrome are considered *candidates for surgery of this type*. Anterior or dorsomedial thalamic lesioning is properly reserved for patients with severe depression or other severe emotional disorders. Lateral hypothalamic stimulation has never progressed beyond the stage of an innovative procedure. The major limitation of this technique is that electrical stimulation of the compact, complex, and functionally potent hypothalamus quite commonly elicits a variety of unpleasant or even dangerous autonomic or emotional responses in addition to the desired "pleasure" responses. Medial thalamic lesioning has been reserved largely for patients with malignant diseases because of a high relapse rate with the passage of weeks or months. Medial thalamic lesions must be made with caution, because they encroach upon the reticular activating system of the brain. Damage to this system may result in loss of consciousness or lasting coma. Perhaps the most promising of these brain-stem surgical procedures has been thalamic, periventricular, or periaqueductal gray stimulation. This technique has been used in several centers in the last few years. In some centers, this form of therapy is now offered to patients with the failed back syndrome who remain in severe pain despite all other efforts at restoration or pain relief.

The chief disadvantage of all of these stereotactic brain-stem procedures is that they involve surgery directly upon the brain. Most patients find this prospect extremely frightening. All of these procedures also have the disadvantage of requiring extremely sophisticated and specialized surgical techniques and extensive, specialized support facilities.

The *advantage of these procedures* is that they have a nonspecific effect on pain and can be used for patients in whom the precise etiology of pain cannot be documented. Furthermore, these procedures are often effective in relieving pain when all other methods have failed.

The *technique of stereotactic brain-stem surgery* will not be reviewed. These procedures are rarely employed in failed back syndrome sufferers. They are extremely specialized and have been adequately covered in the neurosurgical literature.

Complications of all of these procedures include the possibility of brain hemorrhage, meningitis, and brain abscess. Since these electrodes are placed in extremely important or "eloquent" regions of the brain, hemorrhage and infections at these sites—even though they occur rarely—can produce devastating neurologic deficits.

Cingulotomy and Lobotomy

Cingulotomy is currently considered a useful operation for otherwise intractable sufferers from the failed back syndrome. *Prefrontal leukotomy* or *lobotomy* enjoys a more hoary but unsavory reputation. It continues to be an effective means of relieving extreme suffering in patients with terminal malignant disease, but is rarely employed for failed back syndrome sufferers, unless they are also disabled by severe and medically intractable psychiatric illness (Fig. 7.27).

Cingulotomy involves the surgical destruction of the supraventricular cingulum bundles and inferior cingulate gyri.[113-115] These structures are part of the *Papez circuit* or *limbic system* of the brain and mediate the significance of ongoing or chronic pain. Surgical lesioning of this region does not interrupt a conscious awareness of pain but produces rather a habituation to chronic pain. Following this procedure, patients can still perceive acute pain in essentially normal fashion. However, pain that is chronically present gradually fades from consciousness through habituation, in much the same way one gradually loses awareness of cutaneous stimuli that are not emotionally reinforced—such as the clothes

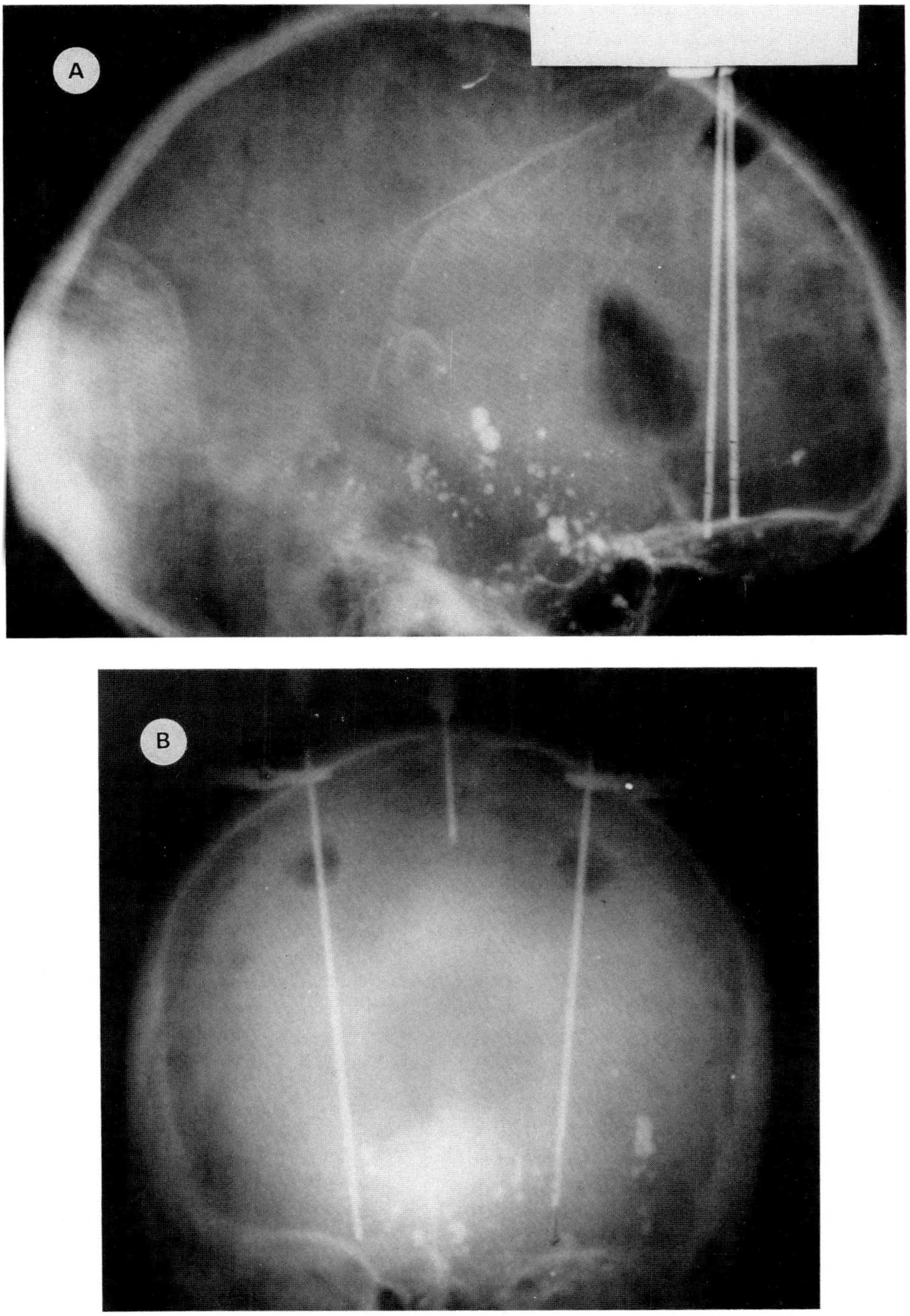

FIGURE 4.27. Bifrontal leukotomy has largely replaced the more extensive frontal lobotomy, but is now rarely performed. It is almost never used any more for psychiatric disease, but is occasionally employed for intractable pain in patients with terminal cancer. It probably has no useful role in the treatment of failed back syndrome patients. This radiograph illustrates bifrontal radiofrequency (RF) lesioning performed on a cancer patient in lateral (**A**) and frontal (**B**) projections.

on one's back or the chair under one's posterior. Following cingulotomy, many patients initially note little change in their chronic pain, yet over the next few weeks or months they gradually become less aware of their pain and less troubled.

Careful *mental status testing* of patients subjected to cingulotomy for pain relief or severe depression (the other principal indication for cingulotomy) has documented unchanged or even improved intellectual performance. The improvement in performance is thought to be due to a reduction in narcotic intake and a release from the distraction caused by pain. A recently completed study at the University of Massachusetts Medical Center of patients who had undergone cingulotomy one to three months earlier did disclose subtle reductions in spontaneity and affect, but confirmed the preservation of cognitive functions.[113]

The *effectiveness* of cingulotomy in relieving chronic, nonmalignant pain has been estimated in the large series published by Hurt and Ballantine as 79% good to excellent results.[115] Cingulotomy is not uniformly effective for patients suffering with malignant disease, because the continuing spread of their disease to new areas continually introduces new episodes of acute pain, and these continue to reach consciousness in full force. My experience with cingulotomy for pain relief has been limited, but only approximately two thirds of my patients have enjoyed good relief, and no patient was totally cured of all pain. Nonetheless, for some patients this procedure can be extremely valuable, such as the patient in the following case:

Case 22

This 48-year-old former industrial foreman came under my care in April 1974 after he had undergone a series of eight back operations over a fourteen-year course. When first seen by me, he was in constant severe pain and could tolerate being out of bed for only brief periods and only while wearing a fiberglass body jacket. He took large doses of opioids every two or three hours, even awakening during the night. He combined these with large doses of various tranquilizers and diazepam (Valium). Previous psychiatric therapy and inpatient pain clinic stays had been ineffective. His major complaint was severe left sciatica. It did not respond to antineuralgia or anti-inflammatory drug therapy, and paraspinal and intrathecal spinal diagnostic blocks suggested that sensory interruption of L5 and S1 roots might provide a useful degree of pain relief. Intrathecal phenol sensory rhizotomy was attempted on two occasions in October 1974, but no lasting sensory loss could be induced despite some mild motor weakness. Surgical sensory rhizotomy in November, 1974, produced a 50% reduction in sciatica, but the patient then complained increasingly of severe back pain. Surgical repair of a postoperative pseudomeningocele was undertaken, but it remained impossible to wean him from his heavy medication intake and constant reliance on an external support.

In April 1976, I performed an open right anterolateral cordotomy. This produced excellent analgesia over the left leg, hip, and lumbar region but failed to improve his activity tolerance. He was, however, able to reduce his narcotic ingestion to a schedule of every four hours.

The possibility of cingulotomy was discussed with the patient, but he professed to be terrified by the prospect of brain surgery. He finally requested cingulotomy after a suicidal ingestion of medication was successful only in producing a broken hip when he fell from bed. At the patient's request, the cingulotomy performed in July 1977 was limited to the placement of smaller than usual electrolytic lesions. Over the next three months, no pain relief ensued, but the patient was extremely relieved not to have suffered intellectual or emotional deterioration. In October 1977, cingulotomy was repeated and lesions of standard size were made. He was somewhat confused for the ten days following this surgery and initially noted no improvement in pain. Over the next few months he continued to complain of pain but gradually reduced his medication intake and increased his activities. Within a year he was no longer wearing his back support and had begun doing light housework and gardening. He had reduced his medication to dihydrocodeinone compound (Percodan), diazepam (Valium), and chloral hydrate. He maintained this level of medication and activity over the next two years, during which he continued to complain of back and leg pain. His wife noted that he was somewhat less spontaneous and more withdrawn than previously, but he continued to be fully alert and brought with him his latest joke to nearly every office visit. At the end of this two-year period, he announced that he was tired of taking medications and abruptly discontinued all further intake.

Potential *candidates for cingulotomy* are those who suffer chronic pain that has failed to respond to protracted restorative and pain-relieving therapy. This operation seems to be particularly beneficial for patients who are markedly distressed by or fixated upon their pain or who seem to be emotionally depressed in addition to having pain. Severe brain atrophy or dementia are relative *contraindications,*

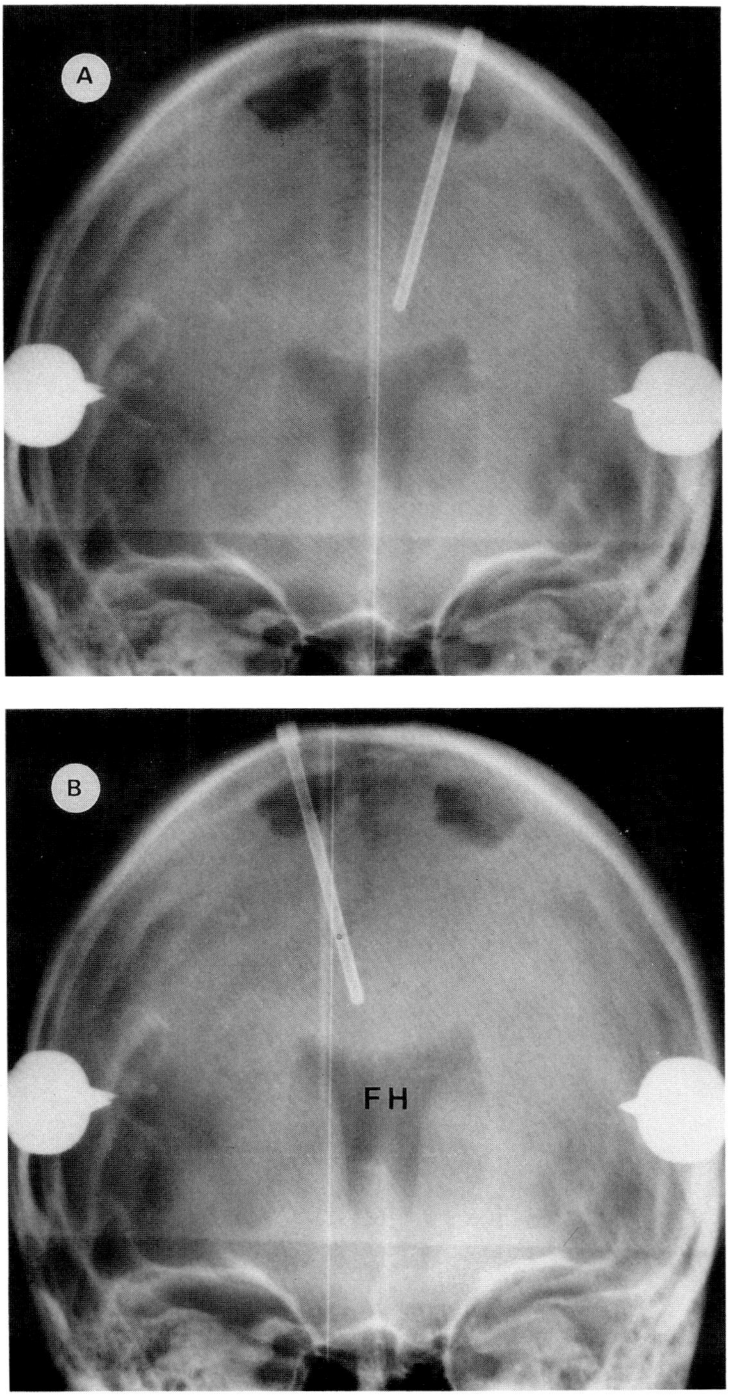

FIGURE 7.28. Bilateral cingulotomy can be quite effective in controlling the pain, suffering, and depression associated with the failed back syndrome. The operation impairs the continued re-enforcement of emotional consciousness of pain and allows chronic pains to slowly fade from consciousness. These radiographs demonstrate radiofrequency (RF) electrodes stereotactically placed into the right **(top)** and left **(bottom)** anterior cingulum bundle and cingulate gyrus in a patient chronically disabled by a failed back syndrome. (FH: Frontal horns of lateral cerebral ventricles.)

since patients with these problems are more prone to develop overt mental or emotional deterioration postoperatively.

One of the main disadvantages of cingulotomy is the same as for stereotactic brain-stem surgery—patients' *fear of brain surgery.* Cingulotomy is also an extremely specialized form of surgery but is much less technically demanding than brain-stem electrode placement. Consequently, cingulotomy is performed by a greater number of neurosurgeons. The cingulate gyrus region of the brain is more superficial than the brain stem, and *hemorrhage* or *infections* that occur here—and these are quite rare in reported series—are less likely to produce devastating neurologic deficits. Long-term follow-up of my own cingulotomy patients has disclosed several who developed the new onset of convulsive seizures, though this is rarely reported in other published series.

As is true of stereotactic brain-stem surgery, cingulotomy has as its chief *advantages* the fact that it has a *nonspecific effect on pain* of many types and all locations and that it can be effective for some patients for whom all other therapies have failed.

The *technique of cingulotomy* requires placement of two parasagittal burr holes just anterior to the coronal suture line (Fig. 7.28). The frontal horns of both lateral ventricles are filled with air for x-ray localization and needle electrodes are placed under x-ray control. Needle placement can be done either with a stereotactic head frame or by hand. The needle electrodes are uninsulated at their distal 1 cm. Ideally, thermistors should be included in the electrode tip to permit monitoring of lesion temperature. The tip of each needle electrode is positioned 5 mm to 7 mm lateral to the midline, 5 mm to 7 mm dorsal to the roof of the lateral ventricle, and 15 mm to 25 mm posterior to the tip of the frontal horn. I generally make the first pair of electrolytic lesions using 80- to 90-degree centigrade temperatures for 180 seconds. The needle electrodes are then withdrawn 1 cm for placement of a second, supra-adjacent lesion. Postoperatively, most patients will be mildly to moderately confused for five to ten days. More anteriorly placed lesions seem to be more effective in relieving pain but also carry a slightly greater risk of urinary incontinence. This rarely lasts more than a few days to a few weeks, but it can be disturbing to families and patients if they were not warned in advance of this possibility.

8

Team Approach or Individual Effort?

Much of what is currently written about treatment of pain patients, including failed back syndrome patients, assumes, recommends, or even proposes to mandate a team approach. In practice, how valuable is this approach? Are those who insist that it is the only valid approach correct in this assumption, or are they merely overly zealous?

The team approach has inherently the same strengths and weaknesses as the committee approach to problems in general. When a complex problem impacts on several special-interest groups or requires expertise from several different disciplines, the committee approach provides an invaluable working vehicle. On the other hand, the inefficiencies of the committee approach are notorious. Common parlance has it that if there is a problem that one wishes to put out of circulation, one gives it to a committee, but if the problem demands a solution, one gives it to a person. In dealing with patients with chronic pain and a complex failed back syndrome, expert input from a variety of disciplines is quite frequently useful. Rheumatology evaluation, pharmacologic management, physical and occupational therapy, orthotics or brace application, psychologic support or psychiatric therapy, social work, vocational rehabilitation, and even marriage counseling can all provide valuable input for many of these patients. But in a group effort or team approach, who actually has final authority? Who actually takes primary control of the patient's myriad problems? Who actually takes responsibility for guiding the patient back to health and happiness? A team approach can work effectively only if the importance of these considerations is recognized and maintained above and beyond the technical operations of the group. When a patient with a problem of this magnitude needs help, he must be able to turn to a person, or perhaps one or two persons, and not be left to contend with an amorphous thing, team, or crowd.

Even if we agree that a well-organized, multidisciplinary team with personalized leadership can be a great asset in the management of failed back syndrome patients, is the team approach actually necessary? As an alternative, is there still a valuable role for individual therapeutic effort? Most patients whose lower back problems result in a failed back syndrome begin their medical treatment in a physician's office or in a community hospital. However, most community hospitals find it difficult to launch a formal and neatly organized team to manage such problems, so most well-organized teams of this sort are centered in larger teaching hospitals. As I have already stated, I feel strongly that shipping a patient to a distant city for treatment of a failed back syndrome can often be severely destructive psychologically and less productive physiologically than thoughtful and conscientious therapy closer to home. The physicians who initially undertake the care of patients with lower back problems should be sufficiently familiar with the complexity of the presenting disease to be able to guide most of their patients to recovery, with as small a number as possible eventually having to face the failed back syndrome. When the unhappy reality develops that a patient undergoes lower back surgery without satisfactory outcome, the initial physician, and especially the operating surgeon, must be sufficiently committed to that patient's welfare, sufficiently knowledgeable of the disease he has undertaken to treat, and sufficiently aware of the complexities of the failed back syndrome that he can and will continue to manage his patient's therapy effectively. This does not imply that he must do so alone, since input from other areas of special expertise is still likely to be of value for these patients. But this expertise may be available through individual referral, and to be optimally effective it should be available close to the patient's home.

I have the feeling that a rallying cry for a team approach too often camouflages a cop-out from the responsibility of caring for a complicated patient. Surgeons are generally expected not only to be capable of dealing with their complications, but also to be responsible to the patient and to see that an ultimate satisfactory outcome is achieved. This same moral or ethical responsibility applies to neurosurgeons and orthopedists who operate on diseases of the lower back; their responsibility to these patients should not end at the time of surgery, and especially should not end if the patient has yet to achieve a satisfactory outcome.

In short, a team approach is valuable in the management of failed back syndrome sufferers but need not be undertaken as a formal effort only. An equally effective team effort can be undertaken under the guidance of one person, so long as that physician is aware of the complexities of the disorders that constitute the failed back syndrome. With this knowledge he can then call on other health care and paramedical specialists whose expertise may greatly aid these unfortunate patients.

References

1. LeBlanc FE (ed): Scientific approach to the assessment and management of activity related spinal disorders. A monograph for clinicians. Spine 1987; 12(7):S1–S59.
2. Wilkinson HA: Unconventional approaches: chymopapain and alternative neurosurgical techniques. In Stanton-Hicks M, Boas RA (eds): Chronic Low Back Pain. New York, Raven Press, 1982, pp 213–230.
3. Wilkinson HA: Failed disk syndrome. Am Fam Physician 1978; 17:86–94.
4. Wilkinson HA: Low back pain with or without sciatica. In Long D (ed): Current Therapy in Neurological Surgery–2. Philadelphia, BC Decker, 1989, pp 269–274.
5. Cantor G: Anti-inflammatory drug therapy for low back pain. In Stanton-Hicks M, Boas RA (eds): Chronic Low Back Pain. New York, Raven Press, 1982, pp 157–169.
6. Burton CV: Lumbosacral arachnoiditis. Spine 1978; 3:24–30.
7. Oppel F, Schramm J, Schirmer M, Zeitner M: Results and complicated course after surgery for lumbar disc herniation. Advances in Neurosurgery 1977; 4:36–51.
8. Mixter W, Barr S: Rupture of the intervertebral disk with involvement of the spinal canal. N Engl J Med 1934; 211:210–214.
9. Calabro JJ, Maltz BA: Ankylosing spondylitis. N Engl J Med 1970; 282:606–610.
10. Engleman EG, Engelman EP: Ankylosing spondylitis: Recent advances in diagnosis and treatment. Med Clin North Am 1977; 61:347–364.
11. Dabezies EJ, Langford K, Morris J, Shields CB, Wilkinson HA: Safety and efficacy of chymopapain (Discase) in the treatment of sciatica due to a herniated nucleus pulposus: Results of a randomized double-blind study. Spine 1988; 13:561–565.
12. Javid MJ, Nordby EJ, Ford LT, et al: Safety and efficacy of chymopapain (Chymodiactin) in herniated nucleus pulposus with sciatica: Results of a randomized double-blind study. JAMA 1983; 249:2489–2494.
13. Saal JA, Saal JS: Nonoperative treatment of herniated lumbar intervertebral disc with radiculopathy—an outcome study. Spine, 1989; 14:431–436.
14. Fager CA, Freidberg SR: Analysis of failures and poor results of lumbar spine surgery. Spine 1980; 5:87–94.
15. Mayfield FH: Autologous fat transplants for the protection and repair of the spinal dura. Clin Neurosurg 1980; 27:349–361.
16. Kabat H: Low Back and Leg Pain from Herniated Cervical Disk: New Method of Diagnosis and Conservative Treatment. St. Louis, Warren H. Green, Inc, 1980.
17. Langfitt TW, Elliott FA: Pain in the back and legs caused by cervical spinal cord compression. JAMA 1967; 200:382–385.
18. Sims-Williams H, Jayson MIV, Baddeley H: Small spinal fractures in back pain patients. Ann Rheum Dis 1978; 37:262–265.
19. Nash CL, Kaufman B, Frankel VH: Postsurgical meningeal pseudocysts of the lumbar spine. Clin Orthop 1971; 75:167–178.
20. Rinaldi I, Reach WF Jr: Postoperative lumbar meningocele. J Neurosurg 1969; 30:504–507.
21. Goldenberg DL: Fibromyalgia syndrome: an emerging but controversial condition. JAMA 1987; 257:2782–2787.
22. Swartout R, Compere EL: Ischiogluteal bursitis: The pain in the arse. JAMA 1974; 227:551–552.
23. Ehni G: Significance of the small lumbar spinal canal: Cauda equina compression syndromes due to spondylosis. J Neurosurg 1969; 31:490–494.

24. Jacobson I, Plewes JL: Sciatica caused by sacral nerve root cysts. Lancet 1970; 2:799–802.
25. Tarlov IM: Sacral Nerve-Root Cysts: Another Cause of the Sciatic or Cauda Equina Syndrome. Springfield, Illinois, Charles C Thomas Publisher, 1953.
26. Fordyce WE, Roberts AH, Sternbach RA: The behavioral management of chronic pain: A response to critics. Pain 1985; 22:113–125.
27. Hendler N: Psychiatric considerations of pain. In Youmans JR (ed): Neurological Surgery, 3d ed. Philadelphia, WB Saunders, 1990, pp 3813–3855.
28. Beck AT: Beck Depression Inventory. Philadelphia, Center for Cognitive Therapy, 1981.
29. Leavitt F, Ganon DC: Low Back Pain Symptom Check List. Wilmette, Illinois, Affiliated Behavioral Consultants, 1980.
30. Mayer TG, Gatchel RJ, Kishino ND, et al: A prospective short-term objective functional measurement. Pain 1986; 25:53–68.
31. Ransford AO, Cairns D, Mooney V: The pain drawing as an aid to the psychologic evaluation of patients with low back pain. Spine 1976; 1:127–134.
32. Wagner GS, Gebe B, Rozen MP, Stead EA, Jr: What This Patient Needs Is a Doctor. Durham, North Carolina, Carolina Academic Press, 1978.
33. Blumer D: Psychiatric considerations in pain. In Rotham RH, Simeone FA (eds): The Spine, Vol 2. Philadelphia, WB Saunders, 1975, pp 871–906.
34. Blumer D: Psychiatric and psychological aspects of chronic pain. Clin Neurosurg 1978; 25:276–283.
35. Burton CV: Lumbosacral arachnoiditis. Spine 1978; 3:24–30.
36. Wilkinson HA: Lumbar adhesive arachnoiditis. In Long DM (ed): Current Therapy in Neurological Surgery. Philadelphia, BC Decker, 1985, pp. 198–200.
37. Mayfield FH: Spondylosis and the lame back. Presented at the annual meeting of the Congress of Neurologic Surgeons, Las Vegas, Nevada, October 9, 1979.
38. Wilkinson HA, Schuman N: Results of surgical lysis of lumbar adhesive arachnoiditis. Neurosurgery 1979; 4:401–409.
39. Caron H, Toomey TC: Epidural steroid therapy for low back pain. In Stanton-Hicks M, Boas R (eds) Chronic Low Back Pain. Philadelphia, Grune and Stratton, 1982, pp. 193–198.
40. Ciric I, Mikhail MA, Tarkington JA, Vick NA: The lateral recess syndrome: A variant of spinal stenosis. J Neurosurg 1980; 53:433–444.
41. Steindler A: The interpretation of sciatic radiation in the syndrome of low-back pain. J Bone Joint Surg 1940; 22:28–34.
42. Scham S, Taylor T: Tension signs in lumbar disk prolapse. Clin Orthop 1971; 75:195–203.
43. Hudgins WR: The cross-straight-leg-raising test. N Engl J Med 1977; 197:1127.
44. Woodhall B, Hayes G: The well-leg raising test of Fajerstajn in the diagnosis of ruptured lumbar intervertebral disk. J Bone Joint Surg (Am) 1950; 32:786–792.
45. Casey KL: Reticular formation and pain: Toward a unifying concept. In Bonica JJ (ed): Pain. New York, Raven Press, 1980, pp 93–105.
46. Melzack R, Wall RD: Pain mechanism: A new theory. Science 1965; 150:971–979.
47. Wall PD: The role of substantia gelatinosa as a gate control. In Bonica JJ (ed): Pain. New York, Raven Press, 1980, pp 205–231.
48. Wall PD, Sweet WH: Temporary abolition of pain in man. Science 1967; 155:108–109.
49. Wilkinson HA: Aseptic inflammatory complications of spinal surgery. Congress of Neurological Surgeons. Audiotape W128–10. Info Medix.
50. Carrera GF: Lumbar facet arthrography and injection in low back pain. Wis Med J 1979; 78:35–37.
51. Williams AL, Haughton VM, Syvertsen A: Computer tomography in the diagnosis of herniated nucleus pulposus. Radiology 1980; 135:95–99.
52. Wilkinson HA: Lumbosacral meningismus complicating subdural injection of "blood patch." Case report. J Neurosurg 1980; 52:849–951.
53. Cuatico W, Gannon W, Samouhos E: A needle designed for myelography, technical note. J Neurosurg 1968; 28:87–88.
54. Dutcher JP, Schiffer CA, Johnston GS: Rapid migration of 111 Indium-labeled granulocytes to sites of infection. N Engl J Med 1982; 304:586–589.
55. Schutz H, Longheed WH, Wortzman G, Averbuck BG: Intervertebral nerve-root block in investigation of chronic lumbar disc disease. Can J Surg 1973; 16:217–221.
56. Deyo RA, Diehl AK, Rosenthal M: How many days of bed rest for acute low back pain? A randomized clinical trial. N Engl J Med 1986; 315:1064–1070.
57. Van Gelderen C: Ein orthotisches (lordotisches) kaudasyndrome. Acta Psych Neurol Scand 1948; 23:57–68.
58. Brunarski DJ: Clinical trials of spinalmanipulation: A critical appraisal and review of the literature. J Manipulative Physiol Ther 1984; 7:243–249.
59. Haldeman S: Spinal manipulative therapy: A status report. Clin Orthop 1983; 179:62–70.
60. Hoehler FK, Tobis JS, Buerger AA: Spinal manipulation for low back pain. JAMA 1981; 245:1835–1838.
61. Ottenbacher K, DiFabio RP: Efficacy of spinal manipulation/mobilization therapy: A meta-analysis. Spine 1985; 10:833–837.
62. Dan NG, Saccasan PA: Serious complications of

lumbar spinal manipulation. Med J Aust 1983; 2:672–673.
63. Edelist G, Gross AE, Langer F: Treatment of low back pain with acupuncture. Can Anaesth Soc J 1976; 23:303–306.
64. Satran R, Goldstein MN: Pain perception: modification of threshold of intolerance and cortical potentials by cutaneous stimulation. Science 1973; 1980:1201–1202.
65. Green LN: Dexamethasone in the management of symptoms due to herniated lumbar disc. J Neurol Neurosurg Psychiatry 1975; 38:1211–1217.
66. Edwards WT, Habib F, Burney RG, Begin G: Intravenous lidocaine in the management of various pain states: A review of 211 cases. Reg Anaesth 1985; 10:1–6.
67. Gildenberg PL, DeVaul RA: Management of chronic pain refractory to specific therapy. In Youmans JR (ed): Neurological Surgery, 3d ed. Philadelphia, WB Saunders, 1990, pp. 4144–4165.
68. Laban MM, Buyck RD, Johnson EW: Sexual impotence in men having low-back syndrome. Arch Phys Med Rehabil 1966; 47:715–723.
69. Hackett GS: Ligament and Tendon Relaxation by Prolotherapy, 3d ed. Springfield, Illinois, Charles C Thomas, 1958.
70. Hirschberg GG, Froetscher L, Naeim F: Iliolumbar syndrome as a common cause of low back pain: Diagnosis and prognosis. Arch Phys Med Rehabil 1979 60:415–419.
71. Naeim F, Frostscher L, Hirschberg GG: Treatment of the chronic iliolumbar syndrome by infiltration of the iliolumbar ligament. West J Med 1982; 136:372–374.
72. Peterson TH: Injection treatment for back pain. Am J Orthop 1963; 5:320–325.
73. Apfelbach HW, Jacobs RL, Ray RD: Chemonucleolysis in the treatment of low back and sciatica. Surg Clin North Am 1975; 55:181–197.
74. Javid MJ: Treatment of herniated lumbar disk syndrome with chymopapain. JAMA 1980; 243:2043–2048.
75. Martins AN, Ramirez A, Johnston J, Schwetschman PR: Double-blind evaluation of chemonucleolysis for herniated lumbar discs: Late results. J Neurosurg 1978; 49:816–827.
76. Parkinson D, Shields C: Treatment of protruded lumbar intervertebral discs with chymopapain (Discase). J Neurosurg 1973; 39:203–208.
77. Sussman BJ, Bromley JW, Gomez JC: Injection of collagenase in the treatment of herniated lumbar disk. Initial clinical report. JAMA 1981; 245:730–732.
78. Braun W: Intradisc injection of Trasylol in lumbar intervertebral disc syndrome. Neurosurg Rev 1979; 1:21–24.
79. Feffer HL: Regional use of steroids in the management of lumbar intervertebral disc disease. Orthop Clin North Am 1975; 6:249–253.
80. Graham CE: Chemonucleolysis: A preliminary report on a double blind study comparing chemonucleolysis and intradiscal administration of hydrocortisone in the treatment of backache and sciatica. Orthop Clin North Am 1975; 6:259–263.
81. Wilkinson HA, Schuman N: Intradiscal corticosteroids in the treatment of lumbar and cervical disc problems. Spine 1980; 5:385–389.
82. Rees WES: Multiple bilateral subcutaneous rhizolysis of segmental nerves in the treatment of the intervertebral disk syndrome. Ann Gent Prac 1971; 16(5):126–127.
83. Boas RA: Facet joint injections. In Stanton-Hicks M, Boas RA (eds): Chronic Low Back Pain. New York, Raven Press, 1982, pp. 199–211.
84. McCullock JA: Percutaneous radiofrequency lumbar rhizolysis (rhizotomy). Can Med Assoc 1977; J 116:30.
85. Shealey CH: Percutaneous radiofrequency denervation of spinal facets: Treatment for chronic back pain and sciatica. J Neurosurg 1975; 43:448–457.
86. Behar M, Magora F, Olshwang D, Davidson JT: Epidural morphine in treatment of pain. Lancet 1979; 1:527–528.
87. Benzon HT: Epidural steroid injections for low back pain and lumbosacral radiculopathy. Pain 1986; 24:277–295.
88. Carron H, Toomey TC: Epidural steroid therapy for low back pain. In Stanton-Hicks M, Boas RA (eds): Chronic Low Back Pain. New York, Raven Press, 1982, pp 193–198.
89. Cuckler JM, Bernini PA, Wiesel SW, Booth RE Jr, et al: The use of epidural steroids in the treatment of lumbar radicular pain: A prospective, randomized, double-blind study. J Bone Joint Surg (Am) 1985; 67:63–66.
90. Gardner WJ, Goebert HW Jr, Sehgal AD: Intraspinal corticosteroids in the treatment of sciatica. Transactions of the American Neurological Association 1961; 86:214–215.
91. Sehgal AD, Gardner WJ: Place of intrathecal methylprednisolone acetate in neurological disorders. Transactions of the American Neurological Association 1963; 88:275–276.
92. Tkaczuk H: Intrathecal prednisolone therapy in postoperative arachnoiditis following operation of herniated disc. Acta Orthop Scand 1976; 47:388–390.
93. Wilkinson HA: Dangers of methylprednisolone ace-

tate therapy by intraspinal injection (letter). Arch Neurol 1989; 46:721.

94. Winnie AP, Hartman JT, Meyers HL Jr, Ramamurthy S, Barangan V: Pain clinic II. Intrathecal and extradural corticosteroids for sciatica. Anesth Analg 1972; 51:990–1003.
95. Goldstein NP, McKenzie BF, McGuckin WF, Mattox VR: Experimental intrathecal administration of methylprednisolone acetate in multiple sclerosis. Transactions of the American Neurological Association 1970; 95:243–244.
96. Archer J: Instrument or impediment: The regulatory monograph in medical communications. JAMA 1972; 220:1440–1477.
97. Wilkinson HA, Mark VH, White JC: Further experiences with intrathecal phenol for the relief of pain. J Chronic Dis 1964; 17:1055–1059.
98. Onik G, Mooney V, Marron JC, et al: Automated percutaneous discectomy: A prospective multi-institutional study. Neurosurgery 1990; 26:228–233.
99. Wilkinson HA: Nerve-root entrapment in "traumatic" extradural arachnoid cyst. J Bone Joint Surg 1971; 53A:163–166.
100. Shikata J, Yamamuro T, Iida H, Sugimoto M: Surgical treatment of symptomatic spinal adhesive arachnoiditis. Spine 1989; 14:870–875.
101. Kumar K, Wyant GM, Ekong CEU: Epidural spinal cord stimulation for relief of chronic pain. The Pain Clinic 1986; 1:91–99.
102. Loeser JD, Ward AA Jr, White LE Jr: Epidural spinal cord stimulation for relief of chronic pain. J Neurosurg 1968; 29:48–50.
103. Ray CD: Percutaneous, peripheral nerve, and spinal cord stimulation for pain. In Youmans JR (ed) Neurological Surgery, 3d ed. Philadelphia, WB Saunders, 1990, pp. 3984–4006.
104. Penn RD, Paice JA: Chronic intrathecal morphine for intractable pain. J Neurosurg 1989; 67:182–186.
105. Penn RD, Savoy SM, Corcos D, Latash M, Gottlieb G, et al: Intrathecal baclofen for severe spinal spasticity. N Engl J Med 1989; 320:1517–1521.
106. Saunders RL, Coombs DW, Harbaugh RE: Central nervous system infusions for pain. In Youmans JR (ed) Neurological Surgery, 3d ed. Philadelphia, WB Saunders, 1990, pp 4121–4127.
107. White JC: Posterior rhizotomy: Possible substitution for cordotomy in otherwise intractable neuralgia of trunk and extremities of nonmalignant origin. Clin Neurosurg 1965; 13:20–41.
108. Hoppenstein R: A new approach to the failed, failed back syndrome. Spine 1980; 5:371–379.
109. Bullard DE, Nashold BS Jr: Brain stem procedures for pain. In Youmans JR (ed) Neurological Surgery, 3d ed. Philadelphia, WB Saunders, 1990, pp. 4070–4085.
110. Hosobuchi Y: Intracerebral stimulation for the relief of chronic pain. In Youmans JR (ed) Neurological Surgery, 3d ed. Philadelphia, WB Saunders, 1990, pp. 4128–4143.
111. Richardson DE, Akil H: Pain reduction by electrical brain stimulation in man. Part 1: Acute administration in periaqueductal and periventricular sites. J Neurosurg 1977; 47:178–183.
112. Wilkinson HA, Mark VH: Surgical relief of pain by intracranial methods. Chapter 34 in Neurology. In Walters W, Ellis FH Jr (eds): Lewis' Practice of Surgery. Hagerstown, Maryland, Harper & Row, 1972.
113. Cohen RA, MacCrae V, Phillips K, Wilkinson HA: Neurobehavioral consequences of bilateral medial cingulotomy. Neurology 1990; 40(1): 171.
114. Hassenbusch SJ, Pillay PK, Barnett GH: Radiofrequency cingulotomy for intractable cancer pain using stereotaxis guided by magnetic resonance imaging. Neurosurgery 1990; 27:220–223.
115. Hurt RW, Ballantine HT Jr: Stereotactic anterior cingulate lesions for persistent pain: A report on 68 cases. Clin Neurosurg 1974; 21:334–351.

Suggested Readings

Caron H, Toomey TC: Epidural steroid therapy for low back pain. In Stanton-Hicks M, Boas R (eds): Chronic Low Back Pain. Philadelphia, Grune and Stratton, 1982, pp. 193–198.

Collis JS Jr: Lumbar Discography. Springfield, Illinois, Charles C Thomas, 1963.

DePalma AF, Rothman RH: The Intervertebral Disc. Philadelphia, WB Saunders, 1970.

Finneson BE: Low Back Pain, 2d ed. Philadelphia, JB Lippincott, 1980.

Macnab I: Backache. Baltimore, Williams & Wilkins, 1977.

Post MJD (ed): Radiographic Evaluation of the Spine. New York, Masson Publishing, 1980.

Rothman RH, Simeone FA: The Spine, Vol I. Philadelphia, WB Saunders, 1975.

Stanton-Hicks M, Boas RA (eds): Chronic Low Back Pain. New York, Raven Press, 1982.

Woolfolk WL, Lehrer PM (eds): Principles and Practice of Stress Management. New York, Guilford Press, 1984.

Index of Case Reports

Subject Index

D

N

O

P